Outpatient Rehabilitation Services

A Guide to Planning and Management

James A. Sliwa, D.O., Project Editor

for the Section for Rehabilitation Hospitals and Programs and the Division of Ambulatory Care and Health Promotion of the American Hospital Association

AHA

AHA books are published by American Hospital Publishing, Inc., an American Hospital Association company

The views expressed in this publication are strictly those of the authors and do not necessarily represent official positions of the American Hospital Association.

Library of Congress Cataloging-in-Publication Data

Outpatient rehabilitation services : a guide to planning and
management / James A. Sliwa, project editor.
p. cm.
Includes bibliographical references.
ISBN 1-55648-075-X
1. Hospitals–Outpatient services. 2. Hospitals–Rehabilitation
services. I. Sliwa, James A.
[DNLM: 1. Outpatient Clinics, Hospital–organization &
administration–United States. 2. Rehabilitation–organization &
administration–United States. 3. Rehabilitation Centers–
organization & administration–United States. WR 320 094]
RA974.5.098 1991
362.1'2–dc20
DNLM/DLC
for Library of Congress 91-22269
CIP

Catalog no. 175710

Printed in the USA

AHA is a service mark of the American Hospital Association used under license by American Hospital Publishing, Inc.

Text set in Palatino
3M–09/91–0302

Marlene Chamberlain, Project Editor
Linda Conheady, Manuscript Editor
Teresa Cappetta-Kroger, Editorial Assistant
Marcia Bottoms, Managing Editor
Peggy DuMais, Production Coordinator
Susan Edge-Gumbel, Designer
Brian Schenk, Books Division Director

Contents

List of Figures v

List of Tables vii

About the Editor ix

Contributors x

Preface xvii

Acknowledgments xix

Part One. Major Factors in Developing Rehabilitation Programs

Chapter 1. The Environment for Outpatient Rehabilitation Services 3

Chapter 2. Market-Based Strategic Planning 31
Sheryl J. Bronkesh, M.B.A., Anne-Marie Nelson, and Steven D. Wood, Ph.D.

Chapter 3. Writing the Business Plan: Operational Issues 57
Suzan D. Boyd, M.S., M.M.

Chapter 4. Patient Management Issues 75
Patricia Lynne McCollom, R.N., M.S., CRRN, CIRS

Chapter 5. Facilities Planning and Renovation 83
Patrick B. Davis, Jr., AIA

Chapter 6. Accrediting Bodies and Their Standards and Processes 111
Carole H. Patterson, M.N., and Mary G. Swope

Chapter 7. Reimbursement and Financial Management 135
Donald H. Ratner, CPA, and Jerry Strum

Chapter 8. Legal Aspects of Outpatient Rehabilitation Services 159
L. Edward Bryant, Jr., J.D.

Part Two. Innovative Programs in Outpatient Rehabilitation

Chapter 9. St. Joseph Hospital Rehabilitation and Fitness Center 177
Suzan D. Boyd, M.S., M.M., and Becky Coven, M.B.A.

Chapter 10. Industrial Medicine Lehigh Valley 187
Lawrence Goren, M.D.

Chapter 11. The Work Hardening Program at the Institute of Physical Medicine and Rehabilitation 197
Lynn Floyd-Decker, OTR/L, CIRS, and Cindy Couri Behrends

Chapter 12. A Vocational Services Program for Brain-Injured Patients at Sister Kenny Institute 209
Carol M. Norris, M.S.

Chapter 13. The Professional Voice Program™ at Schwab Rehabilitation Center 217
Kathleen C. Yosko, M.B.A., M.S.

Chapter 14. Geriatric Rehabilitation at Sister Kenny Institute 225
Nancy E. Rehkamp, M.P.A.

Chapter 15. Pediatric Rehabilitation at the Rehabilitation Institute of Pittsburgh 233
Judith H. Nagy, R.N., M.P.H.

Chapter 16. BackBuilders, Operated by St. Lawrence Rehabilitation Center 243
Sister Janet Henry, R.S.M., and Janice G. Cunningham, OTR/L

Chapter 17. Outpatient Rehabilitation at the Mayo Clinic 253
Gudni Thorsteinsson, M.D., M.S.

Chapter 18. Behavioral Health and Rehabilitation at Advanced Rehabilitation Management 267
Jerry Strum

Chapter 19. The Diversification Strategy of Casa Colina: A Chronology of Change 281
Dale E. Eazell, M.S., F.A.A.M.A.

Annotated Bibliography 295

List of Figures

Figure 1-1. Freestanding Rehabilitation Hospitals in the United States: Growth in Number of Beds, 1980–1989 10

Figure 1-2. Rehabilitation Units in U.S. Community Hospitals: Growth in Number of Beds, 1980–1989 11

Figure 1-3. U.S. Hospitals with Organized Outpatient Rehabilitation Programs, 1980–1989 12

Figure 2-1. The Planning Process 34

Figure 2-2. Sample Referral Physician Survey 40

Figure 3-1. Business Plan Framework 60

Figure 4-1. Interrelationships Affecting Patient Management Issues in Outpatient Rehabilitation 78

Figure 5-1. Freestanding Hospital-Based Outpatient Rehab Center 107

Figure 5-2. Hospital-Based Rehabilitation Center 108

Figure 6-1. Accreditation Outcomes 121

Figure 6-2. Design Elements in Program Evaluation 124

Figure 7-1. Medicare Cost Centers 144

Figure 7-2. Pros of a CORF: General and Hospital-Specific 146

Figure 7-3. Cons of a CORF 146

Figure 10-1. Equipment List for Industrial Medicine/Sports Medicine Lehigh Valley 193

Figure 17-1. Organization of the Department of Physical Medicine and Rehabilitation 255

Figure 17-2. Programs within the Department of Physical Medicine and Rehabilitation 257

List of Tables

Table 1-1. Growth of Outpatient Rehabilitation Programs in U.S. Hospitals, by Census Region, 1980–1989 14

Table 1-2. Growth of Component Rehabilitation Services in U.S. Hospitals, 1980–1989 16

Table 1-3. Outpatient Physical Therapy Service Utilization, Special 1989 Survey 17

Table 1-4. Relative Frequency of Organized Outpatient Rehabilitation Program Types, Special 1989 Survey 18

Table 1-5. Relative Frequency of Outpatient Rehabilitation Services, Special 1988 Survey 19

Table 1-6. Percentage of Gross Outpatient Revenue Attributable to Identified Sources, Special 1988 Survey 22

Table 1-7. Staff Shortages in Medical Rehabilitation, Special 1988 Survey 25

Table 5-1. Small Hospital-Based Outpatient Rehab Space Program 86

Table 5-2. Hospital-Based Freestanding Outpatient Rehab Space Program 87

Table 5-3. Community-Based Freestanding CORF Space Program 88

Table 5-4. Typical Equipment List, Outpatient Rehabilitation Facility 103

Table 6-1. Program Objectives for Stroke Rehabilitation Program . . . 126

Table 15-1. Patient Mix by Acuity, Pediatric Outpatient Services, The Rehabilitation Institute of Pittsburgh . . . 238

Table 17-1. Personnel in the Department of Physical Medicine and Rehabilitation, Excluding Hospital Staff . . . 259

Table 17-2. Referral Sources for Outpatient Clinic, East-10 PM&R, 1985 . . . 260

Table 17-3. Summary of Clinical Conditions Seen at East-10 PM&R in 1985: Arthritic . . . 260

Table 17-4. Summary of Clinical Conditions Seen at East-10 PM&R in 1985: Miscellaneous . . . 261

Table 17-5. Growth in Mayo Medical Center and the Department of Physical Medicine and Rehabilitation . . . 265

About the Editor

James A. Sliwa, D.O., is assistant professor, Department of Physical Medicine and Rehabilitation, at Northwestern University Medical School, Rehabilitation Institute of Chicago. Dr. Sliwa is director of residency training and has taught a variety of clinical topics to medical and rehabilitation residents, including rehabilitation of burn patients, low back pain, and stroke rehabilitation. He is also a consultant to Northwestern Memorial Hospital and for the Health Data Institute of Elmhurst, Illinois. His former positions include serving as director of outpatient services at the Rehabilitation Institute of Chicago and as an attending physician at Mercy Hospital. He has published a number of journal articles and abstracts on rehabilitation medicine and on residency training. He is the current recipient of the Rehabilitation Service Administration Long-Term Training Grant.

Contributors

Cindy Couri Behrends is a registered physical therapist with Associated Orthopaedic Surgeons of Peoria, Ltd. She previously was the area supervisor of the Work Hardening Program for the Institute of Physical Medicine and Rehabilitation, in Peoria, Illinois. She cofounded the Work Hardening Program, developed and presented lectures for industry, participated in the accreditation process of the Commission on Accreditation of Rehabilitation Facilities (CARF). She was formerly on staff at the Jewish Hospital of St. Louis.

Suzan D. Boyd, M.S., M.M., is a research associate professor with the Department of Health Administration, School of Public Health, at the University of South Carolina, in Columbia. Ms. Boyd teaches courses in strategic planning and hospital diversification and medical staff relationships. In addition, she serves as a consultant to the Robert Wood Johnson Small and Rural Hospitals Project for the South Carolina Hospital Association. Previously, she was vice-president of Ambulatory and Ancillary Services at St. Joseph Hospital in Chicago. In that capacity, she worked with Ms. Becky Coven to develop the St. Joseph Hospital Rehabilitation and Fitness Center.

Sheryl J. Bronkesh, M.B.A., is a principal with the consulting firm of Health Services Marketing, Ltd., based in Scottsdale, Arizona. Ms. Bronkesh was formerly the director of marketing for Scottsdale Memorial Hospital. Prior to that, she was director of communications for a multihospital system and director of public relations for a 700-bed teaching hospital. She is a frequent speaker at national meetings in the fields of rehabilitation marketing, hospital marketing, and medical practice promotion. She is coauthor of *Promoting Your Medical Practice,* published by Medical Economics Books (1989).

L. Edward Bryant, Jr., J.D., is a practicing attorney with the Chicago law partnership of Gardner, Carton & Douglas, with whom he has been associated since 1967. He chairs his firm's Health Law Group, which he founded in 1979. His practice is almost exclusively on behalf of corporate and individual health care providers located in 43 states and the District of Columbia. Mr. Bryant speaks and publishes frequently on matters of health law and policy, and he was named one of the nation's outstanding health lawyers in 1985 by the *National Law Journal.* He is on the faculty of the Kellogg Graduate School of Management of Northwestern University and the Loyola School of Law. He has served on many advisory bodies to the American Hospital Association, the Catholic Health Association, and other health industry organizations.

Becky Coven, M.B.A., was director, Ambulatory Services, at St. Joseph Hospital and Health Care Center, Chicago. She managed emergency services, outpatient oncology services, clinic services, and off-site facilities including the Rehabilitation and Fitness Center. Ms. Coven has developed employee productivity standards and done program development, which has resulted in increased ambulatory patient volume and improved quality control. She is currently working as a consultant.

Janice G. Cunningham, OTR/L, is administrative director for the Work Injury Network, a work hardening center in Norristown, Pennsylvania. She is former program director of the BackBuilders Program and the Laurels/Transitional Living Program for Brain Injured Adults in Malvern, Pennsylvania. She held various clinical and administrative positions at the Johnson Institute for Rehabilitation in Edison, New Jersey. Since 1987, she has been providing health care consultation in the areas of planning and implementation of rehabilitation programs. Ms. Cunningham's current affiliations include the American Occupational Therapy Association, the National Association of Rehabilitation Professionals in the Private Sector, and the student division of the American Bar Association.

Patrick B. Davis, Jr., AIA, is vice-president, principal, and director of TRO/The Ritchie Organization in its Sarasota, Florida, office. The Ritchie Organization is an architectural firm specializing in the planning and design of health care facilities and has offices in several states. Mr. Davis has approximately 15 years' experience in the planning and design of health care facilities. He was a consultant to Access Unlimited, an advocacy organization for the handicapped, in Birmingham, Alabama. Mr. Davis has directed, designed, and planned rehabilitation facilities at the Lakeshore Hospital, Birmingham, Alabama; the Venice Hospital, Venice, Florida; and the Baptist Hospital, Miami, Florida. Mr. Davis was a contributor to the book entitled *Outpatient Cancer Centers: Implementation and Management,* published by American Hospital Publishing, Inc., in 1988. He has lectured and conducted workshops with the American Health Care Radiology Administrators Association and the South Florida Health Care Administrators Forum.

Dale E. Eazell, M.S., F.A.A.M.A., is president and chief executive officer of Casa Colina, Inc., a Pomona, California-based health care corporation specializing in comprehensive rehabilitation. Casa Colina includes an inpatient acute hospital; vocational development centers for adults; pain reduction centers; a children's educational, diagnostic, and preschool training center; adult day health services; outpatient medical/vocational rehabilitation services; and transitional living centers. Mr. Eazell has more than 25 years' experience in health care administration, management, and the rehabilitation industry. He is actively involved with the American Hospital Association as a section delegate in the House of Delegates, a trustee for the Commission on Accreditation of Rehabilitation Facilities, and a trustee for the Rehabilitation Nursing Foundation. He is past president of the National Association of Rehabilitation Facilities, past chairman of the Provider Council, and member of the Executive Committee of the National Head Injury Foundation.

Lynn Floyd-Decker, OTR/L, CIRS, is an occupational therapist, registered with the American Occupational Therapy Association, licensed by the state of Illinois, and certified by the Insurance Rehabilitation Specialist Commission. She is currently in private practice in Novi, Michigan. Ms. Floyd-Decker was formerly sectional supervisor of the Return to Work Center, a division of the Institute of Physical Medicine and Rehabilitation, in Peoria, Illinois. She cofounded and developed the multidisciplinary Work Hardening Program. Ms. Floyd-Decker led that program and the vocational evaluation program through the CARF accreditation process, which subsequently resulted in a three-year accreditation.

Lawrence Goren, M.D., is medical director, industrial medicine practice, at Occupational Health Lehigh Valley, Bethlehem, Pennsylvania. His previous experience includes serving as director of the injury care program at St. Luke's Hospital in Bethlehem. He also was assistant instructor in general surgery at Hahnemann University Hospital for two years. His membership affiliations include the American Medical Association, the American Occupational Medicine Association, the Pennsylvania Medical Society, the Philadelphia County Medical Society, and the Samuel Hahnemann Surgical Society.

Sister Janet Henry, R.S.M., is administrator and chief executive officer for St. Lawrence Rehabilitation Center, a comprehensive physical rehabilitation facility in central New Jersey. Previously, she held various administrative positions within the Franciscan Health System and at Mercy

Catholic Medical Center. Sister Henry is involved in state, regional, and national organizations and forums for the health care industry, including the Catholic Health Association. She is a member of the Regional Policy Board of the American Hospital Association. She is also a member of the President's Committee on Employment of People with Disabilities. Sister Henry is a surveyor for the Commission on Accreditation of Healthcare Facilities. She also is a member of the American College of Healthcare Executives, the Catholic Health Association, and the New Jersey Hospital Association.

Patricia Lynne McCollom, R.N., M.S., CRRN, CIRS, has been president and senior rehabilitation consultant for Management Consulting and Rehabilitation Services, Inc., since 1982. The firm is located in Ankeny, Iowa, and Kansas City, Missouri. She also is founder and president of LifeCare Economics, Ltd., Ankeny, Iowa. Ms. McCollom currently serves as chair of the National Task Force on Case Management. She is former president of the Association of Rehabilitation Nurses and was vice-chair of the Nursing Organization Liaison Forum. She authored *Case Management Guide: The Individual with Brain Injury* (ICMA, 1991), has contributed to two editions of *Rehabilitation Nursing Practice: A Core Curriculum* (AMC Publishing, 1985–1987), and has published numerous articles and presentations relating to rehabilitation nursing practice. She has worked as a nursing educator, neurotrauma clinical specialist, and nursing administrator.

Judith H. Nagy, R.N., M.P.H., is director of patient care services at Allegheny Neuropsychiatric Institute (ANI), Oakdale, Pennsylvania. In this role, she is accountable for day-to-day supervision and management of physical therapy, occupational therapy, recreational therapy, speech–language pathology, pharmacy, EEG, volunteer/pastoral services, and physician assistants. Her responsibilities include development of goals and objectives, establishment and implementation of standards of practice and performance, and development and control of the budget. Prior to joining ANI, Ms. Nagy was executive director of the Workplace, director of Outpatient Services, and senior program coordinator, Ambulatory Services, with the Rehabilitation Institute of Pittsburgh.

Anne-Marie Nelson is vice-president of Health Services Marketing, Ltd., Scottsdale, Arizona. Ms. Nelson's previous experience includes serving as communications director for Hillhaven's long-term and rehabilitative care facilities in Arizona. She was also marketing director for a dental firm and director of public relations at Scottsdale Memorial Hospital. Ms. Nelson has extensive experience in health care and rehabilitation marketing, strategic planning, and public relations. She also edited *Promoting Your Medical Practice,* published by Medical Economics Books (1989).

Carol M. Norris, M.S., is director of vocational services at Sister Kenny Institute in Minneapolis. Her previous positions at Sister Kenny Institute include project manager, transitional employment program coordinator, vocational counselor, and placement specialist. Ms. Norris is currently a member of the National Rehabilitation Association, the National Head Injury Foundation, the Minnesota Rehabilitation Counseling Association, and the Minnesota Association of Rehabilitation Providers. She has made many presentations on rehabilitation-related topics and vocational rehabilitation.

Carole H. Patterson, M.N., is associate director for interpretation, Department of Standards, Joint Commission on Accreditation of Healthcare Organizations, Oakbrook Terrace, Illinois, in which capacity she shares responsibility for the interpretation of all Joint Commission standards. She provided staff support for the Joint Commission's Rehabilitation Standards Task Force during the five-year standards review and revision process. Her more than 35 years in the field of nursing include rehabilitation nursing experience while working in academia, clinical practice and administration, consultation, and education. Formerly, she served in a variety of positions with the Joint Commission, including nurse surveyor in the Hospital Accreditation Program, assistant director for the Scheduling Department, and nursing standards specialist.

Donald H. Ratner, CPA, is vice-president of finance with the Rehabilitation Institute of Chicago, a 176-bed tertiary care area hospital for persons with disabilities. His responsibilities include all financial, budgeting, and reimbursement activities as well as all managed care contracts and legislative liaisons. Prior to this, he was with Arthur Andersen & Company for 14 years, where he served as a senior health care manager and a national health care coordinator. He has been a frequent speaker on reimbursement topics.

Nancy E. Rehkamp, M.P.A., is executive director and senior administrator for Sister Kenny Institute and Abbott Northwestern, in Minneapolis. Ms. Rehkamp has been on the Congressional Task Force on Long Term Care Insurance. She has served as chair of the AHA Governing Council on Aging and Long-Term Care. Formerly, she was administrator of a small, rural nursing home/hospital combination facility in River Falls, Wisconsin. Ms. Rehkamp has also served on the Board of Directors for the Voluntary Hospitals of America Long Term Care Foundation.

Jerry Strum is founder of Jerry Strum and Associates, a hospital management consulting company in Statesville, North Carolina. Previously, he was vice-president of finance and president of Advanced Rehabilitation Management, Inc., a subsidiary of Casa Colina, Inc., based in Pomona,

California. He currently assists hospitals that have rehabilitation and psychiatric services subject to the Tax Equity and Fiscal Responsibility Act (TEFRA) limit in recovering additional reimbursement. He also assists hospitals with skilled nursing units and freestanding skilled nursing facilities. Additionally, he does strategic market planning for rehabilitation hospitals, rehabilitation units of hospitals, and rehabilitation outpatient services. Mr. Strum is currently a member of the Healthcare Financial Management Association and the American Hospital Association.

Mary G. Swope is president of American Health Resources (AHR), Zanesville, Ohio, a corporation specializing in consulting and management of comprehensive rehabilitation services. Her firm has constructed two 40-bed freestanding rehabilitation hospitals that are wholly owned and operated by the company. Prior to development of her for-profit company, Mrs. Swope was vice-president of rehabilitation for Good Samaritan Medical Center and Rehabilitation Center in Zanesville. She is a governor's appointee as a commissioner for the Rehabilitation Services Commission in the state of Ohio. She is a national consultant and presenter, a surveyor for the Commission on Accreditation of Rehabilitation Facilities, and a member and past chairman of the American Hospital Association's Section for Rehabilitation Hospitals and Programs. Mrs. Swope is past chairman and secretary of the National Rehabilitation Caucus and served as a member of the CARF Board of Trustees for six years. She served as a member of the advisory committee to the Joint Commission on Accreditation of Healthcare Organizations that established the rehabilitation services section of the *Accreditation Manual for Hospitals.* She is also a member of the national task force to establish a uniform national data base for rehabilitation, and has published on multiple occasions for both the AHA and the Joint Commission.

Gudni Thorsteinsson, M.D., M.S., is chair of the Department of Physical Medicine and Rehabilitation at the Mayo Clinic and Mayo Foundation, Rochester, Minnesota. He is also assistant professor of physical medicine and rehabilitation, Mayo Medical School, also in Rochester. His past affiliations include the following positions within the Department of Physical Medicine and Rehabilitation at the Mayo Clinic and Mayo Foundation: medical director, Rehabilitation Unit, and medical director, Outpatient Department. Dr. Thorsteinsson was also chairman, Department of Rehabilitation Medicine, at the National Hospital in Reykjavík, Iceland.

Steven D. Wood, Ph.D., is professor of Decision Information Systems at Arizona State University. He previously served as dean of graduate programs in the College of Business at that institution. Dr. Wood has been an active researcher, educator, and consultant in the health services industry for more than 18 years. He has published more than 70 articles in professional journals and given more than 150 presentations to various organizations. Dr. Wood writes a regular medical marketing column for the *Journal of the American Group Practice Association* and is one of the authors of *Promoting Your Medical Practice,* published by Medical Economics Books. He is a national vice-president and marketing coordinator of the Decision Sciences Institute and a past president of the organization's Western Region. Dr. Wood has been actively involved with the development and packaging of services and products for health care providers and has developed computer-based expert systems to create marketing strategies for selected services marketing environments.

Kathleen C. Yosko, M.B.A., M.S., is vice-president/administrator of Schwab Rehabilitation Center and vice-president for rehabilitation services at Mount Sinai Hospital Medical Center in Chicago. She serves on the Medical Advisory Committee of the National Association of Rehabilitation Facilities (NARF), is chairman of the Productivity Task Force for NARF, and is a member of the Board of Directors of the Illinois Association of Rehabilitation Facilities. Ms. Yosko has an associate professorship at Rush University. She has received a series of national and local achievement awards for her work in health care planning and marketing and rehabilitation. She was chairman of the Medical Section of the Illinois Association of Rehabilitation Facilities (IARF) for 1986–87.

Preface

For years, *outpatient rehabilitation* was considered an oxymoron by professionals in the field. Many felt that rehabilitation was, by its nature, primarily an inpatient process to improve the functional status of patients disabled by stroke, spinal cord injury, amputation, head injury, or other injuries or diseases. With few time constraints, inpatient hospital stays for rehabilitation were lengthy, progress was at times slow, and discharge occurred when *all* goals were accomplished, teaching was completed, and equipment such as wheelchairs and walkers was obtained.

To make matters worse, rehabilitation in general was not well understood by many physicians, and the concept of improving functional status and adjusting to disability by becoming more independent was not within the scope of medical care, which focused primarily on cure. Consequently, few medical students entered specialty training in the field. Furthermore, not all patients who could benefit from services found their way to rehabilitation units.

Why, then, a book on outpatient rehabilitation? Because within the past decade, many changes have occurred that make this book necessary reading for all who plan to provide a full range of rehabilitation services. Rehabilitation and functional status is now more often than not considered a vital part of comprehensive health care. Awareness and understanding of the specialty have increased. Reimbursement for rehabilitation now requires increasing accountability to health maintenance organizations, peer review organizations, and case managers. As a result, the demand for services has grown and the spectrum of rehabilitation care has broadened. Yet pressures for cost containment have also increased, along with the need to provide care for those not ready to return home directly from inpatient care. The new frontier in rehabilitation has been clearly identified—outpatient services.

The possibilities for outpatient rehabilitation are numerous. Clinically, they span the spectrum from day programs in geriatric rehabilitation to work hardening. Administratively, outpatient services can be provided as part of an inpatient department or as a completely separate entity in an outpatient facility.

The possibilities in outpatient rehabilitation are so vast and uncharted that those venturing into the area must feel much the same way that Lewis and Clark did as they ventured into the land west of the Mississippi River. However, embarking on new territory raises many questions. Which direction to travel? Down what path? And what potential dangers and risks lie ahead?

This book serves as a guide to help those planning and considering outpatient rehabilitation programs answer these questions. It does so by carefully addressing a number of important planning issues. These include developing a business plan for your outpatient program and handling strategic marketing, facility design, reimbursement issues, accreditation, and the legal aspects of outpatient services. In addition, this book provides 11 case studies illustrating in practical terms specific strategies for implementing a broad range of outpatient programs, including ones for pediatric rehabilitation and head trauma.

Outpatient rehabilitation, with the broad range of services available, is the next step in the continued growth of the rehabilitation field. This book will help planners and administrators plan, develop, and implement outpatient rehabilitation programs.

Acknowledgments

The editors of American Hospital Publishing, Inc., would like to thank the following people for their participation in this important publishing effort: Brent England and Diane Howard, formerly of the American Hospital Association, for initiating this project; Susanne Sonik and Shawna Brown of the AHA Section for Rehabilitation Hospitals and Programs, who both evaluated the manuscript during the final stages; and, of course, Dr. James Sliwa, who provided consistent feedback during the manuscript's development.

Part One

Major Factors in Developing Rehabilitation Programs

Chapter 1

The Environment for Outpatient Rehabilitation Services

Introduction

The philosophy and rationale of rehabilitation was probably best explained by Brent England in *Medical Rehabilitation Services in Health Care Institutions:*[1]

> In addressing medical rehabilitation issues, it is important to recognize and accept certain philosophical premises. Rehabilitation is rooted in the belief that the individual has inherent worth. This realization acknowledges that every patient, even the most severely disabled, may possess some physical, emotional, and spiritual resources that can be mobilized to help that individual attain at least some degree of independence.
>
> Rehabilitation requires consistent application of practical, daily therapies to restore and maintain function, to prevent further deterioration, and to train the patient to adjust emotionally to live and work with the disability. Objectives for individual patients will vary. For one patient, the appropriate goal may be self-care and a reasonably satisfactory emotional adjustment; for another, it may be full physical, social, and economic self-sufficiency. The philosophy behind rehabilitation recognizes that even limited improvement is important if it adds some degree of independence. Moving into a wheelchair can be just as meaningful to a previously bedfast patient as walking unaided is to the fracture patient dependent on crutches.

Other industry leaders, including Howard Rusk in a 1978 article entitled "Rehabilitation Medicine: Knowledge in Search of Understanding,"[2] and Edward Eckenhoff in his 1986 lecture "Rehabilitation: Ghosts . . . Images . . . Visions,"[3] have argued the case for rehabilitation eloquently. Unfortunately, although rehabilitation service utilization has increased, rehabilitation is still poorly understood by the medical community, many public and private payers, and the public in general.[4] In *Quality Rehabilitation: Results-Oriented Patient Care,* Brent England states:[5]

> Acute care hospitals and referring physicians frequently do not understand the multidisciplinary process of rehabilitation or the outcomes possible for various patients. This lack of understanding results in inappropriate referrals or, for some persons with disabilities, no referral to rehabilitation at all.
>
> Payers, both public and private, do not understand the cost-effectiveness of rehabilitation and fail to consider the patient and family. Such payers are frugal at the expense of long-term efficiencies and eventual patient independence and productivity. Far too often, employers do not recognize that rehabilitation can successfully return a disabled individual to a former job or to some form of gainful employment. The general public is often not aware that the early intervention of rehabilitation services, coupled with ongoing coordinated rehabilitation resources, can minimize a person's disability and facilitate the attainment of optimal functional capability.

Part of the lack of understanding of rehabilitation may come from the significant differences between rehab patients and acute care patients. Whereas the focus of acute care is on sickness and cure, the focus in rehabilitation is on disability and the reduction of the resulting functional limitations. As Andrew Batavia suggests in *The Payment of Medical Rehabilitation Services:* ". . . conventional medical approaches based on a 'sickness model' are generally not applicable to rehabilitation. Similarly, traditional measures of medical success, such as mortality and morbidity rates, are less appropriate for rehabilitation patients than are measures of functional status and improvement."[6]

There is, however, a growing body of research documenting the efficacy of rehabilitation services. This research has been engendered in large part by the need to examine service utilization as the basis for implementing impending changes in payment methods. For example, a 1988 survey of medical rehabilitation hospitals and units conducted by the American Hospital Association's Section for Rehabilitation Hospitals and Programs found that 70.9 percent of rehab inpatients returned home without requiring further inpatient care. This finding was based on 101,873 discharges in 200 facilities.[7] Other significant studies of utilization include a 1985 study sponsored by the National Association of

Rehabilitation Facilities and conducted by Coopers and Lybrand[8] and one conducted in 1987 by a research team at Tufts University School of Medicine.[9] Another growing body of research is the examination of the cost-effectiveness of rehabilitation services.[10-12]

Beyond refining its ability to demonstrate benefits in relation to costs, the rehabilitation field, like the health care field in general, has redoubled its efforts to define and measure service quality. The initiatives of various accrediting bodies and professional associations to improve high-quality care are well documented.[13]

Perhaps most important to quality measurement is the continuing evolution of a variety of tools for measuring the functional status of patients as they move through the rehabilitation process. These measures are based on a multitude of variables including levels of mobility, level of paralysis, and ability to conduct activities of daily living—all designed to help document the achievement of positive outcomes of rehabilitation interventions. Among these tools is the Functional Independence Measure (FIM), which is an outgrowth of the Uniform Data System (UDS) for Medical Rehabilitation. The UDS is a program begun in 1983 that represents a collaborative effort of major rehabilitation organizations and is administratively managed through the Rehabilitation Data Management Service at Buffalo (N.Y.) General Hospital's Department of Rehabilitation Medicine. The UDS is growing—it is one of the largest data bases in the country, with 100,000 admission/discharge records from 200 facilities in 38 states. The UDS is promising because it is creating a common communication framework among and between providers and among providers, payers, and referral sources. It also helps demonstrate the effectiveness of rehabilitation and helps identify the similarities in treatment and outcome by rehab condition. Ultimately, this program is expected to gather and aggregate FIM data from rehabilitation providers across the United States to help predict outcomes and length of stay based on the age of the patient, the rehabilitation problem, and the level of severity.

The Need for Rehabilitation Services

As evidenced by the data provided in this chapter, both ambulatory care services in general and rehabilitation in particular have experienced dramatic growth in the past decade. Predictions for continued growth of rehab services are supported by a number of demographic trends, including the aging of the U.S. population and the increasing numbers of individuals surviving serious accidents and requiring long-term rehabilitation services. The Society for Ambulatory Care Professionals of the American Hospital Association advises that, to address demographic trends, ambulatory care professionals must:[14]

- Help develop innovative health services to meet the needs of a growing middle-aged population that has strong preferences for wellness and health promotion
- Address the needs of a growing elderly population with hospices, home care, social health maintenance organizations, adult day care, life care communities, and other forms of long-term care services
- Prepare for increased longevity and a growing incidence of chronic illness by investing in such programs as pain management, outpatient rehabilitation, health promotion, wellness, and patient education

The age wave forecast by gerontologists Ken Dychtwald and Mark Zitter is perhaps the best-documented and frequently discussed of the demographic trends.[15] At the turn of the century, only 4 percent of all Americans were age 65 or older. This percentage doubled by 1950, totaling over 12 million people, or 8.1 percent. By 1987, approximately 30 million older Americans were at least age 65, representing approximately 12 percent of the total population.[16] The unprecedented growth in the older population is demonstrated most dramatically among those age 85 and over. In 1950, more than a half million people in the United States were in this age group. By the turn of the century, however, the U.S. Census Bureau projects that the older population will number nearly 5 million. In over a half century, the number of persons age 85 and over will have increased by a striking 700 percent.[17] However, the numbers alone don't tell the full story, as eldercare expert Nancy Persily points out:[18]

> Even though the majority of elderly are functionally independent, the disabled elderly population will continue to grow in terms of absolute numbers. Whatever the functional level or ability, the overall goal of older adults will be to remain as independent as possible. Chronic conditions leading to disabilities will foster the need for long-term care and greater continuity of care. To address this emerging need, the future health care provider will require an interdisciplinary team approach that manages both chronic and acute conditions through an integrated system of care.

Another demographic indicator is the growing population of individuals with severe disability. Stroke, arthritis, accidental trauma involving brain or spinal cord damage, birth injuries, and congenital defects are all conditions that people more often survive, although with sometimes-disabling results that require rehabilitation. The National Institute on Disability and Rehabilitation Research *Chartbook on Disability in the United States* states that an estimated 14.1 percent of 231.5 million noninstitutionalized U.S. residents have an activity limitation. Of these,

8.8 million have health conditions that render them unable to carry out their major life activity, 13.6 million are limited in the kind or amount of major activity they can perform, and 10.1 million are limited in activities other than their major activity.[19] The 8.8 million figure constitutes a nearly 130 percent increase in persons with severe disabilities over the past 25 years, a period in which the adult population grew only 43 percent. This same source points out that more than 20 percent of noninstitutionalized persons age 15 and over (or 37.3 million people) have a physical functional limitation that limits their ability to perform selected physical functions such as getting into or out of bed or going up a flight of stairs without resting. Of this noninstitutionalized population, an estimated 7.5 percent (or 13.5 million people) are severely limited in various functions.[20]

Despite the numbers, disabled adults do not have consistent access to care. For example, the National Head Injury Foundation states that only 26 percent of the 70,000 to 90,000 persons who have severe head injury are receiving specialized care. The National Center for Health Statistics reports that only 20 percent of those with severe head trauma are hospitalized for rehabilitation each year, and 70 percent of head injury patients are still dependent after receiving trauma care.[21]

Interest in rehabilitation services is also fueled by employers' need to balance the needs of employees with work-related injuries against escalating costs to workers' compensation programs. William L. Newkirk, M.D., cites the following statistics:[22]

- Medical benefits resulting from workers' compensation have increased from $3.9 billion in 1980 to $8.3 billion in 1986; these medical benefits represent about 10 percent of the entire medical indemnity market.
- Seventy percent of workers' compensation payments go to wage replacement, providing wages to injured workers unable to return to full-time work. Beyond the $8.3 billion paid out in medical benefits in 1986, companies paid $17.7 billion to workers for missing time from work as a result of their injuries.
- In 1972, there were 10.9 injuries per 100 workers; in 1985, there were 7.9 injuries. However, in 1972, the average injured worker missed 4.4 days as a result of the injury; in 1985, the average injured worker missed 8.2 days.

The emergence of new treatment techniques such as work hardening have improved on previous methods of rehabilitation, which successfully enhanced range of motion and strength but failed to help workers perform their jobs at previous levels. Work hardening is a combination of standard physical and occupational therapy techniques to reduce pain and increase function through work simulation, typically performed in a physical area that resembles the workplace or factory environment. Michael B. Arnall has stated that work simulation, work adjustment counseling, worklike treatment environments, and work hardening programs have yielded return-to-work rates of 50 to 85 percent—even for chronic cases.[23]

The Comprehensive Medical Rehabilitation Model

Addressing the disparate needs of the population with functional impairments (whether those impairments arise from conditions associated with aging, trauma, congenital conditions, or work-related injury) is the concept of comprehensive medical rehabilitation (CMR). *Comprehensive medical rehabilitation* is a program of inpatient and outpatient care that promotes optimum attainable levels of physical independence and functional ability, as well as optimum psychological, social, vocational, educational, and economic adjustment of the individual. To attain these goals and focus on the entire individual, CMR utilizes a multidisciplinary team approach encompassing, among other disciplines, physician services (such as those of *physiatrists,* physicians specializing in rehabilitation medicine), rehabilitation nursing, physical and occupational therapy, speech-language pathology, psychology, social work, vocational rehabilitation, and recreational therapy.

As defined by the American Hospital Association, a CMR program has the following characteristics:[24]

- It is an organizational and physical entity.
- It is *medically directed* by a physician who is knowledgeable and experienced in rehabilitation medicine.
- Services are interdisciplinary, coordinated, and integrated.
- Services for patients are measurable and determined by an individual periodic assessment of basic functional abilities performed by a qualified multidisciplinary team.
- The program accomplishes its rehabilitation goals within appropriate time frames.

Medical rehabilitation programs and services have evolved over time in response to the changing needs and changing demographic composition of the disabled population. As described by Andrew Batavia:[25]

> In the post–World War II era, rehabilitation focused on the needs of individuals with diseases of the neuromuscular and musculoskeletal systems, such as polio and polyarthritis, as well as individuals with amputations resulting largely from war-related and other traumatic injuries. . . .

Due to the virtual eradication of polio and many other previously disabling diseases, and to major advances in emergency and trauma care, medical rehabilitation is now largely focused around central nervous system problems such as spinal cord injury, stroke, and brain injury. It also addresses the needs of persons with a variety of disabilities caused by amputations, hip fractures, burns, polyarthritis, and other disabling diseases and conditions. The common thread among all these patients is that they have functional limitations resulting from their physical impairments.

Conceptually, rehabilitation outcomes may be divided into two types:[26]

- A patient's ability to independently perform self-care, activities of daily living, mobility, and effective communication *(short-term outcomes)*
- A patient's ability to live productively and actively in economic, family, and community life, and to maintain health by avoiding medical complications that result in costly and disruptive medical interventions *(long-term outcomes)*

For many patients, the process of rehabilitation starts with inpatient services, which begin once acute care needs have been met, with the focus on short-term outcomes as described in the preceding paragraph. The inpatient phase of rehabilitation may nonetheless be a lengthy one. Respondents to a special survey of the Section for Rehabilitation Hospitals and Programs of the American Hospital Association reported an average length of stay of 29.2 days for hospitals and units combined.[27] However, the field of rehabilitation has long recognized the importance of follow-up in an outpatient program after a patient has been discharged from the inpatient program. Indeed, accreditation requirements of the Commission on Accreditation of Rehabilitation Facilities (CARF) include the establishment of program evaluation mechanisms that monitor patient status after discharge from the hospital.[28]

It should be noted that some patients may be referred to skilled nursing or extended care facilities rather than to either an inpatient or an outpatient rehabilitation program. Such a referral may be indicated when a patient is incapable of participating in an active program, when a patient has ceased to improve functionally or is improving so slowly as to make continued inpatient care impractical, or when a patient who might normally be discharged to outpatient care lacks the support persons or facilities to care for the patient at home.

Data from the American Hospital Association's *Annual Survey of Hospitals* indicate that utilization of rehabilitation services continues to be significant. Over the course of the 1980s, the number of freestanding rehabilitation hospitals increased from 68 in 1980 to 112 in 1989, and the number of inpatient beds in these hospitals grew from 5,902 in 1980 to 8,726 in 1989 (figure 1-1). The number of community hospitals with dedicated inpatient rehab units similarly increased from 303 units in 1980 to 737 units in 1989, with an increase in the number of inpatient rehab beds from 8,772 in 1980 to 18,135 in 1989 (figure 1-2).

Growth of Outpatient Rehabilitation

The growth in the utilization of inpatient rehabilitation services is evident. At the same time, recent changes in the U.S. health care delivery

Figure 1-1. Freestanding Rehabilitation Hospitals in the United States: Growth in Number of Beds, 1980–1989

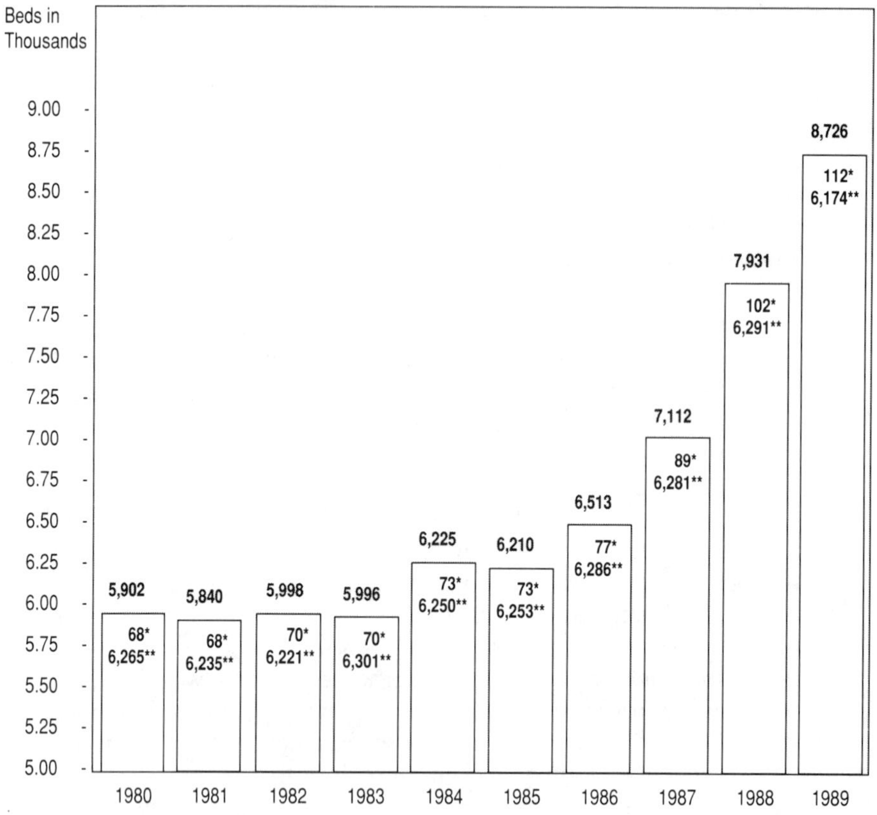

Source: *Hospital Statistics,* 1981 edition through 1990–1991 edition, all copyright by the American Hospital Association. All rights reserved. Data cited are taken from table 13A of each edition, which records data from the AHA *Annual Survey of Hospitals.*

*Number of hospitals identified as rehabilitation hospitals.

**Total number of hospitals of all types reporting.

Figure 1-2. Rehabilitation Units in U.S. Community Hospitals: Growth in Number of Beds, 1980–1989

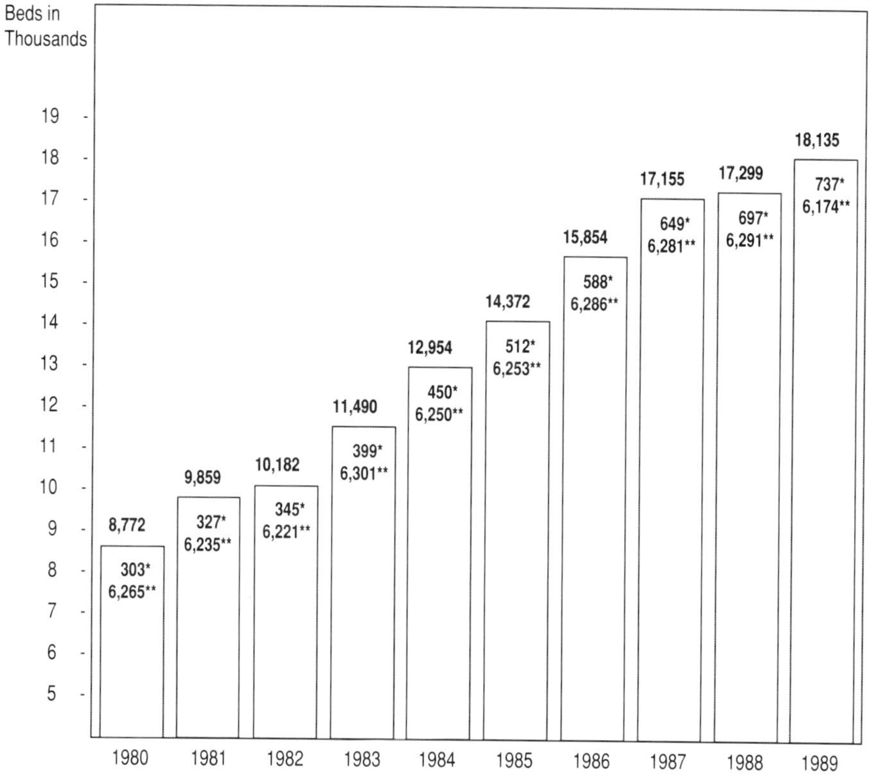

Source: *Hospital Statistics*, 1981 edition through 1990–1991 edition, all copyright by the American Hospital Association. All rights reserved. Data cited are taken from table 13A of each edition, which records data from the AHA *Annual Survey of Hospitals*.

*Number of hospitals that reported having a dedicated rehabilitation unit.

**Total number of hospitals of all types reporting

system brought on by changes in payment systems have led to an increased emphasis on outpatient care, and that emphasis is also reflected in rehabilitation. As Brent England points out:[29]

> For years, the health care field has perceived that outpatient care is the wave of the future. As a way of meeting the challenges of rising capital and labor costs and of increasing regulation, the health care field is banking on substantial growth in outpatient care delivery. Outpatient care is efficient, is easier to cost-control, and can be provided in innovative settings that are less capital- and labor-intensive than inpatient care.
>
> It has taken time for this wave of the future to develop, but at long last purchasers of health care services are discovering

that outpatient services are economical and convenient and are less disruptive to patients' lives than inpatient services. And because third-party payers like outpatient services, they are beginning to demand them and, more to the point, pay for them.

Growth in outpatient programs is clearly evident. For example, according to information from the Health Care Financing Administration (HCFA), as of March 1991, there were 193 Medicare-certified comprehensive outpatient rehabilitation facilities (CORFs) in the United States. As shown in figure 1-3, in 1980, 1,682 hospitals (27 percent of the 6,277 hospitals reporting) had organized outpatient rehabilitation programs. In 1989, 2,830 hospitals (46 percent of the 6,174 hospitals reporting) had organized outpatient rehabilitation programs. This growth does

Figure 1-3. U.S. Hospitals with Organized Outpatient Rehabilitation Programs, 1980–1989

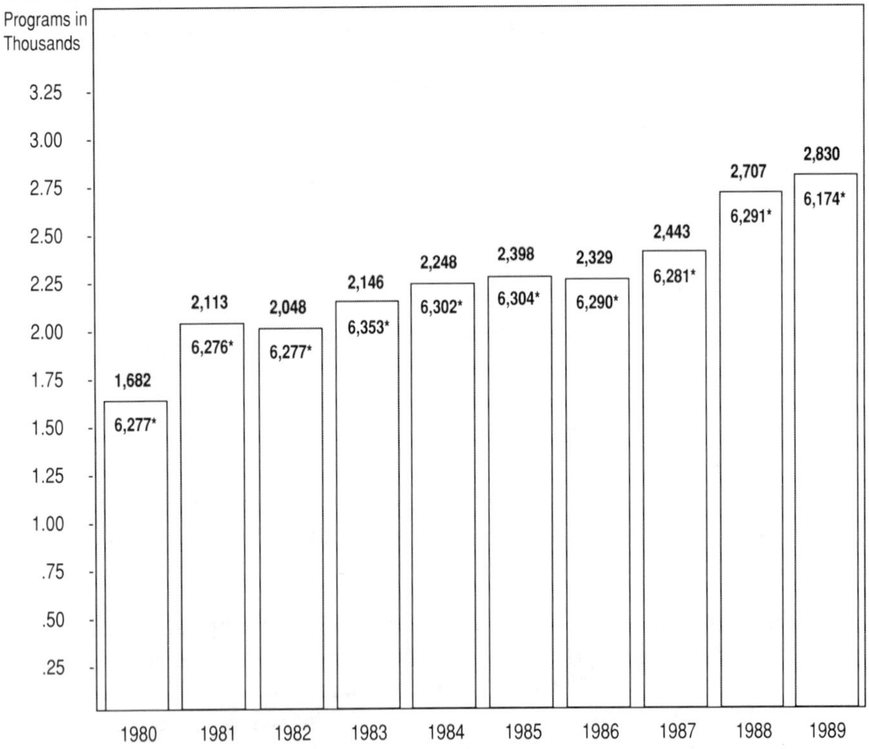

Source: *Hospital Statistics*, 1981 edition through 1990–1991 edition, all copyright by the American Hospital Association. All rights reserved. Data cited are taken from table 12A of each edition, which records data from Section C of the AHA *Annual Survey of Hospitals*. The definition of a program is "provision of coordinated multidisciplinary physical restorative services to ambulatory patients under the direction of a physician knowledgeable and experienced in rehabilitation medicine."

*Total number of hospitals of all types reporting.

not appear to have any regional limitations, with growth (in some cases, dramatic) occurring in all 50 states (table 1-1).

Individual rehabilitation services offered in general acute care hospitals—physical therapy, occupational therapy, respiratory therapy, social work services, and speech pathology services—have generally remained well-utilized services since 1980 (table 1-2, p. 16). The decline in the number of hospitals reporting some of these services may be attributable to the entry of nonhospital providers into the market, but is unlikely to be a reflection of any general market decline given the indicators of rehabilitation growth shown in figures 1-1 through 1-3 and table 1-1. The competitive influence of nonhospital providers is demonstrated in the survey results shown in table 1-3 (p. 17); for those surveyed who used outpatient physical therapy services, hospitals were named as the provider in approximately only one-third of the cases.

The total scope of outpatient rehabilitation utilization is thus difficult to define. One can get some sense of the dimensions of utilization growth in an examination of the numbers of outpatient visits reported by freestanding rehabilitation hospitals in the AHA *Annual Survey of Hospitals:* 706,161 outpatient visits reported by 69 rehabilitation hospitals in 1975; 778,128 outpatient visits reported by 71 rehabilitation hospitals in 1980; and 2,284,053 outpatient visits reported by 127 rehabilitation hospitals in 1989.[30] The average number of outpatient visits per rehab facility increased by 76 percent between 1975 and 1989. The total outpatient growth among the hospitals surveyed was 223 percent, and the number of rehab hospitals increased 84 percent.

Profile of Outpatient Rehabilitation

Outpatient rehabilitation programs include a wide variety of program and service options, which can be provided in a range of different settings. Program planners must examine the potential programs in outpatient rehabilitation and plan services that meet market needs.

Outpatient programs that address the needs of the disabled population may be affiliated with freestanding rehabilitation hospitals, comprehensive multidisciplinary rehabilitation units within community hospitals, or community hospitals that offer rehabilitation services but have no specifically designated rehabilitation beds. Outpatient rehabilitation programs may also be operated by home health agencies, adult day-care centers, freestanding physical therapy centers, and the private practices of physiatrists, physical therapists, occupational therapists, prosthetic providers, and orthotists.

Hospital-based outpatient programs may offer a fairly comprehensive array of services to deal with a variety of medical conditions and functional disabilities. Many outpatient rehabilitation programs address

Table 1-1. Growth of Outpatient Rehabilitation Programs in U.S. Hospitals, by Census Region, 1980–1989

Census Region	1980	1981	1982	1983	1984	1985	1986	1987	1988	1989
Region 1—										
New England	132	163	167	173	178	182	176	184	188	199
Connecticut	28	30	27	29	30	31	36	31	30	33
Maine	11	17	16	16	16	19	18	23	22	21
Massachusetts	69	82	89	94	97	97	82	89	94	104
New Hampshire	11	13	15	15	15	17	21	22	22	21
Rhode Island	7	11	11	10	10	8	9	10	9	8
Vermont	6	10	9	9	10	10	10	9	11	12
Region 2—										
Middle Atlantic	336	387	372	372	383	408	361	382	395	408
New Jersey	65	80	75	71	77	82	76	81	75	78
New York	152	161	157	159	160	167	152	155	166	163
Pennsylvania	119	146	140	142	146	159	133	146	154	167
Region 3—										
South Atlantic	208	263	271	287	302	316	314	340	387	407
Delaware	3	4	3	3	3	3	7	8	6	7
District of Columbia	9	10	13	13	13	12	11	13	14	13
Florida	53	82	83	81	89	95	96	105	125	131
Georgia	36	48	44	47	44	54	50	49	65	63
Maryland	31	35	36	39	35	39	33	31	34	34
North Carolina	21	15	18	27	31	33	33	41	42	44
South Carolina	13	16	15	15	20	21	26	27	26	31
Virginia	31	40	44	47	51	44	39	46	54	59
West Virginia	11	13	15	15	16	15	19	20	21	25
Region 4—										
East North Central	290	370	374	399	422	463	444	466	500	523
Illinois	78	101	99	100	103	113	114	113	116	125
Indiana	39	45	41	42	45	51	44	58	62	75
Michigan	55	75	74	86	89	97	90	94	108	112
Ohio	65	83	87	90	99	108	99	111	123	124
Wisconsin	53	66	73	81	86	94	97	90	91	87
Region 5—										
East South Central	85	103	100	97	108	111	126	139	170	170
Alabama	21	22	22	22	24	29	37	38	37	34
Kentucky	20	26	27	28	28	31	38	36	43	47
Mississippi	15	13	14	7	12	8	13	21	28	27
Tennessee	29	42	37	40	44	43	38	44	62	62
Region 6—										
West North Central	190	242	230	250	265	280	291	284	326	350
Iowa	33	33	29	35	36	39	42	41	44	46
Kansas	22	41	31	35	39	42	42	37	53	52
Minnesota	47	63	59	61	62	66	57	58	68	69
Missouri	50	61	63	71	79	78	88	89	96	106
Nebraska	16	17	20	20	21	26	27	26	29	36
North Dakota	9	11	14	13	13	14	19	16	17	18
South Dakota	13	16	14	15	15	15	16	17	19	23

Table 1-1. (Continued)

Census Region	1980	1981	1982	1983	1984	1985	1986	1987	1988	1989
Region 7—										
West South Central	139	181	167	176	181	192	201	207	260	267
Arkansas	11	14	9	9	12	15	20	20	25	27
Louisiana	27	25	25	28	28	30	33	32	41	42
Oklahoma	19	27	20	21	22	25	24	26	29	33
Texas	82	115	113	118	119	122	124	129	165	165
Region 8—										
Mountain	105	126	115	120	123	145	139	155	173	183
Arizona	28	30	32	35	33	37	37	43	45	48
Colorado	35	45	40	42	41	48	46	48	46	53
Idaho	10	8	10	9	11	15	14	16	18	13
Montana	1	3	3	3	3	4	5	8	6	8
Nevada	6	10	7	6	8	8	5	4	8	10
New Mexico	12	13	11	13	12	15	16	17	22	25
Utah	10	11	8	8	9	9	11	13	16	14
Wyoming	3	6	4	4	6	9	5	6	12	12
Region 9—										
Pacific	197	278	252	272	286	301	277	286	308	323
Alaska	2	1	2	1	2	2	3	4	4	7
California	138	197	179	197	212	222	201	204	217	224
Hawaii	10	11	9	9	8	9	10	11	14	13
Oregon	24	29	28	28	29	29	27	26	28	32
Washington	23	40	34	37	35	39	36	41	45	47
Grand Total	1,682	2,113	2,048	2,146	2,248	2,398	2,329	2,443	2,707	2,830

Source: *Hospital Statistics*, 1981 edition through 1990–1991 edition, all copyright by the American Hospital Association. All rights reserved. Data cited are taken from table 12B of each edition, which records data from Section C of the AHA Annual Survey of Hospitals. The definition of a program is "provision of coordinated multidisciplinary physical restorative services to ambulatory patients under the direction of a physician knowledgeable and experienced in rehabilitation medicine."

not only physiological issues but also psychological, emotional, and vocational issues inasmuch as these issues all have an impact on individual adjustment to disability or loss of function.

As evidenced by the case studies in this book, hospitals have developed a variety of programs that enable them to focus unique expertise and resources on special programs to target specific market groups or develop reputations in specific areas. Larger systems and hospitals may acquire reputations in a number of program areas. The most commonly offered outpatient rehabilitation programs include those shown in table 1-4 (p. 18).

Hospitals may differentiate their programs by focusing on specific age groups, perhaps offering an array of programs and services under such umbrellas as pediatric rehabilitation or geriatric rehabilitation. Depending on internal capabilities, local demographics, and the competition within the hospital's service area, hospitals might specialize services to focus on disabilities such as chronic pain or arthritis programs (for geriatric patients) or burn rehabilitation or spinal cord rehabilitation (for either group). Yet

Table 1-2. Growth of Component Rehabilitation Services in U.S. Hospitals, 1980–1989

Service	1980	1981	1982	1983	1984	1985	1986	1987	1988	1989
Physical Therapy[a]										
Number reporting service	5,353	5,306	5,285	5,418	5,468	5,471	5,407	5,178	5,045	4,900
Total survey respondents	6,277	6,276	6,277	6,353	6,302	6,304	6,290	6,281	6,291	6,174
Percent of total with service	85	85	84	85	87	87	86	82	80	79
Occupational Therapy[b]										
Number reporting service	2,480	2,626	2,604	2,748	2,858	3,032	3,164	3,113	3,151	3,186
Total survey respondents	6,277	6,276	6,277	6,353	6,302	6,304	6,290	6,281	6,291	6,174
Percent of total with service	40	42	42	43	45	48	50	50	50	52
Respiratory Therapy[c]										
Number reporting service	5,374	5,311	5,224	5,351	5,378	5,368	5,300	5,205	5,082	5,006
Total survey respondents	6,277	6,276	6,277	6,353	6,302	6,304	6,290	6,281	6,291	6,174
Percent of total with service	86	85	83	84	85	85	84	83	81	81
Social Work Services[d]										
Number reporting service	5,063	5,048	5,000	5,137	5,209	5,294	[f]	[f]	[f]	[f]
Total survey respondents	6,277	6,276	6,277	6,353	6,302	6,304				
Percent of total with service	81	80	80	81	83	84				
Speech Pathology Services[e]										
Number reporting service	2,723	2,758	2,379	2,602	2,778	2,966	3,135	2,871	2,724	2,740
Total survey respondents	6,277	6,276	6,277	6,353	6,302	6,304	6,290	6,281	6,291	6,174
Percent of total with service	43	44	38	41	44	47	50	46	43	44

Source: *Hospital Statistics,* 1981 edition through 1990–1991 edition, all copyright by the American Hospital Association. All rights reserved. Data cited are taken from table 12A of each edition, which records data from Section C of the AHA Annual Survey of Hospitals.

[a] Defined as "services and use of facilities prescribed by physicians and administered by or under the direction of a qualified physical therapist."

[b] Defined as "facilities for the provision of occupational therapy services prescribed by physicians and administered by or under the direction of a qualified occupational therapist."

[c] Defined as "the equipment and staff necessary for the administration of oxygen and certain potent drugs through inhalation or positive pressure."

[d] Defined as "social services and use of facilities provided under the direction of a qualified social worker."

[e] Defined as "speech therapy provided for inpatients or outpatients by personnel available on a routine basis."

[f] Data not gathered in these years.

Table 1-3. Outpatient Physical Therapy Service Utilization, Special 1989 Survey

Factor	Used a Physical Therapist	At a Hospital	At MD or Therapist's Office	Other Location
Age				
18–24	14.9%	34.6%	35.1%	30.3%
25–34	9.4	36.2	43.3	20.5
35–44	12.2	33.5	45.8	20.6
45–54	11.9	34.4	41.7	23.9
55–64	10.2	37.9	36.6	25.5
65+	34.4	39.5	26.1	
Average	10.5	34.4	39.5	26.1
Income				
Under $15K	8.7%	35.7%	27.5%	36.8%
$15–$25K	10.0	37.7	32.9	29.4
$25–$50K	10.7	34.3	41.8	23.9
$50–$75K	12.9	33.5	46.2	20.4
$75–$100K	14.6	27.4	50.6	22.0
Over $100K	13.8	22.9	55.9	21.2
No response	7.9	37.0	37.4	25.6
Average	10.5	34.4	39.5	25.6

Source: Inforum, Inc., Nashville, 1989. Based on responses from 100,052 households between December 1988 and April 1989. Data table is as published in *Hospitals* 63(23):78 (Dec. 5, 1989).

another common differentiation strategy is to focus the outpatient program on occupational or vocational rehabilitation.

The component *services* available as part of outpatient programs are numerous. Outpatient programs may not include all the services provided in inpatient programs, but there are a number of service possibilities, including those shown in table 1-5 (p. 19):

- *Audiology:* Audiological evaluation, possible aural rehabilitation, and designation of appropriate hearing aids to improve overall communication skills.
- *Bioengineering:* Services applying engineering and technological concepts to improve biological and anatomical systems.
- *Case management:* Assessment, rehabilitation treatment planning, referral, and follow-up to ensure the provision of comprehensive and continuous service and the coordination of payment and reimbursement for care.
- *Dental care:* Services in improving oral communication, mastication, maxillofacial prostheses, and cosmesis related to dental needs.
- *Nutritional counseling:* Dietary assessments, counseling, training, and education on the unique nutritional problems of persons with complex, debilitating illnesses.
- *Occupational therapy:* Services providing assistance to patients in restoring, developing, or maintaining skills necessary to perform work; may

Table 1-4. Relative Frequency of Organized Outpatient Rehabilitation Program Types, Special 1989 Survey (does not include all U.S.-registered hospitals)

	Hospitals (N = 66)		Units (N = 388)		Services (N = 77)	
Program	Adult	Pediatric	Adult	Pediatric	Adult	Pediatric
Amputee	48	28	274	87	42	16
Arthritis	38	22	243	72	42	17
Back program (not SCI)	36	11	258	44	50	11
Brain/head injury	50	29	222	87	23	10
Burn rehab	18	16	115	57	25	12
Cancer/oncology rehab	11	1	129	40	31	12
Cardiac rehab	12	4	198	37	35	6
Chronic pain	33	10	166	31	31	8
Other orthopedic	40	24	253	84	47	20
Pulmonary rehab	16	9	155	42	37	14
Spinal cord rehab	44	24	201	76	20	9
Stroke rehab	46	17	276	68	45	10
Other	8	7	38	14	6	4

Source: American Hospital Association, Department of Special Surveys, *Survey of Medical Rehabilitation Hospitals and Units—1988*, copyright 1990 by the American Hospital Association. All rights reserved.

Note: The universe sampled for this survey was 1,048 institutions, from which 602 surveys were returned. Definitions of the classifications used are:

Hospital—a separate and distinct entity that provides a comprehensive array of multidisciplinary medical rehab services for the disabled on an inpatient and outpatient basis, and provides all of the support services either directly or on a contractual basis.

Unit—a physically distinct unit or department of a hospital or medical complex having designated beds and providing a comprehensive array of multidisciplinary medical rehab services for disabled persons. Some treatment services and all or part of the support services may be provided by the parent entity.

Service—a medical facility providing coordinated multidisciplinary physical restorative services to inpatients and outpatients under the medical direction of a physician knowledgeable and experienced in rehab medicine *but having no separately designated rehabilitation beds.*

include treatment of specific problems that impede the patient's ability to carry out activities of daily living.

- *Orthotics:* Designing, fabricating, and fitting patients with braces and other orthopedic devices as ordered by physicians.
- *Pastoral care:* Services that respond to patients' spiritual needs. Religious professionals with traditional theological backgrounds subsequently may obtain special clinical and pastoral training in rehabilitation services; they are available for counseling.
- *Physical therapy:* Identifying and treating specific problems that interrupt the patient's ability to move normally or carry out activities of daily living. The physical therapist structures a program of therapeutic exercise, functional mobility training, and use of physical agents (heat, cold, electricity) aimed at achieving the highest possible functional level.
- *Prosthetics:* Designing, fabricating, and fitting artificial devices to replace partially or totally missing extremities or other body parts.
- *Psychological evaluation and counseling:* Evaluating and treating patients with problems in coping with daily stresses or adjusting to their dis-

ability. These services may include, but are not limited to, psychological testing, interviewing, counseling, psychotherapy, behavior and biofeedback therapy, and consultation.

- *Recreational therapy:* Services to teach patients interactive social and leisure skills designed to boost morale, alleviate mental stress, facilitate reintegration into the community, and prevent mental and physical deterioration.

Table 1-5. Relative Frequency of Outpatient Rehabilitation Services, Special 1988 Survey (does not include all U.S.-registered hospitals)

	Hospitals (N = 66)		Units (N = 388)		Services (N = 77)	
Program	**In-House**	**Contracted**	**In-House**	**Contracted**	**In-House**	**Contracted**
Audiology	23	21	187	71	30	25
Bioengineering	14	8	101	35	14	4
Case management	32	—	150	3	25	—
Dental care	7	7	107	27	23	3
Nutritional counseling	39	3	255	3	54	—
Occupational therapy	56	1	311	7	67	4
Orthotics	23	25	94	182	21	18
Pastoral care	22	2	207	8	35	1
Physical therapy	58	1	313	9	65	6
Prosthetics	21	27	73	195	11	21
Psychol. eval. & counseling	46	7	217	56	35	5
Recreational therapy	40	1	159	3	20	1
Rehab nursing	41	—	167	3	13	—
Rehab physician	50	5	244	42	30	12
Respiratory therapy	27	9	240	3	58	—
Social work	49	—	252	6	60	1
Speech-language pathology	51	5	281	31	48	23
Sports medicine	15	4	123	7	18	3
Transitional living	13	—	39	13	4	2
Vocational evaluation	29	14	120	77	15	3
Vocational training & placement	21	8	60	69	5	2
Other	7	—	24	3	3	2

Source: American Hospital Association, Department of Special Surveys, *Survey of Medical Rehabilitation Hospitals and Units—1988*, copyright 1990 by the American Hospital Association. All rights reserved.

Note: See table 1-4 for sample size and definitions of classifications. Several facilities checked both in-house and contracted services; thus totals may exceed the number of facilities reporting. A *contracted service* is one in which the general active charge of day-to-day management of one or more departments/functions of an institution is undertaken by another organization under a formal contract.

- *Rehabilitation nursing services:* Specialized nursing services generally under the direction of a certified rehabilitation registered nurse (a designation conferred on RNs who pass an examination established by the Association of Rehabilitation Nurses), with supervised licensed practical nurses and nurse assistants.
- *Rehabilitation physician services:* Medical direction by a specialist in physical medicine and rehabilitation (a physiatrist). Physiatrists are certified by the American Board of Physical Medicine and Rehabilitation after completing a four-year residency (the first year of which includes nine months in internal medicine and three months in an elective field of study such as pediatrics, neurology, orthopedics, rheumatology, or neurosurgery) and passing a two-part examination (the second part of which can be taken only after one year in full-time practice of the specialty). Physiatrists may also have additional certification by the American Association of Electromyography and Electrodiagnosis in those specialties.
- *Respiratory therapy:* Services providing ventilatory support and associated services to patients, such as pulmonary function studies and blood and gas analysis, administration of oxygen and certain potent drugs through inhalation or positive pressure, and the teaching of breathing exercises.
- *Social work:* Services to assess patient and family functioning designed to enhance the individual's ability to return to the previous environment or adapt to a new one. Such services could include financial planning, identification and coordination of entitlement programs and sources for funding/reimbursement, income, planning for environmental modification and placement, discharge planning and preparation, coordination of home or day-care services, and family and patient follow-up and counseling.
- *Speech–language pathology:* Providing evaluation and treatment of communicative deficiencies to improve the patient's overall listening, reading, speaking, writing and cognitive skills.
- *Sports medicine:* Rehabilitation for injuries suffered in athletic endeavors.
- *Transitional living:* Services for those who have been discharged from inpatient care but need a period to adjust to living with a disability before returning home.
- *Vocational evaluation:* Evaluation to prepare individuals to return to work.
- *Vocational training and placement:* Training provided by vocational counselors, occupational skills instructors, and other specialists to prepare individuals for work and placement in a new line of work.

Future Directions

Predictions about the future are most often built on sand. It does seem clear, however, that expansion and development of outpatient programs by hospitals will become a principal line of business, rather than a secondary source of patient care activity. The nature of services delivered along the ambulatory care spectrum will expand with the sophistication in technology that will allow more procedures to be performed non-invasively and that will give rise to new and effective methods of diagnosis and treatment. It also seems safe to predict that the separation of ambulatory care and rehabilitation into discrete disciplines will continue to be blurred, and the areas will be integrated into a continuum of care that also includes acute and long-term care. Such a continuum will have the salutary effect for both patients and payers of assigning patients to the most appropriate and cost-effective level of care.

Beyond changes engendered by demographic trends and emerging technologies, the major issues that will shape the future of rehabilitation are changes in payment mechanisms and the demand for cost accountability, the demand for performance documentation, changes in the competitive environment, and shortages of qualified rehabilitation professionals.

Changes in Payment Mechanisms and the Demand for Cost Accountability

Of the issues facing rehabilitation providers, none has engendered more debate and concern than the question of payment. The Social Security Amendments of 1983 (P.L. 98-21), which created the prospective payment system (PPS) based on diagnostic-related groups (DRGs) for inpatient acute care, granted rehabilitation hospitals and units an exclusion from PPS. The statutory exclusion is contained in section 1886(d)(i)(B) of the Social Security Act, and regulations setting forth the specific criteria that must be met are contained in 42 C.F.R. sections 412.23(b), 412.25, and 412.29. Excluded rehabilitation hospitals and units are subject to the cost limits imposed by the Tax Equity and Fiscal Responsibility Act (TEFRA) of 1982, P.L. 97-248. Programs that do not qualify for the exclusion are paid under Medicare's DRG-based PPS.

This consideration was made because DRGs were not constructed with rehabilitation patients in mind. However, as evidenced by the U.S. Department of Health and Human Services *Report to Congress: Developing a Prospective Payment System for Excluded Hospitals* (October 1987), the press is on to find a suitable substitute for the DRG system to apply to rehabilitation hospitals and units. Although that report indicated that it was premature to advance specific recommendations, it alludes to the possibility of a prospective payment system or a capitation-based system.

The difficulty in arriving at a specific recommendation is due to the great challenge in rehabilitation care of establishing norms and basing payment on averages. Rehabilitation is notable for the number and range of the variables that determine the cost of a case. For example, a stroke patient's length of stay in a rehabilitation hospital or unit can vary from a few days to 25 or 30 days to as many as 70 days, depending on the severity and permanance of the damage incurred. For a rehabilitation patient with severe head trauma, there is no such thing as a typical length of stay—the stay can range from a few days to months or even years. With such extreme variation, averages are meaningless. Beyond severity of the disability, length of the rehabilitation process may vary by reason of (1) medical complications, (2) inherent genetic powers of resistance and recuperation, (3) mental attitude and drive to succeed, and (4) lifestyle factors such as weight, smoking, alcoholism, or, by contrast, physical fitness orientation.[31]

Andrew Batavia makes the preliminary conclusion that, of the possible systems, the models that appear to be "particularly attractive" for the payment of medical rehabilitation are (1) a prospective payment model based on DRGs adjusted for severity of illness, (2) a model based on improvements in functional status, and (3) a per capita payment model.[32] Outpatient rehabilitation program providers might also chart HCFA's physician payment reform initiatives using the resource-based relative value scale (RBRVS) and hospital outpatient services payment reforms using HCFA's Common Procedural Coding System (HCPCS) for evidence of trends that might ultimately be applied to outpatient rehab services.

The demand for cost accountability that underlies the examination of payment methodologies remains significant when one looks at the typical payer mix for rehabilitation hospitals and units (table 1-6), despite their lower percentage of Medicare and Medicaid patients compared to acute care providers. Medicare and Medicaid are significant payers, and

Table 1-6. Percentage of Gross Outpatient Revenue Attributable to Identified Sources, Special 1988 Survey (does not include all U.S.-registered hospitals)

Source	Hospitals (N = 23)	Units (N = 50)	Services (N = 10)
Medicare	19.4%	24.7%	18.2%
Medicaid	10.4	10.5	10.4
Blue Cross	18.1	10.5	18.9
Commercial insurance	25.8	22.8	17.0
Department of Vocational Rehab	1.8	0.2	—
Workers' compensation	11.1	5.9	9.2
HMO, PPO, PPA	3.3	4.4	3.0
Self-pay	7.4	13.5	17.7
Federal, state, local funding	0.6	1.4	1.5
Other	2.1	5.9	4.1
Total Outpatient Billings	$42,875,934	$53,601,730	$6,210,265

Source: American Hospital Association, Department of Special Surveys, *Survey of Medical Rehabilitation Hospitals and Units—1988*, copyright 1990 by the American Hospital Association. All rights reserved.
Note: See table 1-4 for sample size and definitions of classifications.

changes in the demographics of the U.S. population can be expected to elevate the current percentages.

Changes in payment methodologies will also raise questions of access to care, questions already evident for medically indigent populations.[33] Many in health care view Medicare payments for geriatric patients to be inadequate. Families with lower incomes have a disproportionate number of children who require rehabilitative therapies but have no funds to pay for such care. In most states, Medicaid offers no primary reimbursement to outpatient rehabilitation centers, thereby excluding many low-income families from receiving outpatient care. Addressing the current and intensifying questions of access to care will be further complicated by the need to address the ethical and practical issue of the allocation of scarce resources (exacerbated by shortages of physiatrists, rehab nurses, and practitioners of the various therapeutic disciplines) and the influence of competition on the ability of providers to subsidize indigent care. These issues may prompt some degree of regionalization of service delivery, including further development of "hub-and-spoke" network models involving national networks (such as Voluntary Hospitals of America), regional networks (such as SunHealth), and local and physician networks.[34]

Demand for Performance Documentation

Hand in hand with the payers' call for cost accountability is the call from payers and consumers alike for documentation of performance. Rehabilitation, perhaps more than acute care, has historically placed great value on measuring and communicating the outcomes of its services, as evidenced by the accreditation standard for facilities to have a program evaluation system by the Commission on Accreditation of Rehabilitation Facilities (a requirement evolving from CARF's first National Invitational Conference on Rehabilitation and the Measurement of Its Results in 1973). Similar emphasis on outcomes measurement for continuous quality improvement is reflected in the standards of the Joint Commission on Accreditation of Healthcare Organizations (in the "Physical Rehabilitation Services" chapter of its *Accreditation Manual for Hospitals* as well as in such Joint Commission publications as the 1988 *Monitoring and Evaluation: Physical Rehabilitation Services*).

The continuing evolution of program evaluation and quality improvement systems and such initiatives as the Uniform Data System (UDS) for Medical Rehabilitation mentioned earlier in this chapter should help rehabilitation providers meet the challenge to improve performance documentation. Some forms of information gathering and sharing have always been evident owing to the standard practice of holding routine team meetings of the multiple disciplines involved in the treatment planning and monitoring of rehab patients. New demands may help providers refine existing documentation procedures, and strategies for improving the customer-service orientation of providers may extend information gathering to include routinely measuring and monitoring patient satisfaction. The multiple demands for information from the provider's multidisciplinary team, payers, and patients will in turn force a reexamination of existing information systems, and systems built for inpatient programs may not be adequate for outpatient programs.[35]

Changes in the Competitive Environment

The increased demand for outpatient rehabilitation services described in this chapter have brought a wide variety of nonhospital providers into the market. Hospital-based programs must contend with the fact that some nonhospital providers may be able to produce the same patient outcomes at a considerably lower cost, and creative strategies may be indicated, such as spinning off separate corporate entities operating out of freestanding satellite centers or joining forces with other providers under some form of network, alliance, or joint venture. Competition will also force hospitals to reevaluate how they differentiate, position, and market their programs and services.

Above all, competition will force concentrated efforts in market research, planning, and development. Paul Smith and Howard Wodinsky suggest eight reasons why hospitals have had problems in developing a coherent and coordinated approach to ambulatory care:[36]

- *Poor product definition:* In many hospitals, the ambulatory care product remains poorly defined, thereby hampering innovation.
- *Growth pains:* Ambulatory care is still in its infancy. For years, it had existed as a "stepchild" to other areas of health care. Ambulatory care may be celebrated as being the future of health care, but many health care executives still grant it little more than second-best status.
- *Increased competition:* Lately, ambulatory care has begun to feel the impact of managed care and more competition. As managed care proliferates, health care organizations must compete more aggressively for managed care contracts.
- *Internal strife:* Ambulatory care suffers from the internal conflicts present within health care organizations. Many practitioners cling desperately to traditional hierarchies and organizational structures.
- *Executive ambiguity:* Responsibility for ambulatory care is diffuse and unclear. Within some hospitals, a vice-president of ambulatory care controls relatively little of the ambulatory care market. In other organizations, outreach programs may operate out of a variety of corporate structures.
- *"Me-tooism":* Many health care executives remain victims of the "bandwagon effect." Some ambulatory care programs are poorly conceived

and developed. As is said of some health care executives, "If they read it in a magazine, they're convinced they ought to do it." Health care executives have been known to develop a costly women's health center for no reason other than a colleague's success with a similar program. Unfortunately, many of these centers fail to achieve differentiation through specific services or programs of research.

- *Faith healing:* Other health care executives look to ambulatory care for a quick-fix solution. In their urgency to develop a better bottom line, these administrators are more than willing to experiment with ambulatory care. In the process, they often lose sight of how ambulatory care relates to their organization's mission, vision, and values.
- *Customer blindness:* Ambulatory care often is not developed and managed from the customer's point of view. In some institutions, ambulatory care involves a crazy quilt of bewildering and confusing programs. Patients and family members therefore often experience a disjointed array of services.

The need to acknowledge competition and adjust strategic planning to changes in the competitive environment forces planners to evaluate ambulatory care programs that are responsive to customer needs as well as the overall goals and mission of the hospital.

Shortages of Qualified Rehabilitation Professionals

As indicated by the results of the special survey shown in table 1-7, shortages in trained and qualified rehabilitation professionals represent a significant barrier to program growth in many hospitals. To partially offset

Table 1-7. Staff Shortages in Medical Rehabilitation, Special 1988 Survey (does not include all U.S.-registered hospitals)

Position	Number of Vacant Positions under Active Recruitment[a]		Average Number of Weeks to Fill Vacancies	
Physiatrist	71.7	(194)	35.0	(64)
Rehab RNs	952.1	(310)	13.7	(229)
LPN/vocational	271.5	(228)	10.3	(119)
Physical therapist	636.6	(381)	22.5	(293)
Physical therapy assistant	82.0	(205)	14.5	(102)
Occupational therapist	468.0	(353)	16.9	(268)
Occupational therapy assistant	66.1	(173)	14.8	(96)
Speech-language pathologist	91.4	(253)	11.1	(142)
Audiologist	15.6	(94)	9.5	(35)

Source: American Hospital Association, Department of Special Surveys, *Survey of Medical Rehabilitation Hospitals and Units—1988*, copyright 1990 by the American Hospital Association. All rights reserved.

[a]Numbers in parentheses indicate number of respondents answering question.

the problem, hospitals may use an internal float pool (hospital employees with flexible hours used when and where needed) or agency/contracted staff, and many hospitals stretch current staff by granting overtime pay.

The consequences of staff vacancies may be as severe as facing the need to close beds or discontinue selected programs and services. Hospitals have also found the need to adjust patient–staff ratios to less-than-desirable work loads, to create waiting lists for program admissions, and to substitute desired personnel classifications with other types of personnel.

Shortages have also led hospitals to reexamine their recruitment and retention strategies. High among the list of items being reexamined are compensation programs, with recruitment bonuses, enhanced pay scales, and a wide variety of incentive compensation schemes becoming more common, including continuing education and tuition reimbursement.

According to Douglas Shepherd, there are a number of things hospitals can do to address the problem of shortages in general.[37] These efforts include:

- Focus on retention issues rather than staff turnover.
- Establish formal affiliations with training programs in rehabilitation or work with student interns to develop loyal relationships among new personnel about to enter the rehabilitation field.
- Fund-raising efforts must also be directed toward the education of personnel, including tuition subsidies or outside educational programs.
- Hospitals must make efforts to develop new revenue sources, establishing endowments to support continuing education opportunities.
- Hospitals must also establish programs to encourage reentry for those rehabilitation practitioners who have temporarily left the field.

Outlook for Program Innovation

Despite the challenges that lie ahead for the field of outpatient rehabilitation, industry observers see many promising developments. Michael B. Arnall sees 12 developments:[38]

- *Entrepreneurial ventures:* Increasingly, new technologies and treatment models will be available to spin off business units that are small, profitable, cost-effective, and responsive to the market.
- *Compensation schemes:* There will be more opportunities to experiment with different patterns of compensation, such as incentive systems.
- *Revitalization:* Rehabilitation will be used as a strategy to revitalize a hospital that is currently experiencing financial difficulties.
- *Staffing:* Private rehabilitation practices and facilities will provide additional staff to hospitals. Some hospitals are already using staff from independent rehabilitation practices to staff inpatient units.

- *Increased demand:* Because of the aging of the population and other demographic changes, there will be increased demand for rehabilitation services.
- *Innovation:* Newer models of care will be developed and older models will be further segmented.
- *Occupational rehabilitation:* Rehabilitation of injured workers will take place within the factory and involve gradual assimilation into the workplace. Other units will be located in industrial parks to better serve employers.
- *Diversification:* There will be rehabilitation clinics geared to the needs of women, pediatric patients, and arthritic patients.
- *Networking:* Larger institutions or consortiums of institutions will develop smaller, more differentiated rehabilitation units with greater opportunities for cross-referrals among larger institutions, consortiums, and smaller rehabilitation units.
- *Comprehensive care:* Although clinics will be segmented to serve the needs of specific patient populations, they will offer a broader range of services.
- *Product evolution:* Rehabilitation will move away from a generic rehabilitation product such as physical therapy or occupational therapy and toward a more "augmented" product: *health security.* The new thrust of rehabilitation will be minimizing the probability of insult to the body and maximizing measures to control health problems and injuries.
- *Employer involvement:* Business and industry will be more involved in developing health care models. Preferred provider organizations for rehabilitation already exist and may expand in the years ahead. Hospitals will begin to realize the advantages of selling an augmented product to business and industry and to physicians.

Overview of This Book

Against the backdrop of the environment presented in this chapter, the following chapters will invite a deeper exploration of the major factors that influence success in developing a program, whether it is a single-service physical therapy department or a specialized multidisciplinary program designed to treat head trauma patients. These factors include:

- Conducting market-based strategic planning for an outpatient rehabilitation program and fostering a market-driven, customer-first attitude among program staff
- Preparing a business or operating plan for the program that includes definition of the program, determination and resolution of medical staff issues, definition of organizational and staffing structure, determination

of information and data system needs, and formulation of a strategy for working with managed care plans

- Identifying and finding mechanisms to address the major patient management issues of special concern in outpatient rehabilitation
- Addressing specialized design considerations in renovating existing space or planning new space
- Identifying the major accreditation criteria and processes for the Commission on Accreditation of Rehabilitation Facilities (CARF) and the Joint Commission on Accreditation of Healthcare Organizations (Joint Commission)
- Determining the major payers for outpatient rehabilitation and their basic restrictions and requirements
- Identifying the major means of structuring outpatient rehabilitation programs, tax restrictions, and fraud and abuse regulations

The book contains 11 case studies representing the broad spectrum of outpatient rehabilitation, including pediatric rehabilitation, geriatric rehabilitation, and market-specific programs. The annotated bibliography provides pertinent information on selected resources.

References

1. England, B., editor. *Medical Rehabilitation Services in Health Care Institutions.* Chicago: American Hospital Publishing, 1986, p. 7.
2. Rusk, H. A. Rehabilitation medicine: knowledge in search of understanding. *Archives of Physical Medicine and Rehabilitation* 59:156–160, 1978.
3. Eckenhoff, E. A. The 35th John Stanley Coulter memorial lecture. Rehabilitation: ghosts . . . images . . . visions. *Archives of Physical Medicine and Rehabilitation* 67(2): 75–78, Feb. 1986.
4. England, B. *An Agenda for Medical Rehabilitation 1987 and into the 21st Century.* Chicago: American Hospital Association, 1987.
5. England, B., Glass, R., and Patterson, C., editors. *Quality Rehabilitation: Results-Oriented Patient Care.* Chicago: American Hospital Publishing, 1989, p. 12.
6. Batavia, A. *The Payment of Medical Rehabilitation Services: Current Mechanisms and Potential Models.* Chicago: American Hospital Association, 1988, p. 5.
7. American Hospital Association, Department of Special Surveys. Survey of medical rehabilitation hospitals and units–1988. Chicago: AHA, 1990 (unpublished).
8. National Association of Rehabilitation Facilities. *NARF Position Paper on a Prospective Payment System for Inpatient Medical Rehabilitation Services and a Study Regarding a Prospective Payment System for Inpatient Medical Rehabilitation Services: Final Report.* Reston, VA: NARF, 1985.

9. McGinnis, G. E., Osberg, J. S., and others. Predicting charges for inpatient medical rehabilitation using severity, DRG, age, and function. *American Journal of Public Health* 77(7):826–29, July 1987.

10. Johnson, M. V., and Keith, R. A. Cost-benefits of medical rehabilitation: review and critique. *Archives of Physical Medicine and Rehabilitation* 64(4):147–54, Apr. 1983.

11. Johnson, M. Cost-benefit methodologies in rehabilitation. In: M. J. Fuhrer, editor. *Rehabilitation Outcomes: Analysis and Measurement.* Baltimore: Paul H. Brookes Publishing Co., 1987.

12. DeJong, G., and Lifchez, R. Physical disability and public policy. *Scientific American* 248(6):40–49, June 1983.

13. England and others.

14. Flory, J., editor. *Ambulatory Care: A Management Briefing.* Chicago: American Hospital Publishing, 1990, p. 28.

15. Dychtwald, K., and Zitter, M. Changes during the next decade will alter the way eldercare is provided, financed. *Modern Healthcare* 18(16):68–69, Apr. 15, 1988.

16. Special Committee on Aging. *Aging America: Trends and Projections.* Washington, DC: U.S. Government Printing Office, 1989, p. 4.

17. Special Committee on Aging, p. 4.

18. Persily, N. *Eldercare: Positioning Your Hospital for the Future.* Chicago: American Hospital Publishing, 1991, p. 29.

19. National Institute on Disability and Rehabilitation Research. *Chartbook on Disability in the United States* (U.S. Department of Education Contract # HN88011001). Washington, DC: NIDRR, Mar. 1989, p. 2.

20. NIDRR, pp. 3–4.

21. Differentiating the rehabilitation product. *Healthcare Planning and Marketing* 11(2):4–7, Mar.–Apr. 1988.

22. Newkirk, W. L., and Jones, L. D., editors. *Occupational Health Services: A Guide to Program Planning and Management.* Chicago: American Hospital Publishing, 1989, pp. 7–8.

23. Arnall, M. B. Rehabilitation services. In: J. Flory, editor. *Ambulatory Care: A Management Briefing.* Chicago: American Hospital Publishing, 1990, p. 77.

24. American Hospital Association. *Management Advisory: Comprehensive Medical Rehabilitation in the Health Care Setting.* Chicago: AHA, 1990.

25. Batavia, p. 19.

26. DeJong, G. Medical rehabilitation outcome measurement in a changing health care market. In: M. J. Fuhrer, editor. *Rehabilitation Outcomes: Analysis and Measurement.* Baltimore: Paul H. Brookes Publishing Co., 1987.

27. American Hospital Association, Department of Special Surveys. Survey of medical rehabilitation hospitals and units—1988. Chicago: AHA, 1990 (unpublished).

28. Commission on Accreditation of Rehabilitation Facilities. *Standards Manual for Organizations Serving People with Disabilities.* 1990 ed. Tucson, AZ: CARF, 1990.

29. England, *Medical Rehabilitation Services in Health Care Institutions,* p. 68.

30. American Hospital Association. *Hospital Statistics.* 1976 ed., 1981 ed., and 1990–1991 ed. Chicago: AHA, 1976, 1981, and 1990. Table 5A in each edition.

31. England, *Medical Rehabilitation Services in Health Care Institutions,* p. 66.

32. Batavia, p. 117.

33. Flory, p. 79.

34. England and others, pp. 116–17.

35. Matson, T., and McDougall, M., editors. *Information Systems for Ambulatory Care.* Chicago: American Hospital Publishing, 1990.

36. Flory, pp. 7–8.

37. Shepherd, D. The collaborative roles of universities and hospitals in addressing the allied health manpower shortage. *The Journal of Allied Health* 19(4):293–295, Fall 1990.

38. Flory, pp. 80–81.

Chapter 2

Market-Based Strategic Planning

Sheryl J. Bronkesh, Anne-Marie Nelson, and Steven D. Wood

Introduction

Opportunities in rehabilitation are increasing. There is greater interest in returning injured employees to work as soon as possible, more concern about rehabilitation of the elderly and those impaired by brain injury, and increased awareness of the needs of persons with disabilities. However, opportunity also leads to competition. Thus, *strategic planning* in outpatient rehabilitation is of greater importance than ever. Hospitals today regard outpatient services as a means of reducing length of stay and as feeder programs for their inpatient services. Strategic planning helps to ensure that the objectives and activities of the rehabilitation program align with those of the hospital.

The primary objective of strategic planning in outpatient rehabilitation is to develop and support a *lasting* competitive advantage. As M. C. Porter has crisply stated, "The essence of strategy formulation is coping with competition."[1] Above all, the rehabilitation provider must maintain momentum in achieving program growth and success, especially in the face of stiffer competition. To this end, strategic planning is the development of a sense of direction and a definition of what the organization intends to *do* and *become,* in both the short and long term, in order to achieve its objectives.

One of the easiest ways to think of strategic planning is to contrast effectiveness–"Doing the right things"–with efficiency–"Doing things right." Strategic planning involves *selecting the right things to do and to be.*

In this chapter, you will learn how to adopt a marketing orientation in the strategic planning process in order to develop services that meet the wants and needs of the specific customer group(s) for your work hardening program, geriatric rehab program, pediatric rehab program, and any other outpatient rehab program.

The Strategic Planning Process

A strategic plan provides the structure for decision making. When strategies are not planned within an organization, they may be dictated by the competition. For example, a hospital that is considering creating a hand rehabilitation program requested by its hand surgeons may find it impossible once a private group of hand therapists from a nearby community enters the market with a satellite office. Even if the hospital then follows through and quickly implements the requested therapy program, its actions are reactive rather than proactive and are less likely to be initially successful.

Strategic planning in rehabilitation accomplishes a number of key objectives:

1. Forces setting of objectives
2. Clarifies opportunities and threats
3. Defines target markets and appropriate strategies
4. Focuses attention on key issues that will determine project success
5. Establishes a framework for making decisions
6. Provides a basis for measuring performance

In rehabilitation, the therapist has a treatment plan for each patient. This entails setting objectives, determining obstacles to progress, planning the appropriate modalities and treatment intervals, and evaluating patient progress on a daily or weekly basis.

In developing and implementing a rehabilitation program, the *treatment plan* is called strategic planning. Just as the therapist's treatment plan serves the needs of the patient, strategic planning matches the characteristics and needs of potential therapy consumers and referral sources. This is considered a *marketing* orientation as opposed to a *product* orientation; it means you are responding to those who need and will use your planned outpatient rehabilitation service. A strategic marketing plan accomplishes a hospital's objectives by providing the means to generate and retain customers through the efficient distribution of needed rehabilitation services.

These are the elements of the strategic planning process:

- The strategic planning team
- Decision making
- Environmental assessment
- Market segmentation
- Macro objectives
- Strategies and goals
- The marketing mix
- Positioning

- Requirements and benefits of the program
- Plan finalization and review
- Evaluation

The relationship between most of these elements is shown in figure 2-1; all are discussed in the following sections.

The Strategic Planning Team

Strategic planning requires accurate information. Gathering this information in order to develop a realistic action plan requires bringing together a knowledgeable team. This group constitutes the *strategic planning team.* It should be headed by an individual who will be administratively responsible for implementing the program. Most likely, the director of rehabilitative services will be the strategic planning team leader. The team may consist of representatives from the following departments or disciplines:

- Rehabilitation medical director
- Likely referral specialties from the medical staff
- Occupational therapy
- Physical therapy
- Speech and/or other therapies
- Marketing
- Administration
- Financial services
- Planning

The individuals and departments represented on the planning team will depend on the service(s) under discussion. For example, the team planning a back program will not require representation by speech or audiology, whereas a brain injury program will require that almost every clinical discipline in rehabilitation be represented. The planning team should be kept relatively small—no more than six or eight persons—to simplify scheduling of meetings and to allow all participants time to share their views.

Depending on the nature of the project and the medical staff at the institution, one or more influential, politically astute referral physicians should participate in addition to the physiatrist. The type of program may dictate when to involve physicians. A hand rehabilitation program may depend on referrals from a small but busy group of hand surgeons. In this case, their early involvement is crucial. However, planning for a physical capacity evaluation service probably will not require medical staff participation in the initial phases. In many cases, it may be more reasonable to bring key specialists into the planning process when back-

Figure 2-1. The Planning Process

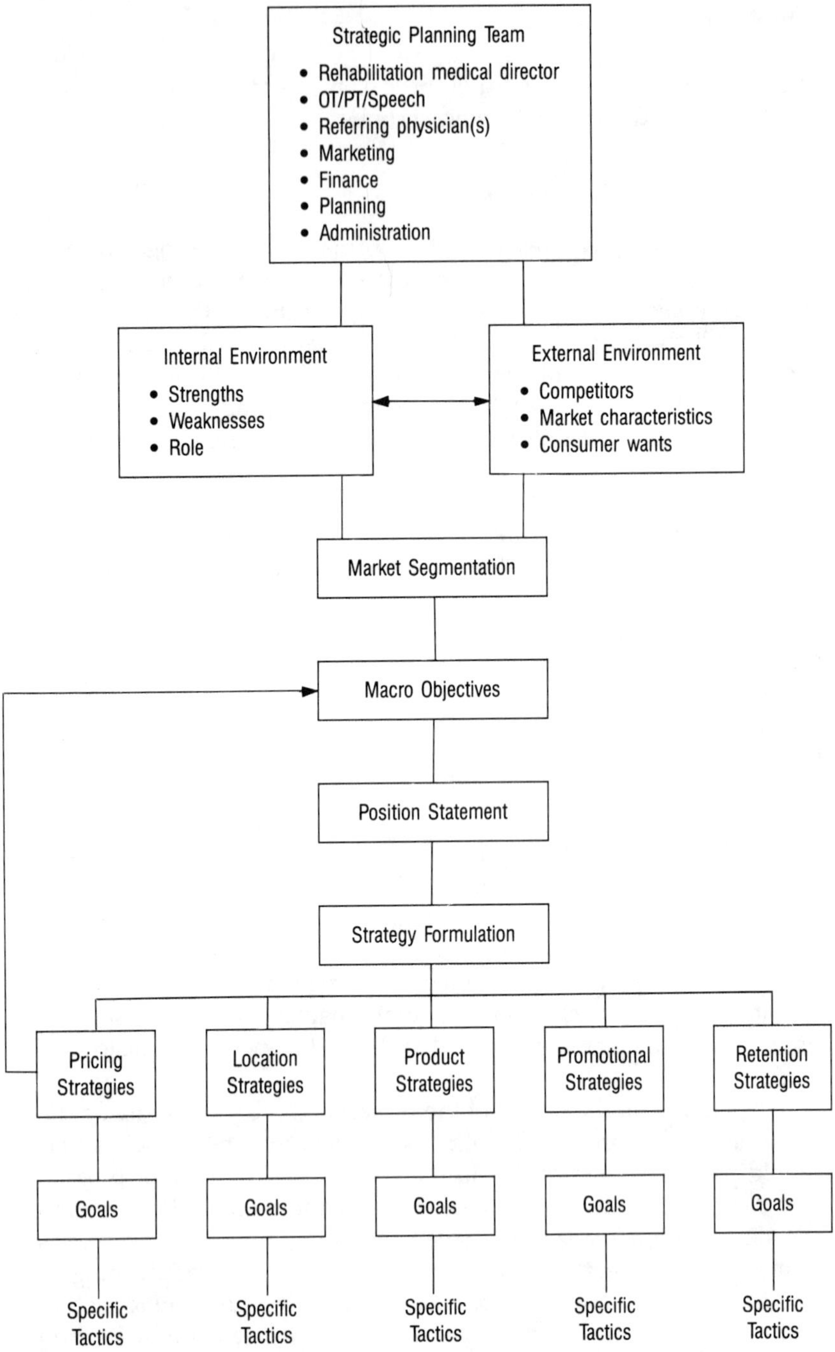

ground work is completed and preliminary objectives are formulated. Others who may be considered for later involvement are a member of the hospital board and, if appropriate, one or two representatives from area businesses.

Accountability must be built in with the planning team's responsibilities. A well-conceived plan identifies individuals within the organization who will be responsible for executing various facets of the plan and spells out accountability through deadlines and expectations. For example, a telephone survey of child neurologists, pediatric neurosurgeons, pediatricians, and family practitioners may be seen as essential to the consideration of a pediatric rehabilitation program. If this responsibility is given to a member of the physical therapy staff, the information required, the number of physicians to be surveyed, and the date by which the survey must be completed should be clearly specified.

Decision Making

Making decisions about rehabilitation program development has the potential to be confusing and time-consuming, especially because a multidisciplinary team is involved. A few key questions will help move along the process of decision making. Each team member—clinical, administrative, and marketing personnel—will approach the situation from a different perspective and with a different set of concerns, but by keeping the following points in mind and working to answer the questions, the team can reach a consensus that will satisfy overall hospital objectives:

- *Why* is the service to be offered?
- *To whom* will the service be provided?
- *Through whom* will patients be referred?
- *What* unmet need exists?
- *What* is the reimbursement source?
- *How* will availability of the service be communicated?
- *Who* will provide the service?
- *Where* will it be provided, and *when?*
- *How* will we know if we are successful?

In the initial discussion stage, all points of view and interpretations should be openly welcomed and reviewed. At this stage, brainstorming is most useful. The riskier, newer, or more controversial the service opportunity, the more review and discussion will be required, and the clearer the decisions must be. Making a decision and advising all members of the team of the decision and the reasons for it may not satisfy everyone, but it moves the process along to the next step.

When a final decision is made, full support is vital. There must be commitment on the part of all team members to fully stand behind the agreed-upon actions and objectives. This also translates to allocating sufficient resources to allow the project to grow in its embryonic stages. Underfunding, understaffing, and underpromoting have resulted in more project failures than have poor project choices.

Environmental Assessment

The strategic planning team seeking to create a successful outpatient rehabilitation program will begin by painting a very clear picture of the total environment, both internally, within the hospital, and externally, in the service area and the rehabilitation field at large.

Internal Environmental Assessment

The environmental assessment begins by analyzing and defining the factors within the organization that may help or hinder development and growth of a program or service. An *internal environmental assessment* entails a comprehensive review of the institution's assets and capabilities, as well as any liabilities and weaknesses that may aid or impose constraints on development of the rehabilitation program(s) under consideration. Areas to include in the internal assessment process are:

- *Organizational strengths and reputation:* A positive organizational reputation, excellent business relationships, and available development capital are assets to the development of a new service. A positive reputation for clinical services, especially those that will feed an outpatient rehabilitation program, or a reputation for rehabilitation services in general, will help foster a positive attitude toward new outpatient rehabilitation services.
- *Existing acute care services:* Is there an internal need or referral source for the planned outpatient service(s)? A driving simulation program may be a pet project of the occupational therapy director, but if the stroke and head injury services in the hospital are weak, a driving program may not be realistic unless strong demand—and patient referrals—from an external source can be demonstrated. On the other hand, lack of a specific acute care component does not necessarily mean a particular outpatient service would not succeed. In a hospital with a good general rehabilitation program as well as a supportive medical director and a skilled staff willing to learn, a postpolio rehabilitation program may be a logical step, especially if the hospital is located in a community with an active Polio Echo (postpolio support group) chapter. The quality and success of acute care units expected to feed patients to an outpatient program should be examined. Strong trauma, neuro, and head injury inpatient programs point to potential success for an outpatient brain injury rehabilitation program.

- *Staff capabilities:* If inpatient therapists will be expected to provide outpatient services, the potential should exist to shift their duties without disrupting the quality of care. The present therapy staff must also have the qualifications, skills, and motivation to offer the intended service(s). If not, can they be trained? If so, how, where, and when? If not, can appropriate staff be recruited? What will recruitment cost? How will existing staff react?
- *Location and space:* Where will the new outpatient service be provided? If in the inpatient rehabilitation gym, is there room to accommodate the expected influx of new patients? Is access convenient for outpatients? Is parking available nearby? Is it convenient? Where will family members who accompany patients wait?
- *Access:* Is transportation available for patients who can't drive? Is it reimbursable? Is it convenient? How will patients get from the transport drop-off point to the rehabilitation service area if they are incapacitated or not ambulatory? Will program hours accommodate patients who work?
- *Competitive factors:* Internal competition may be a factor if (1) potential referral sources (physicians, discharge planners, and so forth) view outpatient care in a negative light or (2) if members of the medical staff already offer some or all of the planned rehabilitation services. Knowledge of the attitudes and clinical perspectives of these individuals will help determine whether internal competition poses a deterrent to the program.
- *Development capital:* Is start-up funding available to ensure that the program is adequately funded, staffed, equipped, and promoted?
- *Commitment:* This is a key factor. If enthusiastic commitment does not exist or develop as the project is given clarity and structure, it will be difficult to ensure success. Support must come from administration, rehabilitation management *and* staff, marketing/public relations, development (for not-for-profit hospitals), key medical staff physicians, and potential users or payers such as health maintenance organizations (HMOs) and employers.

The organization's strengths and weaknesses must be weighed to determine whether a single dominant factor on one side overrides several on the other side, affecting the form or speed with which the service is developed.

The internal assessment should also lead to an understanding of the role of the planned therapy program within the overall objectives and strategies of the hospital. The assessment may show that a CARF-certified day rehabilitation program for stroke patients is not likely to yield many inpatients for the institution, but will solidify the hospital's existing dominance in the marketplace in stroke and head injury care.

In developing an internal environmental assessment, it is helpful to list the hospital's acute care programs and services, rehabilitation therapies and services, medical staff specialties as well as physicians who can be counted as assets (that is, those who are likely to refer patients), the hospital's existing service area boundaries and geographic characteristics, demographic and psychographic characteristics of patients currently served by the institution, area employers, and health plans or managed care for which the institution is a provider.

Also, in reviewing the characteristics of the organization (reputation, capabilities, and so forth), look for specific characteristics that may point to potential in a certain area or service. A hospital may have a general rehabilitation program that is only average, yet it may have assets such as a well-respected, highly regarded neurology group with strong ties to the institution, a serene, parklike setting, and a large Medicare inpatient base. These elements can help the hospital find a service niche that can build on existing strengths.

External Environmental Assessment

The *external environmental assessment* provides a picture of the external opportunities, threats, and constraints that may have an impact on the intended service. It identifies current and future elements that may influence and shape when, how, and where programs are implemented.

In assessing the external environment, it is a good idea to gather demographic data about the community (and surrounding communities, if the service area extends that far), major employers, third-party payers, local health plans and their requirements, and restrictions on outpatient rehabilitation.

By gathering specific data about the marketplace, it is possible to forecast the total market need; that is, the number or proportion of the total population that could benefit from the service. Of course, this number must be leveled somewhat, because not everyone will recognize their need for the service, and those who do often postpone utilization.

If the service is new to the area, total demand may be forecast entirely on the basis of estimated market need. If the service is a substitute for, or another form of, an existing program, demand may be forecast to a certain extent on the basis of the existing service. Forecasting demand usually requires a combination of objective analysis and subjective judgment.

The type of program or service planned will dictate the nature of the information required and the research needed to obtain the information. Defining the size, scope, and characteristics of the proposed service area is a convenient place to start, no matter what the service. The following demographic data will help create a clear picture of the service area:

- Population size
- Household size and makeup
- Growth projections
- Age distribution
- Income distribution
- Educational levels
- Occupation (blue collar/white collar)
- Ethnic or cultural makeup
- Behavioral patterns
- Leisure activities
- Birth/mortality statistics
- Employers
- Employment/job growth rate

This information can be refined or eliminated according to the rehabilitation program being considered. In determining the data needed, try to create a profile of a "typical" patient for the rehabilitation service, then determine how to further define this typical patient. For instance, if a sports/fitness training program is planned, it would be wise to look at leisure activities (Do participative sports rank high?); behavioral patterns (Is there a high percentage of fitness-conscious adults?); and the ages, educational levels, and income levels of those in the service area. This information is helpful because younger, more educated adults with disposable income are more likely to use this health care service.

In rehabilitation, the external factors that may influence outpatient services include the type and number of employers, demographics of the hospital's service area (or of the intended rehabilitation program location), geographic or physical barriers, competitors and their reputations, reimbursement sources, referral sources, and so forth.

Many local businesses and organizations offer quantitative, demographic, and psychographic information free or for a small fee. Places to check include the hospital marketing or planning department, the city planning office, the chamber of commerce or business development agency, school districts, utility companies, local government agencies, the industrial commission or agency charged with compiling worker injuries and claims, insurance companies, banks, the telephone company, major businesses, universities and community colleges, health agencies such as the local hospital and nursing home associations, and, if available, certificate-of-need (CON) applications from your hospital as well as others.

Surveys of potential referral physicians, surveys of patients in current rehabilitation programs, small group interviews and focus groups, and personal interviews with key individuals as well as formal market research are other methods that may be used in gathering data. A sample survey of referral physicians is shown in figure 2-2.

Figure 2-2. Sample Referral Physician Survey

Dear Doctor:

We appreciate your taking time to complete this questionnaire. The feedback we get from physicians and patients ensures that we will provide the best service and care possible.

When you have completed this survey, please insert it in the enclosed stamped envelope. If you could return it by February 10, we would be most grateful.

Thank you again for your help!

Jane Doe, OTR, Director
Hand Therapy Specialists
Smalltown Memorial Hospital

1. Are you familiar with the services and therapists at Hand Therapy Specialists? ☐ Yes ☐ No
2. Approximately how many patients a month do you see with upper-extremity or hand problems that require therapy? ________
3. Please indicate the frequency with which you prescribe the following services and modalities:

	Frequently	Seldom	Never
Upper-extremity evaluation			
Work/physical capacity evaluation			
Range of motion			
Strengthening			
Sensory reeducation			
Activities of daily living			
Joint protect/adaptive equipment			
Work hardening			
Splint fabrication			
Therapy modalities			
Other:			

4. What is your specialty? ________
5. Do you have in-house therapy services? ☐ Yes ☐ No
   If yes, do you ever refer certain cases to outside therapists? ☐ Yes ☐ No
6. Do you ever refer your patients to a comprehensive work hardening program (rehabilitative services that assist an injured worker in resuming former work activity)?
   ☐ Frequently ☐ Seldom or never
7. Would you be willing to spend no more than 10 to 15 minutes with a representative of Hand Therapy Specialists to discuss the services you would find of benefit to your patients? Please indicate below whether you are willing to spend a brief amount of time *at your convenience.*
   ☐ Yes ☐ No Date: ________ Time: ________

If you've agreed to an interview or if you would like more information about Hand Therapy Specialists, we'll need your name:

Name: ________

Thank you! Your response will assist us in meeting your needs and maintaining the high quality of care at Hand Therapy Specialists.

Health Care Trends

Health care trends need to be assessed, especially those that will affect rehabilitation. What are the short- and long-range indicators in rehabilitation that may affect a new program or service? What is on the horizon in the specific modality or therapy area for which development or expansion is considered? Is new equipment, a new procedure, or a modality change anticipated? Is reimbursement expected to increase, decline, or remain the same? For example, with increasing interest in the needs of the elderly, a geriatric evaluation program may be timely if the institution's marketplace will support such a program. Alternatively, a shortage of physical therapists could make recruiting for a new program difficult without strong competitive advantages, benefits, location appeal, and so forth.

Study trends among area employers, other hospitals, and payers. For example, increasing interest by local employers in containing health care costs may be a good indicator for industrial rehabilitation or work simulation programs. Establishment or expansion of a high-tech firm employing several thousand assembly-line workers may dictate potential need for a hand rehabilitation program. Expansion by a nearby children's hospital may bode well for outpatient pediatric rehabilitation. Greater emphasis on outpatient services by local health plans or HMOs obviously is a positive indicator for outpatient rehabilitation.

Potential Referral Sources

Where will patients for the new program come from? This question must be answered early in the strategic planning process by defining referral sources. Use past experience with similar programs to develop a referral matrix, but be aware that a completely new program may yield patients from unanticipated sources. A temporomandibular joint (TMJ) therapy program can be expected to gain a great number of patients from dentists, but women's crisis clinics and shelters may also be a source. If uncertain about a specific program, it is wise to consult with colleagues in a similar program in a noncompeting area to learn the primary referral sources and types of patients. Once referral sources have been determined, it will then be necessary to determine their needs. Each group may have different needs. Your ability to respond to them precisely can help to create a successful rehabilitation program with repeat referrals.

The next step is to develop a profile of physicians who may be expected to refer to, participate in, or compete with the intended program. Include in the profile the physician's specialty, practice focus, ancillary services, office location(s), credentials, hospital and rehabilitation affiliations, and referral potential. In addition, it is valuable to know physician attitudes toward and willingness to support the intended program, as well as their wants and needs from it—for themselves and their patients. This can be done by dividing physicians into specialty categories, because certain specialties will not be expected to refer patients to certain rehabilitation programs (for example, pediatricians to a stroke program). This profile may be obtained through individual or small group interviews with physicians, through written surveys, or by presenting the program concepts to appropriate medical staff committees or medical specialty organizations for discussion. Research may reveal family practice physicians and orthopedic surgeons who are unaware of the benefits of therapy for carpal tunnel syndrome. Alternatively, it may disclose that a multispecialty group practice near the hospital is planning to open a freestanding outpatient rehabilitation clinic.

Area Employers

Information about employers within the service area is of great value, because more and more employers are directing or influencing the source, scope, and type of health care. It will be helpful to know about health benefits provided by targeted employers: Does medical insurance cover the proposed rehabilitation service in an outpatient setting? Is there a limit on the number, type, or length of treatments? What injuries or ailments are indigenous to local industries? Where do employees live? Will your program be convenient and accessible for them? Are they given time away from the job for treatment, or will evening or weekend hours be required? How extensive is employee participation in health plans? Although secondary resources may provide some of this information, surveys or interviews with employers are the best source.

Competition

It is vital to know who else in the marketplace is offering similar rehabilitative services, where they are located, what services they offer, how and when they are available, and at what rates.

In analyzing current and potential competitors, ask knowledgeable rehabilitation staff at your institution, key medical staff, insurance company case managers, discharge planners, and friendly employers to list the top competitive providers for the services you are planning. With a composite list, these same individuals can be asked to evaluate competitor features: technical quality and skill, patient sensitivity, location, practice environment, convenience, communication with referral sources, fees, and other elements that may serve as marketing points or counterpoints for the rehabilitation program under development.

Review the promotional and educational information of other providers to identify their image and market position. If possible, the competitors should be "shopped," at least by phone, to learn about their services, prices, hours, and interaction with the public. (*Shopping* is a technique in which an individual poses as a patient or consumer in order to gain information about services, attitudes, costs, special program features, and so forth.)

Knowing competitor strengths and weaknesses helps in overcoming or avoiding flaws or weaknesses in your own program and in creating a unique positioning strategy or marketing niche for your service, especially when there are one or more strong competitors in the marketplace. For example, a competitor's stroke rehabilitation program may have a long-standing reputation for quality, but perhaps its weakness is that it is located in a hard-to-reach area and does not offer transportation arrangements.

Knowing your competitors also helps in determining the service area of a particular outpatient program. A service area can be defined quite broadly, depending on the program, the reputation of the provider, ease of access, and the availability of competitive services. Mapleton Rehabilitation's head injury outpatient program in Boulder, Colorado, draws patients from Denver, 100 miles away, because of its long-standing reputation and because Mapleton offers flight arrangements from anywhere in the United States.

Reimbursement Potential

It is important to know the reimbursement potential for a rehabilitation program, particularly because reimbursement is in a constant state of flux. Investigate Medicare Part B requirements and limitations for the proposed service, request information from the major private insurers in your area, health plans, and the workers' compensation agency. Consult with the HMOs with which your institution contracts—or which you intend to approach for an outpatient contract—to determine the average treatment or reimbursement cap for your outpatient rehabilitation services.

Income projections allow a realistic view of the viability of the service(s) being considered. A financial review should take into consideration prevailing rates for like or similar programs, reimbursement caps and restrictions, and other data affecting revenues.

Market Segmentation

With data in hand about competitors and potential consumers, it is now time to narrow the focus to target markets, a process called market segmentation. *Market segmentation* is the process of dividing the market into groups of potential customers with common needs, values, and/or ability to pay.[2] Markets can be segmented by any number of variables, such as sex, geographic location, age, employment, past users, and diagnosis. For example, marketing research led St. David's Community Hospital in Austin, Texas, to target out-of-shape, high-risk persons with bad health habits for its Health and Fitness Center. St. David's did not want to compete with other fitness programs for young, usually healthy individuals. It wanted those with actual or potential medical problems. By narrowing the audience or consumer group, a program can be fine-tuned to meet very specific needs. In St. David's case, this approach provided two referral sources: patients who might refer themselves, and physicians concerned about the well-being of their out-of-shape patients.

Before developing marketing strategies, analyze the market segment(s) to whom your program will appeal. Know also which segments will be most profitable or productive. After narrowing the markets to be served, you must know what specific services these markets need or desire and what appeal will be most effective. With this information, the strategy team can develop a competitive position for each market segment.

As previously indicated, there are dual markets, or customers, for outpatient rehabilitation. Both referral sources and end users (patients) must be considered target markets for the services. The makeup and characteristics of each of these groups will vary depending on the service: brain injury rehabilitation; rehabilitation for stroke, spinal cord injury, or dysphagia; general rehabilitation, safety assessment, work simulation, hand therapy, pediatric rehabilitation, and so forth. Customers for a rehabilitation program may include the following groups, which can be further divided by like characteristics into market segments:

- Physicians
- Social workers
- Case managers
- Other hospitals
- Other therapists and rehabilitation programs
- Patients
- Families
- Insurance companies
- Health plans (HMOs, PPOs, and so forth)
- Chiropractors
- Personal injury attorneys
- Home health agencies
- Business and industry
- Rehabilitation nurses
- Unions
- Social service agencies

Macro Objectives

The next step in the strategic planning process is to establish broad, overall objectives in order to set performance targets and measure progress. These are called *macro objectives* because they are the few broad measures that signal accomplishment of overall project goals. For example, a sports medicine program may have as a macro objective to break even financially by the end of the second year.

Macro objectives for a rehabilitation program should relate to, and aid in accomplishing, the hospital's objectives. Therefore, a hospital with an objective of retaining market share in pediatrics should welcome development of a pediatric rehabilitation program whose objective is to reach capacity in patient census within three years.

Strategies and Goals

Development of strategies and goals is the next vital element in the strategic planning process. Strategies are broad initiatives designed to provide a *measurable* means of achieving macro objectives. Strategies answer the question, "How will we accomplish our objectives?"

Strategies must be *attainable;* that is, capable of being achieved within a reasonable time. They must be compatible with organizational objectives and should be *definable* as well as measurable.[3]

Strategies must address key issues that surface during the planning process. These might include recent or planned actions by competitors; programmatic needs of the service area; medical staff attitudes and/or participation; geographic or marketplace barriers to growth; resource availability and requirements; client mix; ways to encourage use of services by physicians and consumers; and ways to initiate the service and/or integrate it with other hospital operations.

As the team settles on strategies to accomplish program objectives, team members should also be thinking of alternatives. What other services might be offered? Are there other ways of delivering the service—for instance, if there is no public transportation to bring stroke patients to therapy three times a week, is it feasible to purchase a van? What are the requirements to implement or operate the alternatives? What special arrangements, such as a joint venture with a neurology or orthopedic group, might be considered? What are the financial or other benefits that can be expected, such as stronger affiliation with the hospital by physicians who see the rehabilitation needs being met for their patients?

Each strategy must have specific goals. These goals are a way to measure progress toward attaining the desired result. Strategic goals may have several dimensions: financial, customer satisfaction, market share, and so forth. For example, a strategy for a cardiac rehabilitation program may be to locate in the medical building where a large cardiology group has its practice. The goal could be to generate a specific number of patient referrals from this group to the rehabilitation program.

Strategic goals must be *SMART:*

- **S**pecific
- **M**easurable
- **A**ttainable
- **R**elevant
- **T**rackable

Each goal should pass the *SMART* test if it is to be useful in measuring progress. Strategic goals for a rehabilitation program should probably be developed for a three-year horizon and updated during the annual planning/review process.

The Marketing Mix

Development of market-based strategies is a more organized process when the *marketing mix* is used. The marketing mix is a key element in a strategic plan for any new program or service. The marketing mix is commonly referred to as the four Ps: *product, price, place,* and *promotion.* Today, with consumers more knowledgeable and more vocal, and with competition on the rise, there is a strong need in health care for a fifth P—*preservation* or *patient retention.*

Product

Product refers to the product or service you offer potential clients. Defining the scope of the product in outpatient rehabilitation will depend on referral sources, the number and type of patients, reimbursement, and other factors. For example, a sports medicine rehabilitation program may be expected to have a modern, youthful environment, the latest Cybex and other equipment, and a friendly, outgoing staff to appeal to its clientele.

The rehabilitation product may range from a specific service (a "work readiness" evaluation, for example) to a comprehensive temporomandibular joint clinic such as that offered at St. Margaret Hospital in Hammond, Indiana. The rehabilitation program employs a dentist and a physical therapist, and also includes diagnostic tests including thermography, blood tests, bone scans, and tomograms, as well as treatment such as biofeedback, surgery, and therapy.

Amenities help define and enhance the value of your product. A pediatric rehabilitation program will be expected to have child-safe, colorful surroundings and provide snacks or even meals for its young patients, and perhaps their parents as well. Alternatively, CARF certification may be viewed as necessary to give credibility to a full outpatient rehabilitation center as well as to ensure adequate reimbursement.

Price

Price refers not only to the actual cost of a service, but also to the alternative payment options, such as submittal of insurance for patients and acceptance of credit cards. The strategic planning team's knowledge of willingness by several major employers to contract for work-site assessments is a key price consideration in developing such a program.

Price can also include *perceptions of value* created by nonfinancial factors such as ambience in treatment areas or transportation services. An example of a successful pricing strategy might be to submit Medicare paperwork for elderly patients in a head injury program, because these patients (or their families) are often confused by lengthy, complex forms.

Place

In marketing literature, the element of place is also known as *distribution*. In health care and in rehabilitation in particular, it may be thought of as *accessibility*. Place refers to the location in which the service is provided as well as the hours, transportation, and other convenience factors. Whether a center should be freestanding or located within the hospital is a place issue. Although a freestanding center may be considered ideal for an outpatient program, this is not necessarily true. Questions that should be asked in determining location and accessibility include:

- *Where do potential patients live or work?* Employer location is likely to be more important than home address for a hand therapy center, back school, or work readiness rehabilitation program, whereas the patient's home address is likely to be a factor for audiology assessment. If transportation is provided by the program, home or work location may not matter.
- *Where are competitor practices located?* A new hospital-based rehabilitation program in the same service area as an existing program may have difficulty attracting patients or referrals, unless the hospital has a strong reputation in the service and/or a commitment from leading, influential physicians.
- *What schedule will best meet patient needs?* Early morning or evening hours, Saturday morning appointments, and full staffing at midday may be required to satisfy strategic goals concerning convenience. A work hardening program that only schedules appointments on weekdays from 8:00 a.m. until 5:00 p.m. and that closes for lunch from 11:30 a.m. to 1:00 p.m. is neither convenient nor accessible for injured

workers who are unable to take time off from their jobs for therapy appointments.

- *How will patients reach the rehabilitation center?* Transportation, parking, and other issues are especially important accessibility matters to consider when planning an outpatient rehabilitation service. A downtown location may be convenient for a majority of patients referred to a pain management program, but if parking is expensive or unavailable, the convenient location means little.

Promotion

Promotion involves all methods of communicating the message about the product or service to potential clients. As we have seen, clients encompass a broad group and may include the hospital's inpatient units, physicians, other therapists, employers, health plans, rehabilitation nurses, and many more individuals and organizations in addition to the patients themselves.

Promotional techniques available in marketing rehabilitation services include brochures, newsletters, educational pamphlets, and other printed material; direct mail; media exposure; personal sales calls; exhibits; special events and speaking engagements; public education forums; billboards; and, of course, advertising.

The promotional techniques used to increase awareness of an outpatient rehabilitation program—and thus to generate patients—will depend on the type of program. Memorial City Rehabilitation Hospital in Houston, Texas, found television advertising effective for its industrial injury rehabilitation program. Research indicated a lack of public awareness that the hospital had a separate, freestanding facility with a variety of rehabilitation programs. Inexpensively produced 30-second spots that ran in the afternoon and late at night featured "patients" using various therapy equipment. The advertising attracted attention and patients. Recognizing that advertising is not the only appropriate promotional strategy, Memorial City also invited physicians to receptions and area high school and junior high school coaches to barbecue dinners at the park in which the facility is located, with equipment demonstrations and tours.

At Waco Rehabilitation Institute in Texas, a new freestanding center was promoted with educational classes and programs for therapists. The well-planned seminars drew therapists from across the country, training them in the use of state-of-the-art equipment and technology. The educational seminars generated national publicity and local credibility for the Institute, which quickly reached near-capacity patient referrals.

A key promotional strategy for almost every rehabilitation program will be personal visits to physicians who may be able to refer patients. Frequently, the person who makes these visits will be a therapist—

someone who can speak the clinical language of rehabilitation, who understands physicians' needs and concerns, and who can tactfully correct misunderstandings about the particular therapy service. Cardiologists do not always understand the benefits of cardiac rehabilitation; rheumatologists and internists are not always familiar with therapeutic modalities available for arthritis patients; endocrinologists may not know of the latest technology for treating diabetic ulcers. A well-informed clinical person with a sales orientation can provide information and stimulate referrals.

More basic bottom-line information as well as therapeutic efficacy of rehabilitation will be involved in promoting the program—through personal visits, advertising, and print material—to insurance companies, HMOs, employers, and others.

Preservation

Although preservation is the least-talked-about element of the marketing mix, it can prove to be the most cost-effective and crucial element. Preservation is simply customer or patient retention. It involves activities to ensure that current customers—referral sources and patients—are satisfied with your rehabilitation service and will continue to use it as long as they need it.

Preservation may involve establishing competitive prices along with delivering high-quality care to ensure that health plans renew your provider contract; responding quickly to physician requests; maintaining the skills of therapy staff; purchasing modern equipment; offering a schedule that ensures appointments for recently discharged inpatients; and extending courtesy and compassion to patients and their families. In reality, preservation involves working to please all audiences and following the four Ps of the marketing mix. Conducting discharge surveys, heeding and responding to patient and physician complaints, and other techniques are excellent ways to monitor customer satisfaction and thus ensure preservation.

The Marketing Mix in Action

How might an institution utilize the marketing mix in developing strategies to fulfill the needs of its market segments for outpatient rehabilitation services? The following example shows how one hospital did it.

Southside Hospital, a 500-bed community hospital in Bay Shore, New York, significantly expanded its rehabilitation services and increased its square footage and therapy staff by sixfold. The outpatient rehabilitation facility, Southside Health Institute, is a freestanding building on hospital grounds. It provides evaluation and corrective therapy for acute and chronic spinal dysfunction, educational programs, and work hardening/industrial rehabilitation.

Research confirmed a need by local industry for high-quality rehabilitation services, so this became the primary target market. Southside positioned its rehabilitation program as the comprehensive center for industrial rehabilitation, placing strong emphasis on the workplace environment, task evaluation, and worker reconditioning and education to prevent similar injuries.

The *product* strategy was to develop a staff with expertise in orthopedic dysfunction and manual therapy. A back school educates workers on the causes of back injuries and preventive techniques. The work hardening component was developed in response to industry demand for a program that could condition employees to return to their original jobs or identify alternative job functions and tasks. To ensure that the work hardening program met clinical and promotional objectives, the hospital purchased EASY STREET ENVIRONMENTS™. Southside's customized EASY STREET ENVIRONMENTS™ re-creates industrial work sites found in the hospital's service area, with a stud wall simulator for the building trade, several factory and heavy industry activity areas, and an office setting. The hospital was first in the marketplace with its industrial rehabilitation/work hardening program and its unique workplace simulation environment.

In New York's highly regulated health care environment, pricing policies are fairly rigid. Southside's *price* strategy is based on the benefits a patient or business derives from its rehabilitation service. Promotion emphasizes the lower overall cost of treatment due to a lower reinjury rate resulting from patient education, as well as more rapid return to the work force as a result of work hardening activities.

To address the *place* strategy, a separate freestanding center was built on the hospital campus to provide easy access for patients, with ample parking close to the entrance. The center is open 12 hours a day, 6 days a week.

The hospital's marketing director has worked closely with the rehabilitation department to develop a multifaceted *promotion* plan. Their efforts include personal calls on physicians, direct mail to local industry, a comprehensive advertising campaign including ads in the business sections of local and regional dailies and business publications, public relations efforts, and a fund-raising campaign. Southside Health Institute's positioning theme is used in all elements of marketing communication: "We'll put more people back to work than most employment agencies."

Patient satisfaction is the key to Southside's success. The professional expertise of the rehabilitation staff and their commitment to treating each patient as an important and unique individual have ensured the *preservation* of the patient and referral base.

Positioning

Positioning is the pathway along which strategies are developed and is another important element in the strategic planning process. Positioning involves creating an image in the mind of the consumer or the referral source–an image that defines and differentiates the perception of the rehabilitation service. Think of positioning as *establishing a reputation.* Effective positioning gives your program an exclusive place or niche in the marketplace from which to compete.

Rebound, a brain injury rehabilitation program with facilities throughout the South, has made its position an image of highly personalized, "don't-give-up" rehabilitation therapy. Very high-quality, well-written print material–brochures, recruitment flyers, and so forth–convey this image. Rebound's outpatient programs, located in the same communities as its inpatient facilities, have been successful because of the carry-over reputation for high-quality, personalized rehabilitation. Occupying the "quality" niche has been a successful promotional strategy for Rebound, generating referrals from a broad spectrum of professionals as well as a high number of patients referred by themselves or their families. However, a positioning effort can be too successful. Rebound's image that it can handle the tough cases occasionally causes potential referral sources to consider referring less-severe patients elsewhere, believing that such patients may be functioning at too high a level for Rebound and therefore may not be worth the staff's time. Planners must know how to establish an image that is flexible enough for the market.

At DCH Regional Medical Center in Tuscaloosa, Alabama, the rehabilitation pavilion features a broad variety of standard therapy services as well as work hardening and sports medicine. Its image is one of comprehensive, innovative care. Promotional efforts throughout the state are aimed at a variety of audiences, including public and professional markets, and they stress the image. Despite competitive programs in Birmingham, the strategic marketing promotional efforts by DCH have expanded its service area for rehabilitation to a 10-county, 1-million-person population base.

In a city with a great many HMOs, the most effective marketing niche for a rehabilitation program may be high-quality care *and* competitive or low fees. In a rural or blue-collar community, it may be a well-trained, friendly staff in an accessible location. An inner-city arthritis program may choose to focus its positioning strategy on the program's convenience and gentle, compassionate care.

Positioning depends to a great extent on the positioning of competitors. In a very competitive marketplace in which consumers may select from four sports medicine centers, one usually dominates. The one that opened first may have the strongest image and the largest share of the market (if it has worked to maintain and upgrade its image). The others need to play catch-up, trying to persuade potential consumers that their services are better than those offered by the first sports center. The provider that will win the battle for loyalty is the one that does the most effective job of positioning its services.

In rehabilitation, dual positioning may be necessary to satisfy dual markets. For an industrial rehabilitation program, high-quality care and modern technology is a good position to occupy in the public eye, but insurance companies and workers' compensation agencies are likely to appreciate a positioning strategy that emphasizes cost-effective, efficient therapy that returns employees to work quickly. Likewise, a manual therapy program may market its highly trained, compassionate therapists to the public, but referring physicians will appreciate a program that is prompt and responsive to them.

To develop a positioning strategy, you will use the information gathered from your internal and external environmental assessments. Focus on the following:

1. Identify your competitors.
2. Determine your competitors' position in the marketplace.
3. Analyze your customers (referral sources and patients) and potential customers, classifying them by similarities (that is, by specialty, occupation or employer, location, age, cultural or economic status, and so forth).

With this information, you can then seek to establish a position for your rehabilitation program that is appropriate for your objectives and consumers. Do not try to be something you are not, target patients you cannot serve, or tailor promotions to the wrong audience. If your patients are primarily blue-collar workers who play football, trying to position your sports medicine program by using testimonials from polo or squash players who have sustained injuries will certainly guarantee failure. Relate your services to your target market.

As a rule, do not attempt to go head-to-head with a competitor. If an industrial medicine program at St. Prestigious Hospital is firmly entrenched in its niche as providing "everything to every employer," it would be unrealistic for Smalltown Hospital's industrial medicine center to try to occupy the same niche. It may be reasonable, however, for Smalltown Hospital to position its program as having the most responsive, well-trained staff—ingredients of great interest to both patients and referral sources. Exploiting a competitive weakness or serving an unserved or underserved market would be wiser for the second provider.[4]

St. Charles Hospital in Toledo, Ohio, used a positioning strategy of "ease of access" to enhance its image and attract patients. It is the only hospital in its service area, which is bounded by a river that acts as a natural barrier to cross-over traffic. Its outpatient rehabilitation services include pain management, cardiac rehabilitation, sports medicine, and industrial rehabilitation as well as the bread-and-butter physical, occupational, and speech therapy programs. When suburban hospitals began taking measurable market share from its outpatient programs, St. Charles reacted by developing satellite facilities in suburban communities and extending its weekday schedule (originally 8 a.m. to 5 p.m.) to 7:00 a.m. to 6:30 p.m.

The strategic planning team recognized that ease of access is a key feature for patients who must receive therapy services several times a week. A strategy emphasizing accessibility to its satellite programs has allowed St. Charles Hospital to position itself as the comprehensive, convenient provider of rehabilitation services. To ensure that user needs continue to be met, every outpatient is surveyed at discharge, and physicians are surveyed annually.

There are a variety of ways a rehabilitation service may be positioned: by attribute or distinctive competencies, price or quality, use or application, association with a user or class of users, or comparison with a competitor.[5] Waco Rehabilitation Institute, mentioned earlier, has sought a niche by product attribute, emphasizing its superior expertise and technology. Salem Hospital in Salem, Oregon, developed a comprehensive inpatient and outpatient rehabilitation program in a new building. The centerpiece of its facility is EASY STREET ENVIRONMENTS™ (mentioned earlier in connection with Southside Hospital), a re-creation of community settings such as the supermarket, bank, restaurant, and other real-world locations. This colorful, realistic program allows Salem Hospital to position its rehabilitation program as innovative and patient-centered. Through comprehensive services and publicity generated by EASY STREET ENVIRONMENTS™, Salem's strategic goal was to stop the flow of patients to larger hospital rehabilitation centers in Portland to the north.

It is important to note that a positioning strategy can only be successful if it is realistic, if it is directed to a fairly substantial market segment (or one with growth potential), and if it involves significant differences between your rehabilitation program and that of the competition. The marketplace position for your program will be realized by effective execution of carefully planned strategies that align with your chosen niche.

Requirements and Benefits of the Program

At some point in a strategic marketing plan, there must be a thorough review of the program's expected requirements and benefits. This should begin with a pro forma financial analysis that outlines the expected income by source category, the capital investment needed to launch the program (again by major category of capital application), the operational expenses to support the activity, and the projected surplus or deficit and return on investment. A narrative discussion should accompany the pro forma, outlining key assumptions for projections of utilization and requirements to succeed. For example, if utilization statistics for a head injury program assume the promised expansion of a 10-physician neurology group, the program's growth would be negatively affected if expansion plans fell through.

Additional discussion should address potential barriers to success and anticipated by-product benefits. For example, if you were to develop a successful hand therapy program that is utilized by orthopedic surgeons, they may be encouraged to send joint replacement patients or amputees to your general OT/PT outpatient programs.

Plan Finalization and Review

Once the plan has been approved by appropriate parties within the hospital, the strategy team leader should convene everyone responsible for accomplishing the action plans and establish regular meetings on the project. This group will evaluate progress, modify strategies, and coordinate activities, with the main objective being to finalize the plan and establish a review process. Quarterly meetings with an expanded group of rehabilitation managers, key physicians, marketing and public relations directors, appropriate inpatient managers, and administrative directors will serve to update assumptions about the environment and adjust strategies and goals as necessary.

Evaluation

Is the rehabilitation program successful? A strategic marketing plan simplifies answering the question by establishing an evaluation process. You need only compare objectives, strategies, and goals with actual results on a monthly, quarterly, or annual basis. If the objective of a general outpatient rehabilitation program is to retain 75 percent of the hospital's discharged inpatient rehab population, a computer review of inpatient medical records can provide the data needed to determine the success rate. A second objective may be to provide high-quality care that achieves a 95 percent satisfaction level with physicians and referral sources. A year-end survey of these target groups will let you know if you have succeeded.

Gathering and reporting results will be a part of the evaluation process and a necessary component of the strategic plan. Evaluation helps the strategy team adjust or revamp a program if needed. Depending on the objectives of the rehabilitation service, evaluation may include a comparison between projections and revenues, number of patients, percentage of market share, referrals by target markets, and similar data.

Evaluation should always include qualitative analysis as well as quantitative data, for the opinions and satisfaction of various users can help to explain quantitative results.

Marketing Philosophy

Marketing is everybody's business. This essential reality is often overlooked. To be successful, marketing must be the responsibility of every therapist, nurse, and cafeteria employee, not just the administrator or marketing department representative assisting in the execution of the marketing plan. In short, marketing is a team effort, and the team has many members.[6]

To explain this philosophy, we need only review the definition of marketing: *the satisfaction of customer wants and needs.* Satisfying the customer–whether it is the health plan administrator, the physician, the rehabilitation nurse, or the patient–should be the goal of all individuals in the organization. This is true whether they encounter the customer directly or indirectly in the performance of their jobs.

To infuse this marketing philosophy throughout the organization, leadership must come from the top. Administrators, the medical director of rehabilitation, and clinical supervisors must demonstrate that marketing–customer satisfaction–is part of everyone's job description. When this orientation becomes infused throughout the hospital, the organization becomes *marketplace-driven,* which is how Peters and Waterman characterize successful businesses in their book, *In Search of Excellence.*[7] They identify *closeness to the customer* by top management as the common denominator of successful companies. They describe firms such as IBM, where members of senior management spend time each month in the field dealing with customers.[8]

Unfortunately, closeness to the customer is not always readily apparent in many health care organizations. It is important for those in health care never to lose sight of customer needs. How many occupational or physical therapy managers lose their patient orientation because stacks of paperwork and monthly reports require the time they once spent working with patients? It is important for the rehabilitation director and the physician relations coordinator to remember that the receptionist practices marketing when answering the phone, scheduling a referral, or accepting insurance forms from a patient. The aide who escorts the patient to the therapy gym and the therapist consulting with the neurologist are both interfacing with the consumer and are integral to the success of the program. If an insurance clerk trying to verify insurance coverage is treated with disdain, if documentation and reports are slow to reach the referring doctor or employer, if employers are kept on hold for long periods when they call to check on an employee receiving therapy, if a physician's nurse is not treated courteously when calling to schedule a patient–these consumers may influence the decision to seek services elsewhere.

Without an organizationwide, customer-first attitude, the most carefully planned, thoughtfully executed strategic plan will be no more than words on paper. When everyone demonstrates their crucial role in marketing, the strategic plan will have achieved a most important objective.

Conclusion

Strategic planning today is as vital a component of outpatient rehabilitation program development as the care plan is to a patient's recovery. Properly carried out, strategic planning is the organization's map; it provides direction and momentum. Once the strategic plan is in place and communicated throughout, it will become clear to individuals and groups exactly what the organization intends to *do* and *become.* With the future clearly defined, it is much easier to gain the commitment of those within the organization, from clerks to administrators. And commitment is the fuel that accelerates progress.

With a strategic plan that identifies the right things to do and to be, an organization can chart the course it selects while meeting the needs of patients and the community it serves.

References

1. Porter, M. C. How competitive forces shape strategy. *Harvard Business Review* 47(2):139, Mar.–Apr. 1979.
2. Nimer, D. Good market-driven pricing is a lot of work. *Healthcare Forum* 30(4):20, July–Aug. 1987.
3. Gup, B. *Guide to Strategic Planning.* New York City: McGraw-Hill, 1980, p. 18.
4. Reis, A., and Trout, J. *Marketing Warfare.* New York City: New American Library, 1986, pp. 68 and 84.
5. Aaker, D., and Shansby, J. G. Positioning your product. *Business Horizons* 25(3):56–62, May–June 1982.
6. Brown, S. Health care marketing: an assessment and look to the future. *Journal of Healthcare Marketing* 2(4):5–6, Fall 1982.
7. Peters, T. J., and Waterman, R. H., Jr. *In Search of Excellence.* New York City: Harper & Row, 1982, p. 12.
8. Reis, A., and Trout, J. *Positioning: The Battle for Your Mind.* New York City: Warner Books, 1982, p. 37.

Chapter 3

Writing the Business Plan: Operational Issues

Suzan D. Boyd

Introduction

A clear, logical, and concise business plan will serve as the basis for the decision to invest in both the development of an outpatient rehabilitation program and its implementation. The plan should provide the hospital's senior management and board with the data they need to evaluate the proposed program and, subsequent to their approval, it should also provide the guidelines necessary to implement the new program.

The parent corporation, be it a hospital, a rehabilitation chain, or a group of private physicians, should have in place a standardized approach to new program proposals that includes an outline for a business plan. The hospital's strategic planning committee should have explicit standards and a clear process for developing and evaluating new programs. A standardized approach to new program planning will ensure that all program proposals are developed according to the same criteria. This will help determine which programs represent the best investment for the parent organization. Each new business proposal under consideration by the hospital should be evaluated according to predefined criteria that cover areas ranging from start-up costs to the impact of government regulation to return-on-investment (ROI), and then it should be compared with other proposals. The data compiled in the business plan will form the basis for this comparison. The planning process should also include a format for choosing among strategic alternatives.

As planners begin to develop a proposal for an outpatient program, they must understand how the proposed business plan will proceed through the internal decision-making system, who will evaluate it, and

The author would like to acknowledge and thank Ms. Becky Coven for her contribution to this chapter through her review and comments.

what criteria they will use. This will require knowledge of the organization's political and structural decision-making process. Although the hospital's board of trustees has ultimate decision-making authority, board approval is usually based on the recommendation of the chief executive officer (CEO). Politically astute planning team leaders will know when to introduce the concept of the program and will be aware of any politics associated with its proposal.

Additionally, planners should have a clear understanding of the hospital's overall strategic plan. Different hospitals will expect business plans to show varying levels of complexity, and decision makers will compare the proposal for outpatient rehabilitation with other new program/service proposals. Thus the new program proposal should assure decision makers that all pertinent and appropriate data are included in the business plan and are clear, accurate, and present a good case. A good proposal should not be returned because of insufficient data.

Generally, the information needed to evaluate a new rehabilitation program should not differ significantly from that needed to evaluate any other diversification option being considered. However, what will differ is the knowledge base and the key variables that are specific to rehabilitation.

A system to compare new business proposals should have both quantitative and nonquantitative criteria. *Quantitative criteria* may include measurement of the ROI, projected utilization, and current market share. *Nonquantitative criteria* can include such considerations as compatibility with the hospital's mission, likelihood of medical staff support, and improvement of the hospital's image. Murphy called this evaluation process "venture profile analysis" and established a system that measures the relative advantages and disadvantages of proposed ventures and assigns a quantified score or value of that venture for the hospital. The criteria recommended by Murphy are reimbursement, market size, capital costs, competitors, staffing, image, positive spin-offs, certificate of need (CON), and compatibility with the hospital's role in the community. Each criterion is assigned a weighted value, and each program is then scored by totaling the values of all the criteria involved. The total scores are then used in the comparison of the new proposals being considered.[1] Murphy and Jennings both outline alternative approaches to evaluating new program proposals, with different key criteria and weights.[2,3]

This chapter will outline a basic approach to developing a business plan for an outpatient rehabilitation facility. The first part of the chapter will provide a framework for the overall business plan.

The Business Plan

Although the key steps to be included in a business plan may vary in sequence and in explicit variables to be addressed, the plan's major factors do not usually differ. These factors include a definition of the new product or service being proposed, its relevance to corporate mission and values, strategy, governance, medical staff and referrals, market definition and market research, regulatory and reimbursement issues, operational issues, finance, and implementation and evaluation. Operational issues of particular importance to rehabilitation will be discussed in detail in this chapter. These issues include defining the program, medical staff issues, supervision, staffing, management information systems and data needs, and managed care contracts.

Health care and business journals and textbooks offer many different approaches to business planning.[4,5] The details of a sample business plan are outlined in figure 3-1. The general factors to be addressed in the business plan include the definition of the new program/service, the mission and the strategic plan, the governance of the new program, market demand and market research, medical staff issues, regulatory and reimbursement issues, key operational issues including supervision, staffing, productivity, financial analysis, implementation, management information systems, and data needs. Managed care contracts are also addressed.

Responsibility for the actual preparation of the business plan will usually fall to the senior manager and the middle manager, who have line-management responsibility for the hospital's rehabilitation department and program. Because later chapters in this book address strategic planning, finance, and legal issues, these topics will not be discussed here.

Definition of the Program

The first step in the business plan is to define the program. This description must include what outpatient program model will be developed. Three major variables will influence this choice: the mission of the organization, the present and potential strengths of existing rehabilitation programs, and the relative importance of rehabilitation within the context of the hospital's overall strategic plan. The program/service definition will in turn strongly influence the subsequent organizational structure of the program.

There are three basic types of outpatient rehabilitation programs:

- Expansion of outpatient service within the physical space and programmatic context of the hospital's current rehabilitation department
- An outpatient rehabilitation program that is geographically separated from the hospital inpatient department but that is still a part of the hospital corporation and appears on financial reports as a hospital cost center
- A freestanding dedicated outpatient rehabilitation facility in a separate but affiliated corporation

Figure 3-1. Business Plan Framework

I. Definition of New Business/Product
  A. Clear description of product/service
  B. Identification of scope of services, service features, and associated technology
  C. Goals and objectives (short- and long-range)
II. Mission and Strategic Plan
  A. Relationship of program to corporate and subsidiary mission
  B. Relevance to corporate and subsidiary strategic plan
  C. Relationship to and synergism with other businesses and/or departments
III. Governance
  A. Relationship to sponsoring organization
  B. Organizational structure
  C. Partners/joint venture structure
  D. Supervision and reporting relationships
IV. Market, Demand, and Market Research
  A. General product market
    1. Historical and projected market size
    2. Relevant trends
  B. Target market
    1. Delineation of size, attractibility of new market, current market share for proposed market, service area
    2. Importance and relevance of product to targeted consumer market
  C. Competition
    1. Identification of key competitors, relative market share, strengths and weaknesses, current and future strategies
  D. Market research
    1. Summary and implications of relevant market research
    2. Requirements for ongoing market research and projected cost
  E. Promotional requirements
    1. Initial plans and cost projections
    2. Ongoing requirements and projected costs
V. Medical Staff Issues
  A. Role of physicians
  B. Impact on medical staff relationships
  C. Physician competition
VI. Regulatory and Reimbursement Framework
  A. Outline of regulatory and licensure requirements
    1. CON
    2. Local, state, and federal requirements affecting start-up
    3. Initial and ongoing licensure requirements
  B. Reimbursement
    1. Medicare and Medicaid payment policy (current and future)
    2. Blue Cross and commercial payer policy (current and future)
    3. Market share information relating to anticipated payment source and policy
VII. Key Operational Issues
  A. Resource requirements
    1. Staffing
    2. System requirements (management information systems and data needs)
    3. Current and future technology
    4. Facility requirements
    5. Program insurance requirements and costs
    6. Collection, billing, and payment procedures

Figure 3-1. (Continued)

- B. Quality assessment
- C. Productivity measurement and requirements
- D. Procedural relationships with other departments

VIII. Financial Analysis
- A. Start-up costs
  1. Planning, operations, capital, and facilities
  2. Source of funding
- B. Determination of pricing policy and set prices
- C. Determination of volume projections and associated payer mix
- D. Pro forma financial statements for start-up and first three years of operation
- E. Financial projections: best-case, worst-case, and most likely scenarios
- F. Financial ratios: operating, net internal rate of return, capitalization rate, debt service rate (if applicable)
- G. Net cash flow and discount cash flow

IX. Implementation and Evaluation
- A. Time frame and detailed plan for implementation
- B. Evaluation
  1. Operational and associated plan and procedure for corrections
  2. Consumer and associated plan for remediation

The off-site and freestanding facility may be developed as either a for-profit or not-for-profit subsidiary of the parent corporation. (Related legal and joint venture issues will be discussed in chapter 8.)

The first two models as defined by Medicare are likely to be categorized as rehabilitation facilities for the purposes of reimbursement, whereas the freestanding model is more likely, though not necessarily, to be a comprehensive outpatient rehabilitation facility (CORF). The range of services in the first two models may be mainly physical and occupational therapy, and speech therapy.

The service mix will be based on the target market that will be derived from patients discharged from the parent hospital and the case mix of their referring physicians. If, for example, the hospital has a large orthopedic service, it is likely that the mix will heavily favor physical therapy, or if the hospital has a large rheumatology service, demand for occupational therapy could be anticipated. However, if the center is located in a medical office building with several ear, nose, and throat specialists, this might increase the need for a speech therapy service. Referring physicians can play a major role in determining service demand. For example, experience at the Rehabilitation and Fitness Center at St. Joseph Hospital in Chicago has demonstrated that a very small percentage of the patients are referred from the hospital itself post-discharge; rather, most are referred from physicians' offices.[6]

By definition, CORFs will serve the same markets as the first two models and, in addition, will provide a comprehensive array of extended rehabilitation services, including vocational rehabilitation, psychological counseling, and rehabilitation nursing. Their target market is more likely to be the posttrauma victim and the long-term multisystem rehabilitation patient.

The mission of the sponsoring organization also affects the model chosen. The institution's mission and values will determine the relative importance of rehabilitation within the context of the organization. Generally, the hospital's mission is reflected in the overall strategic plan. A general community hospital with a DRG-exempt inpatient unit may have an outpatient rehabilitation facility that provides general rehabilitation targeted to meet the postdischarge needs of the inpatient mix it serves or one that is related to particular areas of physician strength, for example, sports medicine or general orthopedics. The CORF that is owned by a for-profit rehabilitation chain will have a program array based on its overall mission. Mission and values will also affect the targeted payer mix that will be acceptable to the program and that will allow achievement of margin or profit objectives.

Chapter 2 discussed the key areas involved in an assessment of the external and internal environment relating to outpatient rehabilitation. The predicted continued growth in rehabilitation is predicated on the impact of advancements in medical technology, which may save lives but may also result in physical disability or impairment. Physical disability or impairment is associated with the need for medical rehabilitation, earlier hospital discharge secondary to prospective payment, the aging of the population as a whole, the need for cost containment achieved by effective management of care over the inpatient–outpatient continuum, and the general shift to ambulatory care as the least expensive, most appropriate level of care.[7]

Medical Staff Issues

Additional topics that must be addressed in any hospital diversification effort are medical staff issues. The medical staff issues associated with an outpatient rehabilitation program need to be specifically identified. The success of the outpatient program will ultimately depend on physicians. Medical staff may have an impact on the facility as its primary referral source, as the source from which to recruit a medical director, in the staff's perception of salaried physicians and consultants, or as a major source of competition. Among the medical staff issues that need to be addressed early in the development of the business plan are medical staff education, referrals, medical direction, and competition.

Medical Staff Education

Medical staff education regarding outpatient rehabilitation and rehabilitation in general will be necessary for two reasons: First, some physicians are relatively unsophisticated in their understanding of rehabilitation. Educational activities via both formal programs targeted toward the medical staff and informal one-on-one educational contacts will need to be directed to physicians who will be referring to the center. Examples of formal activities could be a seminar on temporomandibular joint (TMJ) therapy or a program announcing a new piece of equipment, indications for its use, and associated referral information needs. Second, educational efforts will not only teach physicians about rehabilitation but will serve to market the center and its key programs, its technology, and the skills of the program staff.

Referrals

In many states, state professional licensure laws and/or the medical practice acts continue to ensure physician control of referrals for rehabilitation services. The high-volume services in most outpatient rehabilitation programs are physical and occupational therapy ordered from physician office practices. Thus, both patients and hospitals rely on physicians to determine the need for rehabilitation, and the physician initiates the referral. Consumers do not usually seek or self-select the site for rehabilitation services, albeit fitness and sports programs may be the exception. Even the arrival of managed care has not obviated the physician's role in determining when an outpatient service is needed. In fact, because physicians are at financial risk for the total package of outpatient services that individual patients receive, they will closely review the need for referral to rehabilitation, the associated length of therapy, and the cost of care. Thus, their control over referrals to rehabilitation can probably be expected to increase.

Medical Direction

Medical staff participation and direction is required by Medicare regulation for an organized outpatient rehabilitation program, and by Commission on Accreditation of Rehabilitation Facilities (CARF) and Joint Commission on Accreditation of Healthcare Organizations (Joint Commission) standards for both inpatient and outpatient organized rehabilitation programs.[8,9]

The requirements for a medical director may range from a physician who has experience in rehabilitation and has completed some rehabilitation continuing education programs to a physiatrist who has completed a residency in physical medicine and rehabilitation and is board-certified in physiatry. The former requirements may mean that the position can be sought by qualified individuals on the medical staff.

If this is a new program and a new position, all the political and economic issues associated with salaried hospital physicians and revenues from related ancillary services will need to be addressed. For example, how much will the new physiatrist be paid? Also, will the new physiatrist receive professional fees for ancillary services, such as a percentage of the reading fees for electromyograms that are currently all read by the hospital's private, nonsalaried neurology group? These issues require some knowledge of political and turf issues among the medical staff.

Depending on the definition of the outpatient facility, the scale and scope of the program, and the current medical leadership, the need to recruit a physiatrist will have to be addressed in any major expansion of outpatient rehabilitation. Physiatrists are key to the success of many rehabilitation programs in community hospitals. However, it is not uncommon to find a lack of knowledge among medical, nursing, and administrative staffs as to what physiatrists do, and if they are not already on the medical staff, what value they would add to the program. A physiatrist can help market a new program by working to improve medical staff understanding of the therapies, providing consultation in physical medicine and rehabilitation, contributing to enhanced patient goal setting, and providing a relatively sophisticated appreciation of program needs and patient problems.

Competition

The final and probably most important medical staff issue to be addressed is that of competition. As physicians strive to expand their revenue base, they add those services to their office product line that represent natural extensions of their practice. Entrepreneurial practitioners can be expected to consider adding to their own practice those services that do not need to be provided in an acute hospital environment but are already part of their own hospital activities, that do not require major capital investments, and that are services for which they must continually refer patients outside their practice. Although rehabilitation does have technology and capital equipment requirements, the barriers to entry into outpatient rehabilitation are still relatively low. They are the same low-investment thresholds that may draw independent therapists and hospitals to expanded outpatient rehabilitation.

The business plan must identify all physicians on the medical staff who currently provide rehabilitation in their offices, who own or participate in an outpatient rehabilitation facility joint venture, who have a position on the staff of a rehabilitation facility, or who, because of the volume of their rehabilitation referrals, could be expected to consider developing their own rehabilitation services. It then must be determined what their response will be to expansion of the hospital's competitive role in the outpatient rehabilitation market.

An issue that is a correlate of the medical staff referral dilemma is the growth in number of independent physical or occupational therapy practitioners. Two areas of state law will have an impact on the hospital-affiliated outpatient rehabilitation center: the state hospital practice act and the individual professional licensing act. In Illinois, for example, a physical therapist practicing as an independent practitioner can now evaluate and treat patients without a physician referral. However, due to the requirements of the Illinois Hospital Licensing Act, when the therapist is practicing in the hospital, a physician order is required to initiate the rehabilitation therapy service.

For the freestanding outpatient rehabilitation center this brings up two issues: Can the practitioner in the off-site center receive self-referrals and, if so, how will this affect medical staff relationships and associated referrals? And if the therapist can accept private referrals when in private practice, the center will have to provide a group practice environment equally attractive to experienced, credentialed practitioners who could be in practice by themselves. As will be discussed later in this chapter, this will also require that the center develop innovative approaches to salaries and benefits.

Supervision and Reporting Relationships

Supervisory responsibility for outpatient rehabilitation is directly dependent on the model chosen, its location in the organizational structure, and the size and scale of the operation.

Clinical supervisory responsibility should be located at the service site. This becomes especially important when an organized outpatient rehabilitation program moves outside the geographical boundaries of the hospital rehabilitation department. If the organized program remains at the hospital within the rehabilitation department, the necessity for separate outpatient clinical supervisors is less critical. The need for dedicated outpatient supervision would then depend on the size and scope of the outpatient service.

The second supervisory issue involves a therapist of one discipline supervising individuals from other rehabilitation disciplines. If the outpatient program is off-site and relatively small or in the initial growth stage, it may require that one senior therapist supervise individuals from the other therapies rather than each therapy having a designated supervisor. If there is only one half-time occupational therapist in a small rehabilitation service and a physical therapy supervisor who is responsible for the site, the physical therapy supervisor will have to be clinically responsible for the work of the occupational therapist. Because even the most egalitarian individuals have professional egos, it can be anticipated that this may cause some problems. However, the need for one on-site individual who is accountable and responsible for the program cannot be overemphasized. Both physicians and other referral sources need to know who is providing leadership for the program and can answer questions or solve problems, who is responsible for ensuring the quality of all the services, and who is providing the linkage with the sponsoring organization. Individual specialty therapists in an outpatient program, such as a speech pathologist reporting to the inpatient speech pathology supervisor, would cross the boundaries of responsibility and leave no one really in charge of the outpatient or off-site program.

The importance of detailed and clear job descriptions and performance and productivity standards will provide the support necessary to make cross-supervision of disciplines work. The development and approval of job descriptions and productivity standards should, if possible, include the input and approval of the related inpatient specialty supervisor. If that is not possible, consideration should be given to working with an outside consultant in the particular specialty in order to ensure that job expectations and productivity standards are realistic, understandable, and fair.

If the facility is a CORF, the supervisory requirements will be outlined by regulation. This is not the case in an off-site rehabilitation service that is a cost center of the hospital rehabilitation department, or in a freestanding center that does not choose to provide the range of services required of a CORF or to seek licensure as a CORF.

Staffing

Staffing an outpatient program and retaining staff are challenges for those planning new services. Among the staffing issues that need to be addressed are the staffing mix, recruitment and retention, salaries, continuing education, and rotation and scheduling.

Staffing Mix

The number of start-up and ongoing staff members required should be based on analysis of the historical outpatient rehabilitation treatment base in the hospital, if available; hospital product lines that may affect the referral mix to outpatient rehabilitation; the patient mix of key referring physicians; and the target market to be served by the program.

The patient mix will determine the type of therapists that are needed. The projected number of referrals and treatments must then be calculated to determine the number of full-time equivalent professionals in each therapy. For example, if, historically, 50 percent of the outpatient volume has been orthopedics, it will be necessary to determine the number of projected orthopedic referrals, the average number of visits per referral, and the average number of treatments per visit. This information should be prepared for each anticipated grouping of referrals (that is, ortho, arthritis, and so forth) and then quantified in terms of anticipated treatments to determine initial staffing needs (see chapter 9), utilization, and projections for growth as outlined in the business plan. It might be necessary initially to start with higher staff productivity rates in order to allow for quick responses to referring physicians. The ability to accept all referrals from physicians in a time frame acceptable to them will be critical in establishing the center's initial credibility and reputation. It will be very difficult for the center to recapture physicians' referrals once they have not had their needs met and have had to refer patients elsewhere. However, this need must be balanced with the need to keep start-up costs reasonable.

The procedure for authorizing new staff must be clear to allow for rapid addition of staff. Also, the criteria for adding staff should be agreed on prior to opening so that when the need arises, new staff can be added immediately. Specific criteria can include the inability to accept referrals for evaluations within seven days and the prolonged existence of a waiting list for particular therapies or equipment.

When a new facility experiences rapid growth, its success can be undermined if demand cannot be met; thus, initially it pays to be moderately overstaffed. Overstaffing associated with start-up is not as expensive as ongoing utilization of agency therapists or prolonged recruitment expenses. Agency or temporary therapists should be used when necessary to respond to rapid growth and unanticipated demand, pending the recruitment of permanent staff.

Recruitment and Retention

The market for recruitment and retention of physical and occupational therapists is one of the top problems in health care human resources management, and it is likely to be an ongoing problem that many rehabilitation programs will have to live with. Competition for rehabilitation practitioners is not just with hospitals but also with agencies, freestanding for-profit rehabilitation centers, and private group physician and therapy practices.

The fact that the outpatient rehabilitation center represents a new program serving a nonacute market will help with initial recruitment. Some therapists will view the target market as more enjoyable to work with than the inpatient rehabilitation mix.

The payment package must be attractive and commensurate with the increased independence and autonomy required of practitioners outside the hospital structure. Like most health care professionals, rehabilitation therapists expect a working environment in which they are viewed and treated as important professionals in the health care milieu.

Physical and occupational therapy practitioners expect minimum perquisites of paid leave for professional education with expenses paid by the hospital. Training and completion of neurodevelopmental testing

(NDT), spinal mobilization, and other specialty postgraduate training programs should be sought when necessary to match therapist skills with target markets.

Recruitment efforts should be targeted toward therapists with at least one to two years' experience. If the case mix and referral patterns of the program are not clearly understood prior to opening, the use of physical therapy assistants and certified occupational therapy assistants should be limited. These practitioners can and should be added after start-up and when a clear understanding of the patient mix has been developed. The use of registered nurses, psychologists, and vocational rehabilitation counselors will primarily be in CORFs.

Salaries

The first strategic recruitment decision for the outpatient program is to determine how competitive the center will be in the local or regional salary market for health care employees. This decision will affect both inpatient and outpatient therapists, so it must be viewed in the context of its systemwide economic impact as well as its effect on recruitment. In order to attract qualified individuals and assure therapists of the priority of rehabilitation to the hospital, salaries should be set in the top 25 percent of the local market. Because shortages of therapists show no signs of abating, regular market surveys and market factor adjustments must be anticipated and salary changes made as needed.

Of equal importance to salaries is the need to review *how* rehabilitation professionals are compensated and receive benefits. At present, most therapists are paid an hourly wage with fringe benefits. In order to compete with private practice and agencies, hospitals must develop innovative salary practices. Consideration should be given to hiring therapists as independent contractors based on fee-for-service or hiring them with a base salary and incentive payments based on productivity and collections. Flexible benefit packages will also be important for this group.

Continuing Education

Among other perquisites that may be offered to compete with agencies and freestanding centers is continuing education. Clear financial incentives such as college loan payback programs, payment of American Physical Therapy Association and/or American Occupational Therapy Association dues, and annual paid professional conference leave will not only enhance retention but will also ensure the attainment of state-of-the-art skills.

St. Joseph Hospital in Chicago has worked extensively to develop a model recruitment/retention program. Anticipating recruitment needs, St. Joseph will fund $2,000 for senior-year expenses of one physical therapy and one occupational therapy student each year. In return, the students guarantee one year of professional services at the hospital. They do not have to pay back the money unless they subsequently decide not to work at St. Joseph for one year. In that case, they pay back the money interest-free. Therapists already employed at the hospital are eligible for a cash retention bonus at the end of each year of full-time employment. The bonus is based on the number of years of successful service, with the maximum being $800. Professional membership dues are paid for all therapists. First-year employees are given $300 for conference expenses and are eligible for an increased conference expense contribution with each year of continuous employment. After the first year, therapists are eligible for special monies for more intensive courses such as NDT and spinal mobilization. In locations such as Chicago, where the costs of recruiting a new therapist can be over $10,000, the recruitment and retention program more than pays for itself.[10]

At least once a year, off-site continuing education courses should be combined with monthly departmental in-service education programs. These programs can be conducted jointly with inpatient services. Therapists will provide the leadership role in developing and conducting in-service programs. When individual therapists attend off-site conferences, they may present in-service programs on pertinent therapeutic information. The Joint Commission has very explicit requirements related to both documentation of in-service education and orientation and annual continuing education associated with equipment.[11]

Rotation and Scheduling

Consideration should be given to establishing a regular rotation for therapists from the inpatient department to the outpatient facility. This will help with inpatient recruitment, ensure training of younger therapists, and enhance the role of inpatient therapists in discharge planning. Finally, it will help ensure full staffing of the outpatient program.

The autonomy of therapists in determining their schedules while ensuring coverage of the center during necessary weekend and evening hours is important. This will ensure some comparability with independent practice. Four-day workweeks, ten-hour days, and other flex-time models should also be available, if possible. Evening and weekend hours will require payment of hourly wage premiums.

Productivity

Given the need to be scrupulously cost-conscious for current payers and in anticipation of the shift to prospective payment in the outpatient area, clear productivity guidelines must be included in business planning.[12] Productivity standards for the outpatient program must be specified at the onset. The standards will indicate the center's expectations of the therapists and will be used in hiring, monitoring performance, and assuring appropriate evaluation. They will also be critically important in monitoring cost-effectiveness and profitability of the center as it relates to salary expenses and the need to ensure appropriate staffing in response to changes in demand. Staff should be included in the planning, implementation, and ongoing review and revision of productivity standards.

There are many ways to monitor productivity. One is to integrate the productivity data with the patient charge and billing monitoring system. This will ensure appropriate charging of all services provided, because the incentive for the therapist is to provide an accurate reflection of his or her own productive efforts.

At St. Joseph Hospital in Chicago, a monthly productivity monitoring system was implemented using the hospital patient billing system. The center's director, in conjunction with clinical staff, measured average direct and indirect time spent for each patient evaluation and treatment. Direct time only included actual patient treatment time. Indirect time included setup, cleanup, case management, and documentation time. Thus, an indirect time unit was established for each direct treatment unit. Decimal-point values were then assigned based on hourly units. Each time a treatment charge is keyed into the billing computer, the corresponding point value (time) is automatically credited to the center. At the end of the month, a total productivity level for the center is calculated. A productivity level of 85 to 100 percent is expected. When productivity is consistently over 100 percent, it is necessary to review basic staffing needs.

Management Information Systems and Data Needs

Three data areas should be given priority in planning the management information system (MIS) for the outpatient rehabilitation program: financial and billing data, historical and market data, and productivity data. In start-up planning, the management of the rehabilitation center must work with staff from the hospital finance and management information systems to ensure development of systems that obtain standard hospital patient, financial, and demographic information and that can be integrated with the hospital information system.

Financial and Billing Data

The MIS of the off-site rehabilitation program should be linked to the hospital mainframe and thus directly integrated with the hospital financial and data systems. If this is not possible, the data system at the center should be designed to enable down-loading into the hospital financial and billing system.

Small or start-up outpatient rehabilitation facilities, though responsible for on-site cash collections, will not usually do the billing of third-party payers. This should be handled by the hospital business office.

Historical and Market Data

Initial development of the data systems should also ensure retention of historical data on patients and referral information to assist with marketing and planning.

If a program's opening staff is developed on the traditional hospital outpatient mix, good data will assure monitoring and identify how it is changing during the initial months of operation. Data should also identify shifts in case mix and specific diagnoses that might affect staffing.

Data on referral sources will ensure careful monitoring of any changes in volume from usual referral sources or growth in new sources. Any changes can quickly be followed up by staff to identify any specific satisfaction or dissatisfaction with service on the part of referral sources.

There are new software programs on the market that will enable the center to carefully monitor the activity of physicians and other referral sources. A significant volume decrease from a major physician referral source might also indicate a new competitor in the area.

Understanding the internal markets' and referral sources' receptivity to the program is as important and has as much potential impact on the program as the correct identification of the external markets. It cannot be assumed that the traditional outpatients in the hospital or discharges from the inpatient rehab unit will automatically come to the center. A business plan must clearly profile the potential market and volume of an outpatient rehabilitation program.

In order to ensure a profitable payer mix, data on payment should be gathered that will assist with target marketing. And as the center negotiates for managed care contracts, detailed cost and payer data will be critical. Data on the cost of the therapy by diagnosis will be necessary with the extension of prospective payment to the outpatient setting.

Productivity Data

As previously discussed, productivity data can be measured by a link with the billing system. Productivity information can be used to assess staffing needs, ensure appropriate compensation, and provide incentives to deliver more efficient patient care.

Managed Care Contracts

Managed care offers the potential for reducing the costs of health care to employers, third-party payers, and consumers. The implications of managed care programs are equally important to the CORF and the hospital outpatient rehabilitation program. Both the CORF and the outpatient rehabilitation program can play key roles in the hospital's ability to manage the rehabilitation patient over the inpatient, outpatient, and home care continuum, assuring that the patient is always at the most appropriate and most cost-effective level of care. The outpatient program will enhance the hospital's ability to manage care under prospective payment by facilitating discharge to immediate posthospital care with a resulting positive impact on the hospital's contractual adjustments.

As hospital negotiations with managed care companies have become more sophisticated, the manager of an outpatient rehabilitation program may negotiate directly with the managed care companies. The outpatient rehabilitation program director will work with the hospital managed care director or whoever is responsible for these negotiations, advising that individual on the outpatient rehabilitation component of the contract. Regardless of the role he or she plays in the negotiations, the manager of the outpatient program must participate in decision making with respect to the price of the discounted services to be offered by the center. The rehabilitation manager must provide the cost, market, and utilization data that will ensure that the discounting of care does not result in financial losses for the outpatient program. Without these data, the hospital may indeed sign a contract that could result in such losses.

The outpatient rehabilitation program director is likely to be involved in direct negotiations with managed care programs and businesses relating to specific programs marketed by the center. This will be for contractual arrangements for the provision of specific outpatient services, work hardening and strengthening, or a component of an industrial health program. In this role, the manager again must have a detailed understanding of the program's costs and its overall marketing and pricing strategy.

As contractual arrangements are implemented, the outpatient program data system must be expanded to include the impact of managed care contracts in the monthly financial reports.

Conclusion

In proposing the development of an outpatient rehabilitation program, the importance of a clear, concise, and well-thought-out business plan cannot be overemphasized. The business plan will serve as the basis for marketing the value of the program to internal decision makers. The astute manager will have accurately predicted and planned accordingly for both the operational and financial needs of the program as well as the political determinants that will affect the program's chances for success. The business plan should address those issues of specific importance to developing an outpatient rehabilitation program. These issues include defining the program, determining and resolving medical staff issues, addressing staffing issues including the number and type of staff needed, determining information and data system needs, and working with managed care. How well the business plan addresses these issues and provides guidelines for implementing the program will have a significant impact on the program's success.

References

1. Murphy, R. Venture profile analysis. *Hospital and Health Services Administration,* Nov.-Dec., pp. 81-85, 1985.
2. Murphy, pp. 80–95.
3. Jennings, M. *Guidelines on Evaluating Diversification Strategies.* Chicago: American Hospital Association, 1989, p. 2.
4. Griffith, J. *The Well Managed Community Hospital.* Ann Arbor, MI: Health Administration Press, 1987, pp. 246–47.
5. Howard, D., editor. *New Business Development in Ambulatory Care: Exploring Diversification Options.* Chicago: American Hospital Publishing, 1988, pp. 44–47.
6. Coven, B., director of ambulatory services, St. Joseph Hospital, Chicago, Aug. 31, 1989, interview with author.
7. Cassak, D. Medical rehabilitation: tapping into a growing alternate site market. *Health Industry Today,* Mar. 1988, p. 52.
8. Commission on Accreditation of Rehabilitation Facilities. *Standards Manual for Organizations Serving People with Disabilities.* Tucson: CARF, 1990, pp. 40, 41, 62, 63, and 64.
9. Joint Commission on Accreditation of Healthcare Organizations. *Accreditation Manual for Hospitals,* 1990 edition. Chicago: Joint Commission, 1989, pp. 178, 184, and 189.
10. Coven, interview (see note 6).
11. Joint Commission, pp. 179 and 200.
12. Boyd, S., and others. Productivity considerations in the development of a new program and the ongoing management of an outpatient rehabilitation center. *Journal of Ambulatory Care Management* 11(1):34–40, 1988.

Chapter 4

Patient Management Issues

Patricia Lynne McCollom

Introduction

Approximately 30 million Americans are persons with disabilities resulting from chronic health problems. As the population ages and new and improved technology increases survival rates, the need for rehabilitation services will increase. Those services are also needed to help the thousands of people who experience low back or sports injuries annually.

Rehabilitation treatment on an outpatient basis provides high-quality, cost-efficient care without costly inpatient stays. As the nation focuses on rising health care costs, outpatient rehabilitation service delivery provides a cost-effective alternative to inpatient care for those persons with chronic or acute disabilities. Studies reported by the Family Hospital, in Milwaukee, Wisconsin,[1] and the Coathill Hospital, in Coatbridge, Scotland,[2] demonstrate that outpatient rehabilitation is indeed cost-effective and promotes maintenance of persons with disabilities in the home.

Although the need for rehabilitation services is obvious, the methods for coordinating and managing rehabilitation in the outpatient setting require particular attention. Without the inpatient systems to fall back on, it becomes imperative to establish methods for ensuring that patients receive the outpatient rehabilitation care prescribed and that providers address patient issues that might obstruct care and reimbursement. This chapter addresses a number of issues in patient management that need to be part of the process of coordinating and providing outpatient rehabilitation treatment. These issues include discharge planning from inpatient care and outpatient intake, consistency in patient management, communications methods and documentation, the role of the insurance case manager or care coordinator, and program evaluation/quality assurance.

Discharge Planning from Inpatient Care and Outpatient Intake

Appropriate discharge planning from inpatient care or direct physician care is critical to the success of outpatient rehabilitation programs. A plan for continuing care from an inpatient setting or a physician's office defines the need of each patient to obtain maximum health and function. The American Nurses' Association defines discharge planning as "that part of the continuity of care process which is designed to prepare the patient or client for the next phase of care and to assist in making any necessary arrangements for that phase of care, whether it be selfcare, care by family members, or care by an organized health care provider."[3] A discharge plan defines the need for ongoing health services and establishes a communication mechanism for the next level of care.

Conversely, the outpatient program admitting/intake staff must take steps to ensure that they obtain all critical information about each patient admitted for outpatient treatment. Failure to do so could mean inappropriate treatment plans or other miscommunications of patient needs. To promote continuity of care, each discharge plan for outpatient services should include the following information:

- *Assessment of the individual's status:* This section should include a description of the individual's function and dysfunction at the point of discharge from inpatient care or acute care provision. Because of the individual's disability, this assessment must include the physiological, psychological, cognitive and behavioral, social/family, communication, vocational, and educational components of the patient's situation. A clear definition of functional ability, or the individual's ability to perform specific activities of daily living, must be included.
- *A plan for service provision:* The plan for service is based on the individual's needs, as identified by assessment. It includes the components to be addressed in outpatient treatment. Specific methods of treatment must be noted and specified, and the professionals accountable for plan implementation should be identified.
- *Definition of actual treatment:* Again, based on individualized needs, the *prescriptions* for continuing treatment must be listed. These prescriptions are prepared by the primary physician and any associates who have participated in the individual's acute care.
- *Mechanisms for monitoring progress:* This part of a discharge plan identifies the methods and the time frames for evaluating service and monitoring progress. Often a follow-up examination by the inpatient team that served as the patient's primary care providers will be conducted to assess the patient's progress toward the goals established for continuing treatment.

Although the individual is undergoing continuing care on an outpatient basis, the primary care physicians and other care providers must review the patient's status for their own program evaluation until he or she is released from care. For example, an individual with a spinal cord injury may be discharged with a prescription for outpatient physical and occupational therapy. The primary care providers generally anticipate a three-month follow-up appointment to evaluate the patient's progress and recommend any change in treatment.

- *Goals for treatment:* The goals for rehabilitation treatment are directed toward helping the person with disabilities to achieve maximum potential of function, independence, and reintegration into the community. Individual assessment guides the service providers, as treatment goals are established.

  Ongoing treatment goals identify expected outcomes for the individual, relating to physical, mental, social, emotional, vocational, and economic factors. When full recovery is not possible, treatment goals must address issues of quality of life for both the individual and the family.

  Through a discharge plan, the outpatient rehabilitation service providers receive direction and guidance for treatment, including information on potential barriers to ongoing care.
- *Need for further coordination of community resources:* Community resources respond to the health and social needs of those within the community. The discharge plan must include an assessment to determine which available community resources are necessary to help service providers coordinate transportation, supplies/equipment, financial aid, education, and support for each patient.

With appropriate discharge planning from an inpatient program or from acute care, the outpatient rehabilitation program staff then assumes accountability for implementation of the discharge plan and its extension or revision based on the patient's progress.

Consistency in Patient Management

Outpatient rehabilitation programs serve the varying needs of patients referred. A number of interrelationships must be coordinated to ensure that patients obtain the required outpatient care (see figure 4-1). Because particular situations and problems vary widely from patient to patient, consistency is the only assurance that patients will receive the care they need. Consistent methods for intake, planning, scheduling, and patient management in general must be developed to ensure patient compliance with the health care plan.

Figure 4-1. Interrelationships Affecting Patient Management Issues in Outpatient Rehabilitation

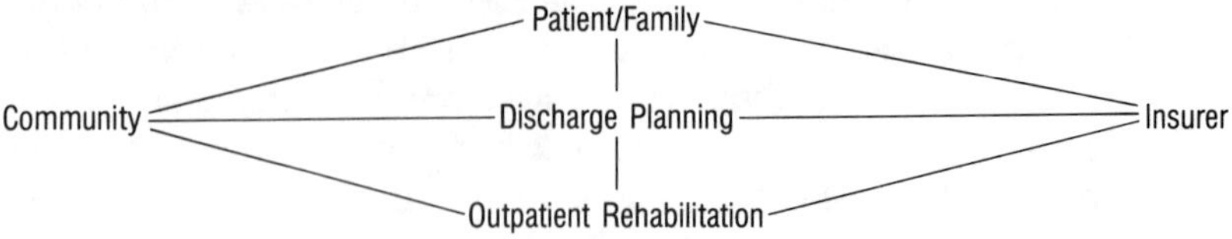

The following case example demonstrates complications that may occur in patient care when a lack of consistency exists:

> A sixty-year-old female industrial worker sustained a severe low-back injury. Following acute care, she was referred to an outpatient pain management program with a physician's prescription for full program participation. The discharge plan from acute care did not note the woman lived in a rural area and was unable to drive. No one person in the outpatient program was assigned responsibility for intake or scheduling. The outpatient treatment scheduling was handled by non-medical personnel and the woman was assigned physical therapy at 9:00 a.m. and again at 1:00 p.m., and counseling from 4:00 p.m. to 5:00 p.m. After one week, she discontinued participation because of inability to secure transportation for several trips a day.

Clearly, neither adequate records transfer, assessment, planning, monitoring, nor community coordination took place to allow the individual to comply. The patient in this example may have been better served by a primary care coordinator within the outpatient setting, who is assigned responsibility for intake and scheduling.

A four-step process is suggested to ensure successful management of the individual participating in outpatient rehabilitation:

1. Responsibility for acceptance/transfer of an individual from inpatient care to outpatient rehabilitation must be assigned to one person who may be designated the *primary care coordinator.* This individual may be a nurse or a social worker. The coordinator must review acute care records and the discharge plan for continuity of care. Gaps noted in the discharge plan, such as transportation needs, must be addressed with the patient and/or family at intake.
2. Planning for ongoing services is initiated by the primary care coordinator, based on the discharge plan and the services prescribed.
3. The primary care coordinator must identify factors at intake that may affect a patient's full participation in the outpatient program. As the

case example showed, the lack of transportation and long time lapses between the different services contributed to the failure of that particular outpatient treatment. Additionally, the use and coordination of community resources must be established.

4. Time frames for monitoring and communicating patient progress to all parties concerned must be established at intake. Third-party payer limits may define parameters for monitoring and communication, and these should be met.

Communication Methods and Documentation

Outpatient rehabilitation programs must establish effective and innovative techniques for coordinating activities and exchanging information.

The outpatient interdisciplinary team, led by a physician with rehabilitation experience, coordinates patient care and includes the patient and family in its planning. The team functions to exchange information, define ongoing rehabilitation needs, develop an integrated plan for continuity of care, and evaluate the effectiveness of rehabilitation care.

For outpatient rehabilitation programs, as with inpatient rehabilitation, the regular patient care conference, including all team members, is the base for both internal and external documentation.

Documentation must include the actions taken and their relationship to patient needs, define outcomes, and indicate what further intervention is planned. Standards for documentation are well known through the Commission on Accreditation of Rehabilitation Facilities (CARF) and the Joint Commission on Accreditation for Healthcare Organizations (Joint Commission). However, as health care insurers become more involved in care provision through approval mechanisms, a more consistent and concise method for documentation and external reporting is needed. For example, insurance claim reviewers often review hundreds of claims daily, and deciding to approve claims for services often must be done with limited knowledge of the insured individual. To facilitate communication with insurers, a one-page report that includes the following data should be submitted monthly or at regular intervals as specified by the insurer:

- Patient name, address, and age
- Diagnosis and brief statement of etiology
- Summary of current treatment
- Patient status as of date of report
- Further treatment planned
- Goals for continued treatment
- Extended timetable for services
- Variables affecting the rehabilitation plan
- Date of next report

The Role of the Insurance Case Manager

A new member to be welcomed to the patient care team is the insurance case manager or care coordinator. Both workers' compensation carriers and health care insurers find case management/care coordination increasingly necessary in the dynamic health care system. Case management is the balance between care providers and care payers that coordinates benefits and ensures that limited dollars are spent wisely.

The book *Hospital Administration Terminology* defines case management as "a system of assessment, treatment planning, and follow-up that ensures the provision of comprehensive and continuous service and the coordination of payment and reimbursement for care."[4] In outpatient rehabilitation, the insurance case manager/care coordinator serves as a direct communicator to third-party payers to provide information on the patient's status. In the role of communicator, the insurance case manager/care coordinator facilitates the most appropriate use of available health care dollars in cooperation with treatment providers.

Program Evaluation/Quality Assurance

Ongoing program evaluation in outpatient rehabilitation, as with other health care programs, systematically monitors program effectiveness and efficiency. Performance must be reported, on a regular and continual basis, with regard to the program's mission, goals, and objectives.

Program evaluation thus supports overall quality assurance, which identifies potential problems or care issues and their causes and solutions, and evaluates their remedies. Quality assurance (QA) programs aim to improve and maintain excellence in health care services delivery.

Necessary components of QA programs are:

- *Standard development:* A standard is defined as "a norm that expresses an agreed upon level of practice that has been developed to characterize, measure, and provide guidance for achieving excellence."[5]
- *Problem identification:* Identification of problems that affect patient care is completed through interdisciplinary staff discussion or systematic review of medical records. It is related to the standards for care provision of the treatment plan.
- *Problem study:* Those involved in the problem determine alternative solutions and collect necessary data.
- *Action for problem resolution:* The action to resolve the problem is defined and implemented; time frames for completion of activities must be established.
- *Evaluation of action:* Those involved in care delivery need to determine the effectiveness of the selected action and its impact on care provision, and then review the plan of action as indicated by results.

Each outpatient rehabilitation program must develop a QA program within its own structure. Methods of reporting outcomes to the entire staff must be developed to promote coordination of program changes.

Conclusion

Outpatient rehabilitation programs face challenges for patient management activities. The responsibility exceeds scheduling for treatment and includes participation in and extension of the discharge planning process.

Communication mechanisms must be developed creatively to meet the needs of quality assurance, program evaluation, and documentation for insurers.

Collaborative efforts among care providers, the community, and payers can result in high-quality outpatient rehabilitation services to meet the needs of our changing health care system.

References

1. Day rehabilitation program proves cost effective. *Hospitals* 58(20):60, Oct. 16, 1984.
2. Campbell, A. J., and Mehta, A. J. Outpatient rehabilitation center keeps many elderly living at home. *Hospitals* 55(2):101–102, 105, Jan. 16, 1981.
3. American Nurses' Association. *Continuity of Care and Discharge Planning Programs in Institutions and Community Agencies* (Pub. Code NP-49, 3000). Kansas City, MO: ANA, 1974, p. 3.
4. American Hospital Association Resource Center. *Hospital Administration Terminology.* 2nd ed. Chicago: American Hospital Publishing, 1986, p. 8.
5. American Nurses' Association and Association of Rehabilitation Nurses. *Standards of Rehabilitation Nursing.* Kansas City, MO: ANA, 1986, p. 13.

Chapter 5

Facilities Planning and Renovation

Patrick B. Davis, Jr.

Introduction

Prior to 1980, many hospitals providing rehabilitation services had little in the way of facilities that differentiated outpatient and inpatient care. Many organizations soon realized the revenue potential of outpatient rehabilitation as a way of retaining patients who had been inpatients at their facilities and continuing their care, postdischarge. Networking with physician referrals provided for a continuum of service from trauma to hospital, to outpatient care, to home health care.

For most rehabilitation patients, the transition from hospital to home is an emotional and a conflicting experience. Feelings of joy about leaving the hospital are often mixed with apprehension and a lack of confidence about being able to adapt to their previous lifestyle with the physical limitations resulting from injury or illness. The transitional phase is an important element in the long-term recovery of many persons with disabilities. The development of facilities specifically designed for outpatient rehabilitation allows patients to psychologically recognize their own physical, emotional, and social progress. For example, most patients can easily comprehend a progression from the hospital bed to the wheelchair, then to a walker, and finally to discharge. Shifting the emphasis from full-time inpatient rehabilitation to a transitional phase during which outpatient treatments are integrated into the patient's own schedule facilitates the patient's reentry into the "real world."

A freestanding outpatient rehabilitation center basically has two forms: One is a hospital-based facility that is attached to the hospital, and even to its inpatient rehabilitation department, but has separate facilities expressly for the use of outpatients; the other is a facility that is both physically and administratively separated from the main hospital. Obviously, the latter facility is the one that most clearly meets the definition of *freestanding.* It could be located anywhere on the hospital campus or off-site within the community. The users of either a hospital-based facility or a separate facility rarely encounter inpatients. They arrive, often using their own resources, and undergo treatment utilizing facilities and equipment specifically designed for outpatients. Additionally, they work with therapists specializing in treatments that are tailored specifically to their physical problems and diagnoses.

Freestanding outpatient facilities must present a clear image or identity to outpatients and provide confirmation of each patient's rehabilitation progress. This is important to help patients adjust to their outpatient status, and to ensure that they are less likely to see inpatients and thus be reminded of the trauma they are trying to put behind them.

It is the hospital-based inpatient/outpatient care facility located within the hospital's rehabilitation department that still appears to be the predominant form of outpatient rehabilitation service. This facility utilizes the personnel resources of the inpatient rehabilitation department by cross-training therapists to effectively treat both inpatients and outpatients. However, separate facilities are usually provided for the outpatients and, for the reasons already mentioned, this is preferred.

This chapter discusses the critical factors involved in designing a new outpatient facility or renovating existing space for an outpatient program. Among the factors discussed are the scope of the outpatient rehabilitation program, the program's goals, the planning process, the design process, site selection, renovation, equipment considerations, facility design, and facility maintenance considerations.

Scope of the Outpatient Rehabilitation Program

The scope of the rehabilitation program to be offered to an outpatient population drives the size of the facility. The services that are offered depend on:

- Unmet needs of the community
- Revenue potential
- Reimbursement sources of the potential population
- Demographics
- Budget for the program
- Availability of trained staff

A full outpatient rehabilitation program offers more comprehensive services to the patient than isolated therapy programs do and therefore requires more space than a typical outpatient physical therapy program. A menu of services that could be provided in an outpatient rehabilitation program includes the following:

- Physical therapy
- Occupational therapy
- Speech therapy
- Physiatry services
- Respiratory therapy
- Prosthetic/orthotic services
- Nursing services
- Social services
- Psychological services
- Pharmacy/equipment/supply services

A facility space of less than 4,000 square feet would generally be insufficient to provide the full scope of rehabilitation services. Instead, a space of this size might offer isolated or specific services such as physical therapy, occupational therapy, speech therapy, and social services, either alone or in combination. A smaller program would probably not provide the services required to meet the definition of a Comprehensive Outpatient Rehabilitation Facility (CORF).

The small program is more vulnerable to problems associated with expansion of services, changes to services offered, and responses to changes in patient base, reimbursement, or new equipment demands. Consequently, the facility designed for a small program is extremely crucial. Its space should be flexible and adaptable to accommodate changes. An architectural space program delineating the square footage requirements for a small hospital-based rehabilitation program is shown in table 5-1; table 5-2 (p. 87) shows the space requirements for a freestanding hospital-based facility.

Large programs and/or CORFs may have space requirements in excess of 20,000 square feet. The minimum service components required of a CORF often dictate the minimum square footage for this type of facility. Although it is possible to have various-sized CORFs, for the purposes of this book we will draw the line at CORF guidelines or minimum requirements. The rationale is that the greater the number of program components, the more space needed. Of course, there are additional related services that could be included in the facility, such as cardiac rehabilitation and sports medicine, which could enhance a large program. An example of the architectural space program needed for a CORF is provided in table 5-3 (p. 88).

Table 5-1. Small Hospital-Based Outpatient Rehab Space Program

Space	Number Required	Net Square Feet	Net Square Feet Extended	Subtotal for Zones (square feet)
I. *Treatment Areas*				
Voice disorder	1	100	100	
Speech pathology	1	150	150	
Hydrotherapy	1	650	650	
Modality treatment	1	600	600	
Exercise area	1	800	800	
Gait training functional	1	750	750	
Patient change/locker	2	110	220	
Patient toilet/shower	2	45	90	
				3,370
II. *Support Areas*				
Clean supply	1	100	100	
Soiled utility	1	80	80	
Storage	1	90	90	
Wheelchair alcove	1	20	20	
				290
III. *Administrative Areas*				
Receptionist (2 people)	1	80	80	
Waiting (12–15 seats)	1	225	225	
Public toilet	2	55	110	
Director office	1	120	120	
Clerical work	1	80	80	
Conference	1	180	180	
Staff lounge/locker	1	180	180	
Staff toilet	1	30	30	
PT director office	1	30	80	
PT staff office	1	200	200	
				1,285
IV. EASY STREET ENVIRONMENT™	Proprietary System—Adjust to Needs			
Home Life				
OT supervisor				
OT workstation				
OT hand table				
OT bathroom				
Bedroom				
Kitchen/laundry				
City Life				
Market				
Cafe				
Car				
Bus				
Bank				
Work Life				
Work Hardening				
Key station				
Work simulator				
Testing				
				1,950
		Total Net Square Feet		6,895
		Departmental Grossing Factor		× 1.3
		Total Departmental Gross Square Feet		8,964

Note: PT = Physical therapy; OT = Occupational therapy.

Note: Hospital-based outpatient rehab program in renovated hospital space.

Table 5-2. Hospital-Based Freestanding Outpatient Rehab Space Program

Space	Number Required	Net Square Feet	Net Square Feet Extended	Subtotal for Zones
I. *Treatment Areas*				
Open exercise (PT)	1	1,100	1,100	
Open activity (OT)	1	720	720	
Hand				
Neuro/perceptual				
Splint				
ADL kitchen	1	140	140	
Sensory stimulation	1	130	130	
Driver's education	1	200	200	
Modality	7	80	560	
Hydrotherapy	1	180	180	
Patient toilet	2	45	90	
Speech	3	70	180	
Exam	1	90	90	
Fitness exercise	1	1,200	1,200	
Dressing	3	25	75	
				4,665
II. *Support Areas*				
Clean supply	1	80	80	
Soiled holding	1	60	60	
Storage	1	110	110	
				250
III. *Administrative Areas*				
Reception	1	120	120	
Waiting	1	180	180	
Medical records	1	60	60	
MD consult	1	130	130	
Work conference	1	190	190	
Staff toilet	1	30	30	
Lockers	1	30	30	
				740
		Total Net Square Feet		5,655
		Departmental Grossing Factor		×1.4
		Total Departmental Gross Square Feet		7,917

Note: Freestanding outpatient rehab facility constructed in hospital-based doctor's office building tenant space.

The Program's Goals

The beginning of any planning process requires that the planning group meet to agree on program goals and objectives. The mission statement with its goals for the outpatient rehabilitation program is the foundation on which the functional planning process is based. Without a list of goals, it is likely that problems will develop later in the planning process, or worse, during facility start-up and/or operation.

Table 5-3. Community-Based Freestanding CORF Space Program

Space	Number Required	Net Square Feet	Net Square Feet Extended	Subtotal
I. *Treatment Areas*				
Biofeedback	1	100	100	
Psychologist	1	100	100	
Speech	1	120	120	
Open activity area (OT)	1	800	800	
Open exercise area (PT)	1	1,200	1,200	
Hydrotherapy	1	260	260	
Dressing	2	35	70	
Activities for daily living (ADL)	1	180	180	
Exam	1	125	125	
Hi-lo mats	6	100	600	
Patient toilet	2	45	90	
				3,645
II. *Support Areas*				
Soiled utility	1	80	80	
Clean supply	1	80	80	
Storage	1	135	135	
Janitor	1	35	35	
				330
III. *Administrative Areas*				
Reception (6 waiting)	1	210	210	
Business office	1	155	155	
Director office	1	110	110	
MD office	1	110	110	
Staff conference	1	140	140	
Staff toilet	2	30	60	
Staff charting	1	300	300	
				1,085
		Total Net Square Feet		5,060
		Departmental Grossing Factor		×1.3
		Total Departmental Gross Square Feet		6,578

Note: Basic space program for freestanding CORF in tenant space in existing office building.

Program goals should be oriented toward patient care as well as revenue potential. The following goals and objectives provide a sound foundation for considering the development of an outpatient rehabilitation facility and will guide facility planning:

- Provide the services that will fill voids that currently exist in the facility's market
- Preserve patient dignity through privacy and respect
- Maintain a sense of optimism/cheerfulness through facility design
- Provide flexibility in design
- Promote a sense of well-being
- Develop a sense of achievement for each patient

- Provide service that is economical to the patient and profitable to the hospital

It is important to point out that some of the preceding goals are architectural in nature, some are patient- and user-group oriented, and others focus on the provider. Regardless of their individual focus, the goals of the facility should merge with the needs of the group to be served as well as with those of the provider. Although this author does not advocate design by committee, he does recognize that in order to achieve a successful facility, the needs of the user groups and patients to be served must be identified.

The Planning Process

The planning process begins with an idea to develop a freestanding outpatient rehabilitation program, extend the scope of existing inpatient services to include outpatient services, or redirect an existing outpatient program. The planning process includes development of the functional program, selection of the architect, and development of the architectural space program.

As pointed out in chapter 2, a planning team must be formed. The planning team formed to develop the facility may be different from the group involved in market-based strategic planning, but there will be some overlap. This group need not be large. For example, a 300-bed community hospital might appoint a planning team consisting of the chief operating officer, the chief financial officer, the hospital planner, the rehabilitation department director, and the chief of medical staff or the medical director of the rehabilitation department. Later in the planning process, other expertise may be brought to bear in the form of therapists, architects, and/or facility planners.

Development of a new service is a major undertaking for a community hospital without existing rehabilitation services. For these hospitals, it may be necessary to acquire the expertise of a hospital planning consultant or a specialist in the development of rehabilitation services.

The planning team should first carefully review the hospital's strategic plan. This review is necessary to determine whether an outpatient rehabilitation program is feasible within the parameters of the strategic plan. The chief financial officer should advise on the funding or availability of resources needed to develop the program and plan the facility.

Initially, the planning team must agree that (1) the service is viable, (2) the funding is available, and (3) all resources including staff are available to begin the program. Without this consensus, the planning process will become hampered further down the line.

Development of the Functional Program

The planning committee's first responsibility upon reaching consensus is to develop a functional program. A *functional program* is a document that sets down in writing the foundations for the development of the balance of the planning process. It is called a functional program because it indicates how the facility should operate and perform. It will guide the facility planning and design process, and is the basic document for any decision making involved in planning a new facility or renovating existing space. The functional program should contain the following elements:

- Mission statement
- Goals and objectives
- Rehabilitative services program
- Specific services
- Operational plan
- Personnel/staffing plan
- Marketing plan
- Potential sites
- Time frame
- Budget/financial plan

Although functional program components may vary, at minimum they include the basic elements necessary to get the planning process off to a good start: goals, the services to be offered, an operational plan, and a budget. If any of these four components are missing at the beginning of the facility planning and design phases, problems will likely develop.

A prime objective of the functional program is to develop a list of services to be offered. The following list is considered a master menu from which planners may select services that are most appropriate to their service area and program needs:

- Physical therapy
- Speech therapy
- Sports screening
- Employee health screening
- Occupational therapy
- Functional work analysis
- Work hardening
- Vocational rehabilitation
- Specialized fitness groups/health clubs/group exercise
- Aquatic therapy
- Driving assessment for persons with disabilities

- Driver's education
- Home life activities of daily living training
- Temporomandibular joint (TMJ) therapy
- Hydrotherapy
- Splinting
- Wheelchair assessment and fitting
- Educational classes (nutrition, body mechanics, and so forth)
- Orthotic/prosthetic assessment/fitting
- Counseling (individual and group/family)
- Training in self-care
- Community integration/transition training

The list of services offered is not a basis for any type of market forecasting; rather, it supports the facility's potential size and design, its staffing needs, and its potential for revenue, income, and profit. These are all critical elements that affect facility planning.

Selection of the Architect

The successful completion of the functional program phase allows the planning process to proceed to the next stage of development, which is selection of the architect.

The selection of an architect for the facility is a crucial step in the planning process. It is important that this activity occur early in the process so that the necessary expert input can be obtained to verify that the budget, time frame, and initial projections regarding space needs or potential sites are accurate and viable. Criteria for selecting the architect should include:

- Previous successful experience, specifically with rehabilitation facilities
- A previous working relationship with the hospital and/or user group
- An understanding of the rehabilitation program and its goals and objectives
- Knowledge of local building codes
- Knowledge of particular site characteristics
- Demonstration of sensitivity to providing a high-quality environment
- Commitment to meeting schedule and budget

The most important criterion is that the architect possess prior successful experience in developing rehabilitation facilities. Finding an architect who meets all the listed criteria may be difficult. It is not unusual for a provider to first select a planner to develop the functional program and space program and then an architect to develop the facility design, contract documents for work, and administer the construction process.

As discussed later in this chapter, the space needs of the rehabilitation facility are generally based on a working knowledge of the equipment and treatment procedures to be provided within the facility. Thus, the architectural firm should demonstrate that the proposed project architect possesses this working knowledge to ensure the success of the final plan.

At the onset of the working relationship with the architect, the hospital/provider must clearly delineate the responsibilities of each party and those of other consultants involved in planning. This is particularly important when the provider selects an outside planner and architect. Often the services of the architect and the planner will overlap, and some overlap is beneficial. However, the limits of responsibility and service to be provided by both parties should be clearly defined from the onset to avoid duplication.

Development of the Architectural Space Program

Upon completion of the functional program and selection of an architect, the actual facility design process takes place. The first step in the process is development of an architectural space program.

The *architectural space program* takes the information generated by the functional program and user group meetings and transforms it into a document that will be used to create an initial design drawing, more commonly referred to as a *schematic design,* for the proposed outpatient rehabilitation facility. The architect begins the process by reviewing the functional program and then meets with a committee of designated user groups. The content of the architectural space program is as follows:

- Scope of the project
- List of resources, including participants and user groups
- Design problem statement (what is going to be built)
- List of spaces and square footage requirements
- Review and analysis of potential sites
- Recommendation of optimum site (best location for the facility)
- Zoning and site constraints
- Project cost
- Time frame
- Block diagrams indicating functional and spatial relationships (small-scale diagrams showing how the various program components relate)
- Applicable building codes
- Review and approval process (working with the people who will administer and use the facility)

Architectural space programs are usually listed by room or space, with the net square footage needed for each. *Net square footage* is the usable area of a room exclusive of walls. The sum of the total net square footage is then multiplied by a factor that provides for wall space and corridors (departmental grossing factors) equaling total departmental gross square footage. Total departmental gross square footage must then be multiplied by a building grossing factor to provide for exterior walls and mechanical, electrical, horizontal, and vertical circulation, such as stairs and elevators. This sum equals the total building gross square footage.

Total number of net square feet	×	Departmental grossing factor	=	Total departmental gross square footage
Total departmental gross square footage	×	Building grossing factor	=	Total building gross square footage

$$\begin{array}{r} \text{Total NSF} \\ \times\ \text{DGF} \\ \hline \text{Total DGSF} \\ \times\ \text{BGF} \\ \hline \text{Total BGSF} \end{array}$$

It is important to not only list the spaces required that will generally forecast the total size of the building, but also to begin to address the other components of the program, because these may affect the project cost, square footage, orientation to existing facilities, and configuration. Programming an outpatient rehabilitation facility requires careful coordination among the facilities manager or director, the rehabilitation manager or director, and the equipment planning consultant (see "Equipment Considerations" later in the chapter).

Space will be planned for each *space generator,* or major piece of equipment, including circulation space around, to, and from each space generator. Circulation or access space is an often-overlooked element in space planning, and it is vital to keep in mind that each piece of equipment must be accessed from three or even four sides.

It is very important that the staff working with the architect identify the equipment and treatment areas required to carry out the proposed rehabilitation service early in the architectural programming phase. This is necessary before the architect can begin to accurately program the center's space needs.

There are no truly accurate general rules of thumb that can be used for forecasting space needs for rehabilitation departments, because each facility has its unique program aspects. However, for general planning purposes it may be useful to consider projected annual patient volume, visits, or number of square feet per bed. It is possible to verify a square foot area projection by the following comparative analysis. Obtain data on four or five facilities and compare the following information:

- Total number of licensed beds
- Number of dedicated rehabilitation beds
- Total square footage of all rehabilitation space
- Square footage of inpatient treatment space
- Square footage of outpatient treatment space
- Number of annual inpatient admissions
- Number of annual outpatient visits

These data will allow the planner to forecast or verify initial planning assumptions, such as the following:

- Square footage of outpatient treatment space per inpatient rehabilitation bed
- Square footage of total rehabilitation space per licensed bed
- Number of inpatient admissions as a factor of outpatient visits

A facility generally requires the following minimum treatment areas, which vary in size depending on equipment selection and the number of treatments projected for each area:

- Physical therapy (and related modalities)
- Occupational therapy (and related modalities)
- Hydrotherapy
- Speech therapy and audiology

There may be additional considerations, of course, based on proposed services, such as recreational therapy, driver's education, pediatrics, transitional living, activities of daily living, and so forth. The objective is to allocate appropriate space for all the equipment and/or treatment areas to support the rehabilitation services to be provided and identified in the functional program.

In addition to actual treatment areas, there are administrative, clerical, and support areas needed in each facility, including the following:

- Waiting and reception
- Clerical
- Administrative
- Staff offices
- Equipment storage
- Staff charting/lounge areas

The space requirements needed for these areas are generated by projected patient volume, the number of personnel or staff required to meet the volume, and management policies and procedures. The space forecast depends on the identification of staff and a management plan early in the process, and is then spelled out in the functional program.

Always evaluate the percentage of clerical and administrative staff office and support space against the necessary clinical or revenue-generating space. No more than 25 to 30 percent of total departmental square footage should be devoted to these functions.

The rehabilitation department is one of the more difficult departments in a health care facility to program for space because of the number of program components, the need for activity space, and the program's different priorities. Without a projection of patient visits, volume, or activity, it is difficult, and perhaps impossible, for the architect to accurately forecast the rehab department's space needs.

Most planning errors occur because of the lack of a functional program, the provider's failure to forecast patient volume based on sound marketing strategies, or an oversight in addressing the management and staffing needs of the rehabilitation program.

The Design Process

Upon completion of the architectural space program, the architect and the user groups may begin the design process. The *design process* is an orderly progression of tasks that leads from loosely organized sketches developed during the schematic design phase to hard-lined, detailed construction documents upon which pricing for the facility is obtained. The process involves the architect, the architect's consultants, and the user groups. The user groups' input is considerable in the early stages of the design process but decreases in intensity as the process continues.

Schematic Design

Schematic design involves the translation of the architectural space program into sketches and drawings that illustrate the site and the proposed building's relationship to existing buildings, parking lots, streets, zoning-required setbacks (distances from the property line), and other site requirements. During the schematic design process, the architect will also sketch various floor plan configurations and explore alternatives. The massing and exterior elevations of the building will be sketched, and the floor-to-floor height and its relationship to the existing facility will be investigated.

Upon completion of the schematic design, the provider should review the drawings with the various user groups to determine whether the design is compatible with the outpatient rehabilitation program's goals and objectives, the project budget, and the facility master plan guidelines.

Design Development

After approval of the schematic design phase, the architect begins the design development phase. Any revisions of the schematic design drawings will be incorporated into the design development documents. The structural columns will be set, and a structural system agreed on. The building footprint (area of the building at ground level) will be determined, and the architect will begin to incorporate the equipment items into the floor plan to determine their best configuration and relationship to their spaces.

Preliminary decisions regarding the building's mechanical and electrical systems will be made at this time. Mechanical and electrical engineering consultants will begin to determine the location of the various pieces of mechanical equipment, such as air handlers, chillers, boilers, electrical switchgear, and panels. Preliminary lighting layouts will also be investigated and incorporated into the design development drawings. It is at this point that the architect, the consultants, and the provider must carefully review the documents to determine whether the project is still within the designated budget allocation.

Upon the provider's approval of the design development documents, the architect may begin the construction documents. Construction documents are the final step of the design process. These documents are used to obtain contracting bids and to actually build the facility. They are highly technical and will provide the specific information needed to obtain approvals from the local building authority as well as accurate price estimates from bidders.

Site Selection

Selection of a site for an outpatient rehabilitation program is driven by a priority determinant—*access.* The site must be accessible to the outpatients. Although there could be a lengthy discussion regarding the various types of access, simply stated, the site must be easy for the patient to get to and leave after treatment.

A vital component of accessibility is parking, which must be immediately available. It is preferable to provide parking within 100 feet of the front door of the facility. If accessible parking becomes a problem, other options should be considered, such as valet parking and/or a van service that would transport patients from their homes to and from the facility for treatment.

Good principles of site analysis and selection are constant, whether a site is being selected for an addition to the main hospital building, an on-campus freestanding facility, or an off-campus freestanding facility. The following pages focus on scenarios for selecting either a hospital-based site or a community-based site.

Site Selection for Hospital-Based Freestanding Outpatient Facilities

Hospital-based freestanding outpatient rehabilitation facilities normally are designed as additions to the main hospital building, as tenant infill of space in a doctor's office building, or as freestanding structures elsewhere on the campus. Regardless of the facility's structure, the following factors should be measured:

- *Convenient access:* As already described, this is the prime design determinant. Convenient parking, a large covered area for arriving and departing patients (a canopy could be used), and a site clearly identifiable and visible from the main hospital entrance and/or access road should be provided.
- *Adequate and convenient parking for outpatients:* Parking areas should contain more than the minimum required number of dedicated spaces for persons with disabilities, as well as for high-top vans. Parking should also reflect the fact that many of the patients entering the facility will have some type of physical disability; many will be in wheelchairs. In laying out the parking lot for an outpatient rehabilitation facility, adjusting for the size and configuration of parking spaces is as important, if not more important, than meeting the number of required spaces. Some drivers may not have the best command of their vehicles, and vehicles such as vans and ambulances need sufficient space to maneuver.
- *Space for future expansion:* Projections for an outpatient facility should indicate a steady increase in patient use. Some degree of oversizing of a department is necessary in order to meet projections; however, adequate space should exist on the site for future expansion as a result of program growth.
- *Availability of utilities:* Water, power, sanitary sewer, storm sewer, natural gas, and telephone should all be accessible.
- *Soil suitable for facility construction:* A geotechnical investigation will verify that the soil conditions at the site will not pose any unusual and/or difficult construction techniques that may either cause the facility additional building expense or compromise the project altogether.

Site Selection for Community-Based Outpatient Facilities

Site selection requirements for community-based freestanding outpatient rehabilitation facilities are similar to those for hospital-based facilities. However, some additional factors should be considered:

- *Zoning:* Zoning problems can be costly and time-consuming. The proposed site should be properly zoned for the medical activity being proposed. Only sites zoned for medical facilities or medical offices should be considered. As a rule, a site that is not properly zoned should not be considered. The dollars saved in purchasing a "bargain" site, which is not properly zoned (but perhaps hoping to be rezoned) may result in a far greater expense to the facility than originally budgeted.
- *Location:* The site should be located so that it is easily accessible and highly visible from the roadway. Locations providing direct access from arterials and/or feeder streets are preferred because they generally meet these criteria.
- *Size considerations:* A question arising early in the design process is, "How large a site do we need?" An adequately sized site is one that provides enough area for the structure itself, parking, vehicular circulation, setbacks (distance from the property line), landscaped areas, and future growth. It is important that a site be selected that is large enough to accommodate all functions and activities on one floor. Two-story facilities usually do not work very well for freestanding outpatient rehabilitation facilities. They may require that the outpatient rehabilitation program be located on separate levels and thus experience staffing inefficiencies, loss of operational control, and even difficulties in providing treatment. In addition, two-story facilities are more often expensive to construct because they require elevators and stairs.
- *Easements, rights-of-way:* The existence of unusual setbacks, easements, rights-of-way, and so forth for utilities, roadways, and adjacent properties should be verified, as these could prove to make the site unusual and/or difficult to build on. Easements, rights-of-way, and setbacks are specified in zoning requirements, local building codes, and deed restrictions. They represent areas of the site that must not be occupied by the building.
- *Cost:* The cost of the site is a significant line item in the projected budget for a freestanding rehabilitation center. Typically, the property will be a prime piece of real estate. However, building the facility off-campus may make it physically more accessible and more usable for the outpatients, which could eventually increase both patient volume and revenue generated and thus justify the cost of the site. This is particularly true if the current campus is congested and/or parking is not readily available. The hospital campus simply may not offer a suitable site for a 7,000- to 10,000-square-foot building.
- *Appearance and image:* A good site is readily visible from the adjacent roadways and projects an image of a high-quality health care facility. Attractive landscaping and natural landscape features are a consideration; large, mature trees project an image of longevity and stability.

Renovation

Many freestanding outpatient rehabilitation centers have been developed on sites that have existing buildings. The existing buildings have often been renovated and adapted to the new use. This is an attractive option because it allows a favorable site to be acquired, with an existing building that may be renovated in less time than it would take to construct a new one. A number of factors, however, must be considered in making the decision to renovate. These include proper zoning; structural integrity; heating, ventilating, and air-conditioning considerations; demolition considerations; and adaptive reuse and renovation of existing structures.

Proper Zoning

The existing facility must be properly zoned for an outpatient rehabilitation facility. Local zoning and building codes often allow an existing building to be renovated or retrofitted for a new use to occupy a greater portion of the land than is usually allowed. The setbacks, floor area ratios, and parking requirements of a 20-year-old building may have been less restrictive 20 years ago than they are today. If so, the facility could get more for its money than if it had started with an undeveloped site, because existing facilities are often allowed to be renovated without having to comply with regulations for new construction.

Structural Integrity

The structural soundness or integrity of the building should be verified by an architect or a structural engineer. An important consideration is determining whether the existing building is suitable for its intended use or whether the structure needs to be reworked at significant additional expense.

Buildings with steel or concrete structural frames are best for renovation. Buildings with wood frames and/or roof structures should be avoided. Wood may deteriorate unless the facility has been properly maintained, and it is difficult to fireproof wood structures to meet today's building codes. As previously mentioned, multistory structures should be avoided, if possible. If a multistory building is the best alternative, consideration should be given to using the second floor for administrative offices and so forth.

Ground or grade-level access directly into the outpatient rehabilitation facility is important. The existing building should provide adequate floor space for the space requirements of the outpatient rehabilitation center on the first floor. It may be necessary to add on to the existing building to accomplish this.

A minimum floor-to-floor or floor-to-roof height of 12 feet is normally acceptable, assuming an interior ceiling height of 8 feet. The gym or exercise area, however, should be provided with a ceiling height of 9 to 10 feet. The 8-foot ceiling height allows approximately 2 feet for the structural system to support the floor or roof and 2 feet of clear space between the ceiling and the bottom of the structural members for items such as ductwork and light fixtures.

Interior column spacing is the space between the vertical structural elements. Interior column spacing (also known as the structural grid) of 25 to 30 feet is desirable. Structures with irregular column spacing and/or unusual structural systems may be less efficient, requiring an increased amount of space in which to provide services.

Flat-plate concrete floor slabs are ideal because they provide greater height between the building floors and the structural members.

Exterior walls consisting of brick, stucco on concrete block, and in some cases precast concrete are also ideal because they are adaptable to new openings for windows, doors, and so forth.

Heating, Ventilating, and Air-Conditioning Considerations

Heating, ventilating, and air-conditioning (HVAC) equipment, as well as electrical equipment (wiring, wiring devices, and light fixtures) in existing buildings, usually must be completely replaced. The impact of new energy codes may render existing systems obsolete if they are more than 10 to 15 years old. Existing equipment such as chillers, boilers, transformers, and electrical switchgear in good condition should be investigated for reuse.

Demolition Considerations

In considering a structure for renovation, investigate how much of the existing space may be reused or adapted without demolition. Often it is better to completely demolish or gut the interior of an existing building and start over. This allows you to design space to fit your program and achieve the spatial adjacencies and functional requirements necessary. It does not make sense to compromise functional spatial relationships just to save a few construction dollars. A piecemeal approach to patching up walls, ductwork, wiring, and lighting and plumbing systems could create myriad problems with regard to obtaining approval by local building code authorities. In the end, piecemeal work could cost more than either building a new structure or gutting the old one and completely replacing its interior and building systems. The architect's assessment of the building's condition and its suitability for renovation to meet the program's space needs is paramount.

Adaptive Reuse and Renovation of Existing Hospital Structures

Adaptive reuse and renovation of existing hospital structures has been on the rise. This is generally because inpatient use of hospital-based facilities has decreased, particularly with respect to inpatient beds. This has freed up space for other uses. More and more facilities are being renovated to convert space once used solely for inpatients to outpatient use.

The degree of difficulty can be a significant factor in the cost of renovation. Renovation costs are not always easily identifiable and may be difficult to project. The following questions should be answered before embarking on a renovation program:

- Will existing operations within the facility be disrupted by the renovation?
- Are the building and its systems sound?
- Are there major problems that need to be corrected to meet building codes?
- Will there be enough space for the contractor to stage building operations and store materials?
- Can debris from the demolition be removed easily?
- What is the real cost of the renovation after all the above has been considered?

The two prime problems to consider in renovating an existing facility are (1) the potential disruption of existing operations and (2) the inconvenience caused to patients. Physician frustration and a lengthy renovation process caused by complex phasing may not be worth the effort or the dollars saved if the hospital loses physicians, nurses, or patients, or ends up spending more money than anticipated in order to remain operational during the renovation.

Equipment Considerations

As stated in the discussion on the architectural space program, each piece of equipment used in the treatment of patients is a space generator. Planning for equipment space needs and the utility requirements for the equipment is important. Architectural programming and space forecasting or planning cannot be completed without a relatively accurate equipment list. The list should include the minimum equipment necessary to achieve the program's goals and all the items that are optional (those that would be nice to have but are not necessarily required). This allows the architect to project minimum and maximum space requirements.

Planning the equipment needs for a proposed outpatient rehabilitation department may be beyond the skills of the hospital planning committee. This is particularly true if the hospital is embarking on a new service. Thus the hospital will probably not have the staff expertise aboard and may need to acquire the services of an equipment planning consultant.

The equipment planning consultant should demonstrate successful experience in planning an outpatient rehabilitation department. He or she will work closely with the user groups and the architect to develop the preliminary equipment list. The list and the cost of each piece of equipment will be a factor in the project budget. It is at this point that the project cost may require adjustment in either the equipment category or the construction cost category. If necessary, the entire project cost budget may need to be adjusted. A list of typical equipment for a freestanding outpatient rehabilitation center is found in table 5-4.

Utility considerations for equipment were a minor factor in departments designed a little more than a decade ago. Equipment that was once completely mechanical is now much more sophisticated and may require electricity. The equipment list must indicate space and utility requirements for all equipment used in rehabilitation treatment.

Facility Design

Facility design should ensure that space allocations allow areas that are similar in function to be located adjacent to each other. Circulation and patient flow, therapeutic treatment areas, staff work areas, and the development of an environment conducive to the patient's sense of well-being and achievement should be studied early in the design process. The architectural program should delineate areas such as hydrotherapy, waiting and reception, exercise spaces, and administration and staff work areas. The facility design should address zoning within the department, circulation and traffic flow, and patient environment.

Zoning within the Department

Two major treatment zones are required for outpatient rehabilitation programs: the active treatment zone and the passive treatment zone, or specialty areas. A third zone provides support space for the department's management and administration and includes staff offices and waiting, reception, and clerical areas. The zones usually overlap to some extent.

The Active Treatment Zone

The active treatment zone includes the gym and/or exercise areas that contain most of the treatment-related equipment and incorporates both physical and occupational therapy needs.

Table 5-4. Typical Equipment List, Outpatient Rehabilitation Facility

Description	L × W × H Dimensions		Notes
1. Aqua pans			
2. Back table			
3. Bioconditioner unit			
4. Biofeedback unit			
5. Assignment board			
6. Computer			
7. CRT with keyboard			
8. Cybex II			
9. Dishwasher			
10. Garbage disposal			
11. Double shoulder/chest machine			
12. EMS units (crash cart)			
13. Ergometer			
14. Ergometer, upper-body exerciser			
15. File cabinets			
16. Firm illuminator, single			
17. Film illuminators, 2 over 2			
18. Finger/shoulder ladder			
19. Fluid therapy			
20. Hydrocollator, master unit			
21. Iso tech			
22. Mat table (Hi-lo)			
23. Floor mats			
24. Wall-mounted mirrors			
25. Paraffin bath			
26. Parallel bars			
27. Printer			
28. Refrigerator, under counter			
29. Refrigerator/freezer			
30. Rowing machine			
31. Sewing machine			
32. Storage, high density			
33. Shoulder wheel			
34. Staircase			
35. Stove/oven/microwave unit			
36. Supinator pronator			
37. Table (Hi-lo)			
38. Table, adjustable (princess)			
39. Table, exam			
40. Table, standing			
41. Table, traction			
42. Tilt table			
43. Total gym			
44. Treadmill			
45. Stainless steel tub (Lo-Boy)			
46. TV, console			
47. TV, patient, with wall bracket			
48. Typewriter			
49. Ultrasound			
50. Universal gym			
51. Whirlpool, upper extremity			
52. Wrist roll			
53. Lockers			
54. Linen hamper			
55. Hand whirlpool			

Physical and occupational therapists often require separate spaces in which to conduct their patient treatment activities. Although this may not always be necessary, it is necessary that all spaces within the department be designed to be flexible or adaptable to meet new equipment or treatment needs. A flexible design is extremely important for a hospital undertaking rehabilitation as a new service. Inaccurate projections with regard to patient volume or type of service to be offered can be costly. They may result from a lack of experience in rehabilitation or inaccurate marketing analysis. Consequently, it is desirable to have fewer fixed walls and more movable partitions that can be adjusted to reapportion space as needed.

To define treatment areas requiring patient privacy, movable partitions and cubicle curtains are recommended. This is particularly true in spaces where mats and examination tables are used. Although the need for flexibility and openness is important, fixed wall space must also be provided so that items such as finger ladders, shoulder wheels, pulleys, and the like can be properly mounted and used by patients and therapists.

The introduction of high ceilings, natural light, specialty illumination, and cheerful color is important in these areas. Special attention must be given to storage space for the myriad small items used in rehabilitation such as crutches, walkers, canes, splints, and other durable products, as well as the consumables used in physical and occupational therapy. The architect may be required to design specialty casework and storage systems for these items or involve the equipment planner in the purchase of this type of storage system. Storage areas are required for other large items of movable equipment that normally are not stored within the treatment and work space. These include wheelchairs, carts, weights, and other items that are not used on a daily basis but must be conveniently accessed by therapists.

The Passive Treatment Zone, or Specialty Areas

The passive treatment zone provides spaces that are required to provide relaxed, quiet, or private environments in which special activities may be conducted. Specialty areas within the outpatient rehabilitation department requiring special design include hydrotherapy spaces, staff work spaces, transitional living, home life/activities of daily living, sensory perception/speech/audiology treatment areas, modality spaces, and pediatrics, to name a few.

Hydrotherapy is an area in which patient privacy and dignity is paramount. Adequate toilet and changing facilities must be provided. It is recommended that the changing facilities, including lockers, be provided within the hydrotherapy area itself.

Room finishes within the hydrotherapy department should be designed to resist the high moisture content of the air. Floor surfaces are extremely important; they must resist constant wetness and provide a nonslip surface to avoid patient and staff accidents. Special attention should be given to the ceiling grid, light fixtures, and air diffusers, as these items will rust quickly unless they are constructed of nonferrous metals. Gypsum wallboard used for ceilings and/or walls should be moisture-resistant. Wall surfaces should include ceramic tile and/or vinyl wall coverings that have been treated to resist fungus and bacteria.

Humidity and temperature control in this space will allow the therapist to adjust the environment to meet the comfort and needs of each patient. Each closed space within the hydrotherapy department must have individual temperature control devices to control the temperature of the air. It is just as necessary to control the air temperature as it is to control the temperature of the water in which the patient is immersed.

The equipment planner should verify that the plumbing is designed to accept the desired hydrotherapy equipment. Tanks used in this area must be properly plumbed and grounded in order to ensure the patient's safety. Pay particular attention to devices that regulate the water temperature.

Staff work spaces are normally areas that require considerable planning by user groups and administrators. Space for staff charting should be provided within the treatment areas. This area should be designed to allow the therapist to monitor patient activity during charting as well as provide a medium degree of privacy for note taking and consultation between therapist and physician. Many departments provide fully enclosed staff offices for department directors or occupational and physical therapists. These spaces are necessary for private conversations between staff and directors of service or for conferences with visiting physicians. A conference/lounge area conveniently located near the treatment areas is recommended to provide appropriate space for chart reviews, in-service sessions, meetings, and staff break times.

The design of transitional living/home life activities of daily living spaces are the environments that have undergone the greatest change in the past five years. Many outpatient rehabilitation departments contain bedrooms, kitchens, and bathrooms that are very similar to those found in a standard residential environment. These facilities are not specifically designed for use by persons with disabilities, but contain fixtures and appliances that are found in most homes. The objective is to enable posttreatment patients to return to their own homes and perform many activities of daily living, such as cooking and personal hygiene.

A transitional system called EASY STREET ENVIRONMENTS™ is currently available for use in outpatient rehabilitation departments. This space system allows physical, occupational, and speech therapists to train patients to adapt to a normal, everyday environment by providing scenarios such as an automobile, a bus, a market, a laundry, a bank, a movie theater, and even bowling alleys. These alternative high-quality therapeutic environments are more stimulating and useful for outpatients learning to negotiate the obstacles found in the everyday world than is standard physical and occupational therapy equipment. If a patient is having difficulty negotiating changes in step heights, for example, it may be more practical for the patient to practice stepping onto a bus, onto a curb, or into a restaurant than to work on a training stair.

EASY STREET ENVIRONMENTS™ normally requires between 800 and 2,500 square feet of space. It is adaptable to both new construction and renovation. It is extremely important that this system be integrated into the outpatient rehabilitation department itself and not provided as an add-on or stand-alone feature. This will ensure its use by therapists as well as provide a distinct and attractive environment for outpatient users.

Sensory perception areas normally require a closed, soundproof environment. This environment can be designed with mirrors on all four walls, specialty interior illumination, and a wall-to-wall floor mat. The therapist may work with the patient within the room, allowing the patient to focus on balance, reflexes, and his or her relationship with the space.

Modality bays are a common space found in all outpatient rehabilitation departments. These passive treatment spaces normally require closed, private cubicles for patient treatment. They are normally between 90 and 120 square feet each, and are used for TMJ therapy, massage, electrostimulation, biofeedback, and the variety of modalities deployed by the rehabilitation therapist. The space should have individual room climate control as well as adjustable illumination.

Pediatric rehabilitation areas are usually separated from adult treatment areas. These areas will include space for toys and play.

Circulation and Traffic Flow

Circulation and traffic flow should be designed to avoid inpatients and outpatients mixing, particularly if the facility is an addition to an existing inpatient rehabilitation department.

The flow of patients, staff, and paperwork through the department requires careful study and analysis during the initial design phases. This is necessary in order to provide the most efficient layout with regard to adjacent spaces and the amount of traveling necessary for patients and staff to access those spaces.

The traffic flow should be simple and allow for ease of mobility. For example, the path of an outpatient should be through the front door to the reception area, where his or her record is within close proximity. The patient may be directed to a waiting space or directly to the treatment area, usually accompanied by the therapist. In the treatment area, the patient may be required to change in either a private dressing cubicle, placing his or her belongings in a locker, or a passive treatment room.

Clerical spaces should be located so that patients do not walk through them on their way to the treatment areas.

The medical director's consultation office and exam room should be located off the main reception/waiting area. This would allow new patients to enter the facility and be directed to the physician area and exam room without passing through the treatment zone.

Speech and audiology areas are generally separated from the active treatment zone to ensure privacy and avoid the intrusion of sounds. These spaces should also be located near the main reception and waiting area and provide easy access for those patients receiving only speech/audiology treatment.

Figure 5-1 shows the design of a freestanding hospital-based outpatient rehabilitation center. Figure 5-2 shows a hospital-based rehab facility.

Patient Environment

The design of the department must take into consideration the age group of the patient population being served, whether geriatric, middle-age, or pediatric. Consideration should also be given to the patient population's socioeconomic characteristics. If there is a specific population identified, the facility should respond to that group. This is normally in consideration for privacy, comfort, and the image the facility wishes to project to its users.

It is very difficult to identify a typical patient type or user of an outpatient facility without a great deal of demographic/market research.

Figure 5-1. Freestanding Hospital-Based Outpatient Rehab Center

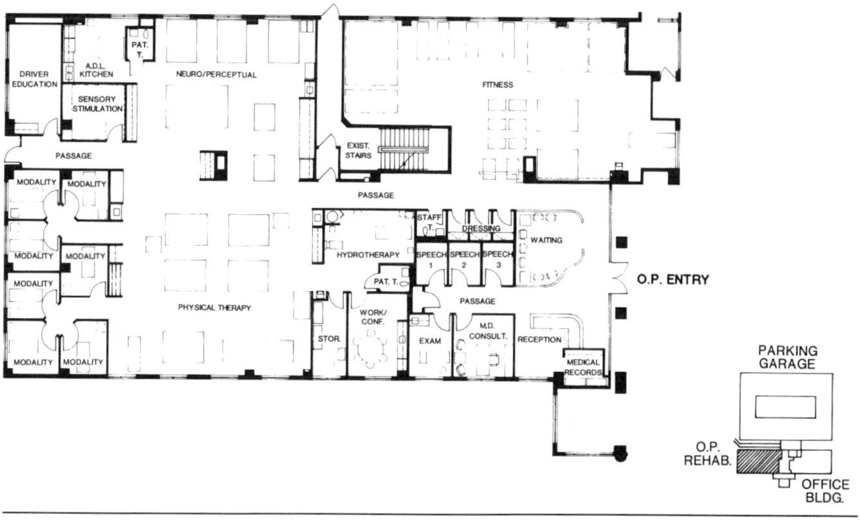

Figure 5-2. Hospital-Based Rehabilitation Center

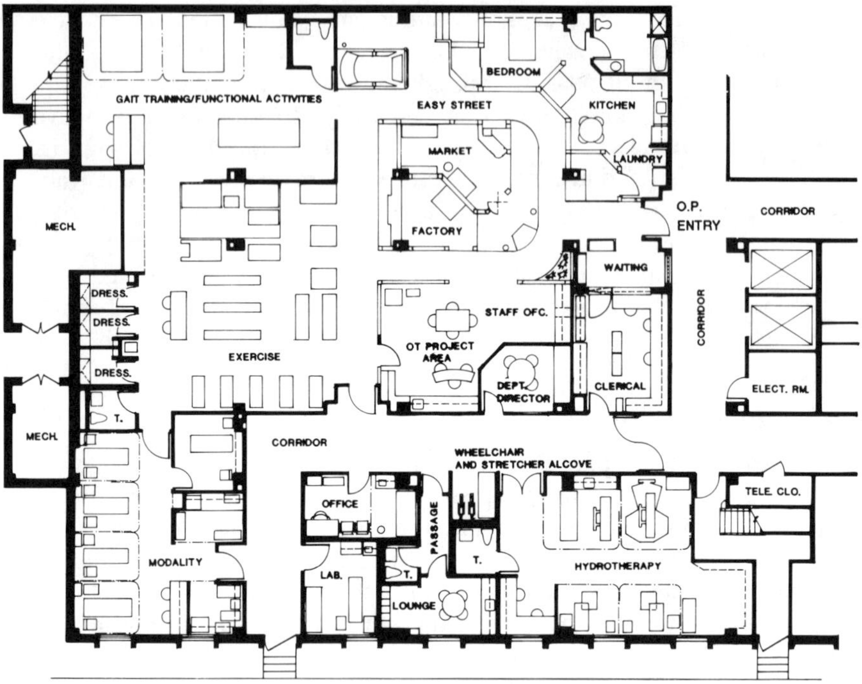

However, this research is necessary in order to identify who would be using the department and what their particular needs or feelings may require.

As already mentioned, patient comfort is of primary importance. Individual room control of air-conditioning and heating will ensure that patients will be comfortable and not complain to the referring physician. The aesthetic appearance of the facility must include concern for a cheerful environment as well as ensure that the area does not present too much of a hospitallike experience.

The quality of the lighting in the patient areas requires thought and planning. Do not overlight spaces. Take care to provide an adequate amount of light with which to conduct treatment but not so much as to intimidate or cause discomfort. Provide controls to vary the brightness appropriate to the treatment. Provide a balance of natural, incandescent, and fluorescent lighting. Discuss lighting quality with architects and lighting engineers during the design process.

Facility Maintenance Considerations

The maintenance of a rehabilitation facility is less intensive than that of an inpatient clinical environment, because there may be fewer high-tech items requiring specially trained maintenance personnel than, say, cardiology or neurology.

The specifications for the interior finishes should be thoroughly reviewed by the architect and user groups. Finishes should be attractive, durable, and easy to clean. Floor finishes should be tactile or nonslip, yet should not present difficulty for walkers or individuals improving their gait. Carpeting is recommended only in specialty areas such as waiting, reception, and offices because of the difficulty it may pose for wheelchair patients. If carpeting is to be used, it should not be provided with a pad but, instead, should be of a level-loop, direct glue-down type.

The use of specialty floor finishes to resist stains, acids, and so forth is normally not a concern within the rehabilitation facility. However, residential-type finishes, though projecting a more homelike environment, may not be durable enough to withstand the heavy use they are likely to receive in outpatient rehabilitation treatment.

Conclusion

To guarantee the success of a freestanding outpatient rehabilitation center, a great deal of work must be done by the planning team prior to the employment of an architect. This work, consisting of developing a functional plan or program, will ensure that the service is necessary and provide the facility with a return-on-investment. The employment of an experienced architect who is sensitive to the user groups' needs and patient population will ensure that the facility will be designed to meet the needs of the hospital and its patients.

Sources

1. Special recognition to Jane Snecinski, chief operating officer, Guynes Design, Phoenix, AZ, for her help in clarifying CORF facilities versus hospital-based outpatient rehab centers.

2. David A. Guynes, Guynes Design, Phoenix, AZ, proprietary use of the EASY STREET ENVIRONMENTS™ facility concept.

3. Janice Guzman, director of rehabilitation, Baptist Hospital of Miami, FL, consultation in postoccupancy evaluation of facilities designed by author.

4. Rehabilitation Center, Venice Hospital, Venice, FL.

5. Baptist Outpatient Center, Baptist Hospital of Miami, FL.
6. Good Shepherd Hospital, Allentown, PA.
7. Garry Woollard, AIA, vice-president, Cannon Design, St. Louis, MO, personal consultation regarding planning and facility programming of rehabilitation facilities.
8. Eileen Philips, director of rehabilitation, Venice Hospital, Venice, FL, personal consultation regarding operational concerns.
9. Earl L. Meyer, Earl Meyer Associates, Birmingham, AL, personal consultation regarding equipment planning issues.
10. Steve Evers, AIA, vice-president, The Ritchie Organization, Boston, MA, personal consultation regarding the planning, programming, and design of rehabilitation facilities.

Chapter 6

Accrediting Bodies and Their Standards and Processes

Carole H. Patterson and Mary G. Swope

Introduction

Outpatient rehabilitation facilities strive to provide high-quality services to persons with disabilities who do not require continuous inpatient care in a rehabilitation hospital or a hospital-based rehabilitation inpatient program. Patients able to benefit from outpatient rehabilitation are those who require services to continue improving upon the functional gains made during their inpatient stay or those who do not require concentrated inpatient services and are able to make functional gains entirely within an outpatient program. In either case, quality of care is an important issue for patients, physicians, and employers or third-party payers.

Many outpatient rehabilitation programs obtain some type of voluntary accreditation to help them maintain a quality of care and project a high-quality image.

Voluntary accreditation of health care organizations has a long history. It began with the accreditation of acute care, hospital-based services in 1917 with the Hospital Standardization Program sponsored by the American College of Surgeons. This program was merged into the activities of the Joint Commission on Accreditation of Hospitals (JCAH) in 1951 and continues today as part of the activities conducted by the Joint Commission on Accreditation of Healthcare Organizations (Joint Commission).

Currently, two major organizations provide accreditation for outpatient rehabilitation facilities. One is the Joint Commission. The other, the Commission on Accreditation of Rehabilitation Facilities (CARF),

---

Portions of this chapter were reprinted or adapted from *Quality Rehabilitation: Results-Oriented Patient Care*, coauthored and edited by Brent England, Rita M. Glass, and Carole H. Patterson, American Hospital Publishing, Inc., Chicago, 1989.

provides standards and surveys for rehabilitation programs offered in the acute care hospital setting, the long-term care facility setting, and the freestanding ambulatory care setting. In addition to granting accreditation, these two organizations also provide additional services to their clients, including consultation, education, and development of health care standards.

In nearly every outpatient rehabilitation organization, competent, qualified professionals and administrative personnel believe that they and their organization are capable of providing high-quality care and functional improvement services to patients and their families. But other than *saying* that their outpatient health care organization is providing its patient care in a high-quality and appropriate manner, the outpatient rehabilitation organization cannot prove this belief or statement. One of the best ways an organization can gather information about patient care quality is through standards-compliance activities, voluntary external review, and survey visits leading to accreditation by a nationally recognized accreditation organization, such as the Joint Commission or the Commission on Accreditation of Rehabilitation Facilities (CARF). It is one way that organizations with outpatient rehabilitation programs can demonstrate that they are meeting nationally validated and published stated requirements or standards.

The administration of the outpatient rehabilitation facility usually makes a decision to seek accreditation because it wishes to voluntarily prove to the external reviewing body (CARF or the Joint Commission) that the facility provides rehabilitation services that are equal to or exceed the national standards set by their peers in both the ambulatory care and rehabilitation fields. The administration also may seek accreditation to have an overview of their program based on these national standards of excellence. Once accreditation is achieved, the outpatient rehabilitation organization is then able to hold itself out to patients and their families, the community at large, governmental and other third-party insurance agencies, and their competition in the health care marketplace as a provider of high-quality health care that meets the requirements for that designated hallmark of excellence represented by the accreditation certificate.

There are still other accreditation organizations that provide services to ambulatory care organizations, but at this time, they do not directly address the provision of rehabilitation services in the ambulatory care setting.

The accredited outpatient rehabilitation organization has the right to:

- Promote its accredited status on its official papers, promotional brochures, and marketing literature
- Seek status with the various case managers working for insurance companies

- Meet reimbursement regulations (This is also true for CARF, for example, in those approximately 14 states where patient referrals must be made to CARF-accredited organizations in order for each organization to receive payment for patients on state assistance programs.)
- Defend its practices and outcomes in risk management and other legal situations
- Hold itself out to other health care organizations (such as referring hospitals) and professionals who would refer patients for outpatient rehabilitation as an organization that has actually demonstrated the level of excellence of its care and services through the achievement of voluntary accreditation

The accreditation of groups of health care professionals working in an outpatient program to serve patients in rehabilitation programs and other types of health care delivery systems, such as hospital-sponsored ambulatory programs and clinics, freestanding ambulatory programs and clinics, and comprehensive outpatient rehabilitation facilities (CORFs), has a relatively short history. This chapter presents an overview of the benefits and general requirements of accreditation by the two major accrediting organizations for outpatient rehabilitation facilities and discusses the relationship between quality of care and accreditation. Even though it is widely recognized that high-quality health care cannot be provided without a qualified professional staff, this chapter does not address the process of certification of those care providers through such national professional associations as the American Occupational Therapy Association (AOTA), the American Speech-Language-Hearing Association (ASHA), or the Association of Rehabilitation Nurses (ARN).

The Joint Commission on Accreditation of Healthcare Organizations

By 1991, the Joint Commission had diversified its accreditation activities into five programs:

- Hospital care formalized and published by the JCAH (1951)
- Skilled and intermediate care offered in long-term care facilities (1966)
- Mental health care offered in settings other than hospitals (1970)
- Ambulatory health care that is freestanding (1975)
- Home care services (1988)

The major areas of focus for achieving Joint Commission accreditation are the development and use of standards of care and the Joint Commission's accreditation process itself. Because standards form the basis for accreditation, it is important to understand the development process and the types of standards. The major levels of accreditation outcomes will also be discussed.

The Development and Use of Standards

It is through the use of standards for acute physical rehabilitation services published in the *Accreditation Manual for Hospitals*[1] that both freestanding rehabilitation hospitals and acute care hospital-based rehabilitation programs and units are surveyed and accredited. The Joint Commission also publishes and uses standards from its *Ambulatory Health Care Standards Manual*[2] for the accreditation of ambulatory (outpatient) health care organizations. Compliance with these standards provides the basis for accreditation, and the degree to which standards are complied with results in various levels of accreditation.

The University of Michigan–Ann Arbor was the place where Avedis Donabedian, M.D., developed and published much of his original work and research on the measurement of quality in health care. Dr. Donabedian's use of the "structure, process, and outcome" construct has been widely replicated in the health care accreditation standards development process. These three types of standards are the basis for measuring the overall quality of a rehabilitation program for Joint Commission accreditation.

Both CARF and the Joint Commission develop accreditation standards for the assessment of organizational performance in the delivery of high-quality patient care by convening panels of experts to advise them on what should be included in either new or revised standards. These expert practitioners (either clinical or administrative, or both used in combination) are convened to define the current and projected state-of-the-art principles, practices, and standards of organizational performance.

Once defined, debated, and field-tested, the standards are used in surveys that include among other things the assessment of an organization's performance in the delivery of patient care to determine whether care is both appropriate to the assessed needs of the patient population being served and is of high quality.

The use of standards in the survey process allows the organization to demonstrate its ability to meet the full letter as well as the intent of the stated requirements, or the standards. The assessment of total organizational performance against the full set of published standards relates to all the structures, processes, and outcomes of the rehabilitation organization's performance, and judgments are made about the effectiveness of specific operations. It does not matter whether a particular standard is directly related to an organizational structural element, a care delivery process, or a requirement related to patient or process outcomes. It is the survey of the organization's *overall performance* against the total set of standards by the Joint Commission surveyor team that determines the degree of compliance with the standards. And that degree of compliance, when substantially complete, results in the organization's full accreditation.

A listing of the Joint Commission chapters of standards from the *Ambulatory Health Care Standards Manual,* 1990 edition, follows:

- Administration
- Educational activities
- Emergency services
- Governing body
- Infirmary
- Laboratory services and pathology
- Medical records
- Pharmaceutical services
- Plant, technology, and safety management
- Quality assurance
- Quality of care
- Radiology services
- Research activities
- Rights and responsibilities of patients
- Surgical and anesthesia services
- Teaching and publication activities

What follows is a discussion of the three types of standards used by the Joint Commission in examining organizational compliance.

Structure Standards

Structure standards generally relate to how the organization is governed, managed, and organized to deliver patient care services. There are numerous "structures" spelled out in an organization's bylaws, for example, that define the ways in which the oversight functions of the organization's governing body are structured and carried out. By way of example, a short, partial listing of the governing body structural requirements from the Joint Commission standards manual includes the following items.[3]

The governing body:

- Adopts a statement of the mission, goals, and objectives of the organization
- Sets policy
- Makes full disclosure of ownership
- Establishes a system of financial management and accountability
- Establishes a policy on the rights and responsibilities of patients
- Meets at least annually

- Makes initial appointments and reappointments and grants or curtails delineated clinical privileges based on documented peer advice and recommendations from appropriate professional staff

Process Standards

Process standards outline the configuration of or the activities used by patient care providers to assess patient needs for rehabilitation care and services, plan care activities or interventions, and evaluate each patient's or group of patients' progress or lack of progress. In rehabilitation, care providers have a great advantage over many of their colleagues in other health care fields because there are various functional improvement measurement tools available that help document each patient's progress during a planned course of treatment.

Outcome Standards

Outcome standards describe the results or patient outcomes achieved through the use of rehabilitation treatment. In a rehabilitation program, the degree of improvement expected is stated as a "functional outcome goal," and the degree of success the organization experiences in achieving those stated goals becomes the objective of the rehabilitation program.

Joint Commission standards do not state what specific patient outcomes should be. However, the standards do specify the requirements on *how* the organization is to set functional improvement goals and how it is to monitor the degree to which it is able to help patients achieve predetermined functional goals.

In a rehabilitation service, the goal is not the short-term acute treatment of a patient's illness, but rather the long-term improvement and maintenance of functional ability. To achieve this goal, staff members must use measurements of functional outcomes as indicators of the quality and appropriateness of rehabilitation care. The monitoring of long-term functional outcomes helps in assessing how well the outpatient rehabilitation program or treatment team is meeting the goals established for and with the patients. However, measures of long-term outcomes alone may not be sensitive enough or specific enough to the *levels of quality* of daily activities of care. If measurements are not sensitive enough, they cannot alert the treatment team to opportunities for improving rehabilitation care or help team members identify the specific areas in which problems may be occurring.

The Joint Commission Accreditation Process

There are a number of elements in the Joint Commission's accreditation process. They include the preaccreditation and compliance activities, and then the survey visit.

Preaccreditation Activities

The preparation or preaccreditation activities required to seek accreditation are as important as the actual survey activities. When a rehabilitation organization decides to become accredited, it should begin that process at least a year in advance. This is because the organization must engage in an in-depth internal review of its patient care and support service activities using members of its own governing body, professional staff, and administrative and management staff *before* it can undergo the actual survey process required by the Joint Commission. This internal review requires the organization to study its own policies, procedures, and practices for completeness and to review its documentation policies.

In addition, a quality assurance (QA) program must be defined in writing and implemented for a specified period of time, usually 12 months or more. The information and data generated by implementing this QA program *prove* that the outpatient rehabilitation program and staff are concerned with improving patient care activities and demonstrating that the program has the capability to meet the accreditation organization's standards.

A guide for developing a QA program is the Joint Commission 10-Step Model. This model is a reference for helping all those involved in quality assurance to meet all requirements for any QA programs. This list is from the preamble for Standard QA.3 in the *Accreditation Manual for Hospitals,* 1991 edition.[4,5]

- *Step 1:* Assign responsibility for monitoring and evaluation activities.
- *Step 2:* Delineate the scope of care provided by the organization.
- *Step 3:* Identify the most important aspects of care provided by the organization.
- *Step 4:* Identify indicators for monitoring the important aspects of care.
- *Step 5:* Establish thresholds (levels, patterns, or trends) for the indicators that trigger evaluation of care.
- *Step 6:* Monitor the important aspects of care by collecting and organizing the data for each indicator.
- *Step 7:* Evaluate care when thresholds are reached in order to identify either opportunities to improve care or problems.
- *Step 8:* Take actions to improve care or to correct identified problems.
- *Step 9:* Assess the effectiveness of the actions and document the improvement in care.
- *Step 10:* Communicate the results of the monitoring and evaluation process to relevant individuals, departments, or services and the organizationwide quality assurance program.

The outpatient rehabilitation organization continues to engage in the extensive self-evaluation of its own performance against Joint Commission standards during the preparatory preaccreditation phase, and engages in the in-depth comparison of its performance against the standards required prior to preparing and submitting an application for the accreditation survey. The Joint Commission works with the applying organization by answering questions about how to comply with the published standards, offers educational seminars and training for the organization's staff to attend, and is flexible in scheduling the first, or initial, survey visit.

Various members of the organization's staff may need to bring in expert consultants to assist in their preparation, or they may decide to try to prepare on their own by attending the educational seminars sponsored by the Joint Commission prior to completing the preparatory phase. A final self-evaluation of compliance with the standards determines the organization's readiness to seek status as an accredited ambulatory (Joint Commission's term) or outpatient (CARF's term) rehabilitation organization.

Compliance Activities

The decision to seek accreditation requires the outpatient care organization to commit itself to *compliance activities* in order to establish a pattern of high levels of or full compliance with the standards prior to the on-site visit by the survey team.

Compliance activities include ensuring that at least the following documents are up-to-date and accurately reflect the way the organization carries out its stated functions:

- Mission statement
- Organizational program description(s)
- Quality assurance plan
- Program evaluation plan
- Governing body bylaws, rules, and regulations
- Administrative policies, procedures, and practices
- Patient care policies, procedures, and protocols
- Rights and responsibilities of patients
- Quality control programs for the laboratory and/or radiology service
- Medical and patient care records
- Safety management plans for patient care equipment and utilities
- Records of safety plan implementation (for example, fire drills)
- Staff educational records of in-service and continuing education
- Staff license/certification verification procedures and records
- Personnel policies and employee handbook
- Job descriptions and performance evaluations
- Clinical privileges files
- Teaching or educational facility contracts
- Research protocols (if any)
- Occupational and business licenses
- Contracts

The Accreditation Survey Visit

The next step in the Joint Commission's accreditation process is the actual on-site review of the outpatient rehabilitation facility's documented and observable compliance with the standards—the survey visit. The survey visit is carried out by consultant surveyors (or field representatives of the accreditation organization) who are currently practicing professionals and administrators or managers actively engaged in providing outpatient rehabilitation services, and who are also employed as consultants by the accrediting organization to serve as its surveyors and representatives. These surveyors are selected because they are also expert educators and reviewers who are able to teach and consult with the organization's managerial and clinical staff on how to achieve full or at least substantial compliance with the standards set and published by the accreditation organization.

The survey process verifies the outpatient rehabilitation organization's degree of compliance with the published standards of the accreditation organization. This process begins with the application for survey. Once the accreditation organization determines that the rehabilitation organization is indeed eligible for survey under its standards and is ready for the survey, survey dates are mutually agreed on, a team of expert surveyors is assigned, and the survey itself is conducted over a period of two to three days.

The surveyors look at the rehabilitation organization's key documents to determine what its stated patient care mission is and how it operates to achieve that mission. Samples of all the documents listed in this chapter under "Compliance Activities" are studied, patient care records are reviewed, and interviews with members of the rehabilitation team are conducted.

The surveyors are particularly interested in reviewing the QA, program evaluation, and quality control program reports. It is in these areas that the focus of the accreditation process comes closest to answering the question: "Is this organization able to deliver patient care that is both appropriate and of high quality to its patients?" The proof of organizational effectiveness should be documented in the various QA and program evaluation management reports. The surveyor(s) spends a large portion of the survey asking questions in this area, reviewing the indicators and data collection tools used, and interviewing the rehabilitation program staff members to determine their degree of involvement in the entire process of ensuring high-quality patient outcomes.

In the areas where the organization or a particular patient care service is found to be less than substantially compliant with a standard, the surveyor provides consultation on how to better achieve compliance, drawing on his or her background and survey experience to make suggestions for improvement. For example, the outpatient rehabilitation facility may not have a good system for verifying physicians' and other professionals' credentials. The surveyor may show key personnel how to comply with the requirements by providing an example of forms and policies and procedures used in another outpatient rehabilitation program that has successfully demonstrated compliance with the standards. If problems appear to be systemic throughout the outpatient rehabilitation organization, the surveyor may conduct a full consultation with key members of the staff, hold a teaching conference with staff members, and/or provide samples of other documents or publications that might help the staff move toward full compliance within the problem area(s).

Once the actual survey of the organization is completed, the survey team fills out several volumes of survey report forms documenting their findings and mails the forms to the Joint Commission for analysis. The surveyor's documentation is reviewed against rules approved by the accreditation organization's governing board. At the Joint Commission, all the survey documentation is entered into a large mainframe computer, and the results of the survey are compared against the approved rules by the computer in order to generate a final decision. Expert survey report analysts review the surveyor's documentation and enter specific references at the end of each validated standard recommendation for future compliance activities. These *specific references* tell the rehabilitation organization exactly what was not in substantial compliance at the time of the survey and, when possible, the degree to which noncompliance existed at the time of survey. When the report is completed, the computer once again provides an aggregate summation of those key areas of compliance and noncompliance and recommends an accreditation decision, again based fully on board-approved rules. These completed reports are reviewed by the Accreditation Committee, and when the decision is confirmed, a letter is prepared stating the outcome of the survey visit.

Accreditation Outcomes

Beginning in January 1991, under Joint Commission requirements, four outcomes are possible: "accreditation with commendation," "accreditation," "summary nonaccreditation," and "conditional accreditation." Figure 6-1 is adapted from the "General Administrative Policies and Procedures" section of the Joint Commission's *Ambulatory Health Care Standards Manual*, 1990 edition,[6,7] and Appendix B: "Accreditation and Appeal Procedures" section. For a full explanation of these procedures, contact the Joint Commission.

The receipt of the accreditation itself is the final outcome of the long process that progressed from the initial decision to seek accreditation to preaccreditation, standard compliance activities, and the survey itself. Once achieved, the receipt of the earned accreditation award letter and certificate gives the outpatient health care organization the option to exercise several rights, including those described in the introduction to this chapter.

Figure 6-1. Accreditation Outcomes

Joint Commission staff evaluates the results of the survey, the recommendations of the surveyor(s), and any other relevant information, such as documentation of compliance with the standards, documentation of plans to correct deficiencies, or evidence of recent improvements. Using decision rules approved by the Accreditation Committee of the Board of Commissioners, staff uses a computer to determine whether the outpatient rehabilitation organization should be accredited, with or without type I recommendations.

A type I recommendation is a recommendation or group of recommendations that should receive the highest priority in the outpatient rehabilitation organization's plans for improvement. The outpatient rehabilitation organization's progress will be monitored by the Joint Commission through focused surveys or written progress reports at stated times during the accreditation cycle. In addition, if staff decides to recommend that the outpatient rehabilitation organization be conditionally accredited or nonaccredited, that recommendation is reviewed by the Accreditation Committee, which then makes the decision.

If the Accreditation Committee conditionally accredits the outpatient rehabilitation organization, the outpatient rehabilitation organization will be asked to submit a plan of correction addressing the deficiencies outlined in the survey report. The plan must be submitted within 30 days from the date of the outpatient rehabilitation organization's receipt of the notification. The outpatient rehabilitation organization will indicate what action will be taken to address the recommendations and the time frame in which the actions will be taken. This time frame cannot exceed six months. If the plan is acceptable, the outpatient rehabilitation organization will be advised that a follow-up survey will be conducted in the sixth month following Joint Commission staff's approval of the plan. The follow-up survey can be conducted sooner, if indicated by the time frames outlined in the plan of correction.

At the conclusion of the follow-up survey and analysis of the findings, Joint Commission staff will make a recommendation to the Accreditation Committee regarding the outpatient rehabilitation organization's accreditation status. The recommendation can be for accreditation, with or without type I recommendations, or nonaccreditation, depending on the outpatient rehabilitation organization's status as determined by the decision rules of the Accreditation Committee.

The above procedures do not apply when a surveyor identifies any condition that poses a threat to public or patient safety. In such cases, the president of the Joint Commission, or a designee, promptly recommends to the Accreditation Committee that the outpatient rehabilitation organization be denied accreditation. This action by the president is reported by telephone and in writing to the outpatient rehabilitation organization's chief executive officer and in writing to the authorities having jurisdiction. The Accreditation Committee then acts on the recommendation of the president of the Joint Commission or of Joint Commission staff.

When it is found to be in substantial compliance with Joint Commission standards, an outpatient rehabilitation organization is awarded accreditation for three years, with or without type I recommendations. The final decision to accredit an outpatient rehabilitation organization becomes effective as of the first day after completion of the outpatient rehabilitation organization's survey. Approximately 18 months from the date of its survey, each accredited outpatient rehabilitation organization receives a letter from the Joint Commission stressing the importance of ongoing self-assessment and reminding the outpatient rehabilitation organization that correction of any recommendations it received in its last survey should be completed or well under way to avoid jeopardizing the accreditation award for the next full survey.

Accreditation is not automatically renewed. An outpatient rehabilitation organization must undergo another full accreditation survey, and survey findings must warrant accreditation, with or without type I recommendations. Approximately seven months before an outpatient rehabilitation organization's accreditation is due to expire, the Joint Commission sends the outpatient rehabilitation

(Continued on next page)

Figure 6-1. (Continued)

organization an Application for Survey. Following receipt of the completed application, a survey is scheduled. The Joint Commission ordinarily schedules the survey as near as possible to the outpatient rehabilitation organization's survey anniversary date. However, to allow latitude, surveys may be scheduled within a 90-day period surrounding the outpatient rehabilitation organization's anniversary date. With an outpatient rehabilitation organization's consent, the Joint Commission may schedule the survey more than 90 days before accreditation is due to expire.

Following a survey, an outpatient rehabilitation organization's previous accreditation status remains in effect until a final decision is made to accredit the outpatient rehabilitation organization or to deny accreditation.

An outpatient rehabilitation organization that is not granted accreditation, that has its accreditation withdrawn by the Joint Commission, or that withdraws from the Joint Commission accreditation process with unresolved type I recommendations is considered nonaccredited. The outpatient rehabilitation organization's nonaccredited status remains in effect for six months from the nonaccreditation decision. The outpatient rehabilitation organization may use formal appeal procedures (described elsewhere in this manual) to challenge an adverse decision.

The Joint Commission provides each accredited outpatient rehabilitation organization with a certificate of accreditation. The certificate and all copies remain the property of the Joint Commission and must be returned to the Joint Commission if the outpatient rehabilitation organization is issued a new certificate reflecting a change in name, or if its accreditation expires or is withdrawn or denied for any reason.

Source: Adapted from the "General Administrative Policies and Procedures" section of the *Ambulatory Health Care Standards Manual,* 1990 edition, and Appendix B, the "Accreditation and Appeal Procedures" section, published by the Joint Commission.

Commission on Accreditation of Rehabilitation Facilities

Many rehabilitation facilities seek accreditation from the Commission on Accreditation of Rehabilitation Facilities (CARF) either in addition to or independent of Joint Commission accreditation. Accreditation from CARF is required in some states for licensing and for outpatient programs to be reimbursable under some state compensation laws such as workers' compensation and Medicaid. A couple of states also require CARF accreditation for certificate-of-need (CON) approval of rehabilitation programs.

A long-held central theme of CARF is the need for the organization to serve as a "quality control intermediary." This belief is reflected in the CARF mission statement, its standards development process, and the specified goals an organization would need to meet to obtain accreditation.

The CARF standards development process is a product of nationally recognized professionals in the specific fields who are convened on a regular basis to review and develop standards that characterize high-quality programs and to define the input processes. It is important to understand the foundation of CARF's standards and criteria before seeking CARF accreditation. This foundation of standards of practice is heavily weighed or judged by the program's levels of compliance during the accreditation process itself.

Program Evaluation

The concept of program evaluation is central to the CARF accreditation process. *Program evaluation* is a recognized method of determining the effectiveness and efficiency of the rehabilitation program service delivery. The rehabilitation organization evaluates the results of its services and the effects the outpatient rehabilitation program has had on persons served. This information is used in the organization's decision-making process, planning, budgeting, and then determining program needs. As defined by CARF, program evaluation has three main elements: design elements, program objectives, and management reports.

Design Elements

The design elements of program evaluation are definitions of markets, mission, and programs (figure 6-2). The design elements first describe the *influencers,* or the external controllers of programs. These include the outpatient rehabilitation markets, third-party payers, and referral sources.

Another design element is the mission statement. Mission statements should speak to three criteria:

- Whom the organization serves
- What service it provides
- What accomplishments or goals it expects from service delivery

The final design element is the description and definition of how the outpatient rehabilitation program achieves its mission. The four aspects of programs are as follows:

- *The program goals:* These are statements that define specific programs, and their expected results are derived from the mission statement.
- *Admission criteria:* These criteria can be inclusionary or exclusionary, but they should facilitate goal accomplishment.
- *Patients served:* The patients served can be defined according to their injury or illness or specific rehabilitation need, such as physical therapy; whether they are dual-diagnosis patients; or any special-market categories.
- *The services provided:* The services provided should describe all medical, vocational, and other services of rehabilitation treatment offered within the program/facility.

Figure 6-2. Design Elements in Program Evaluation

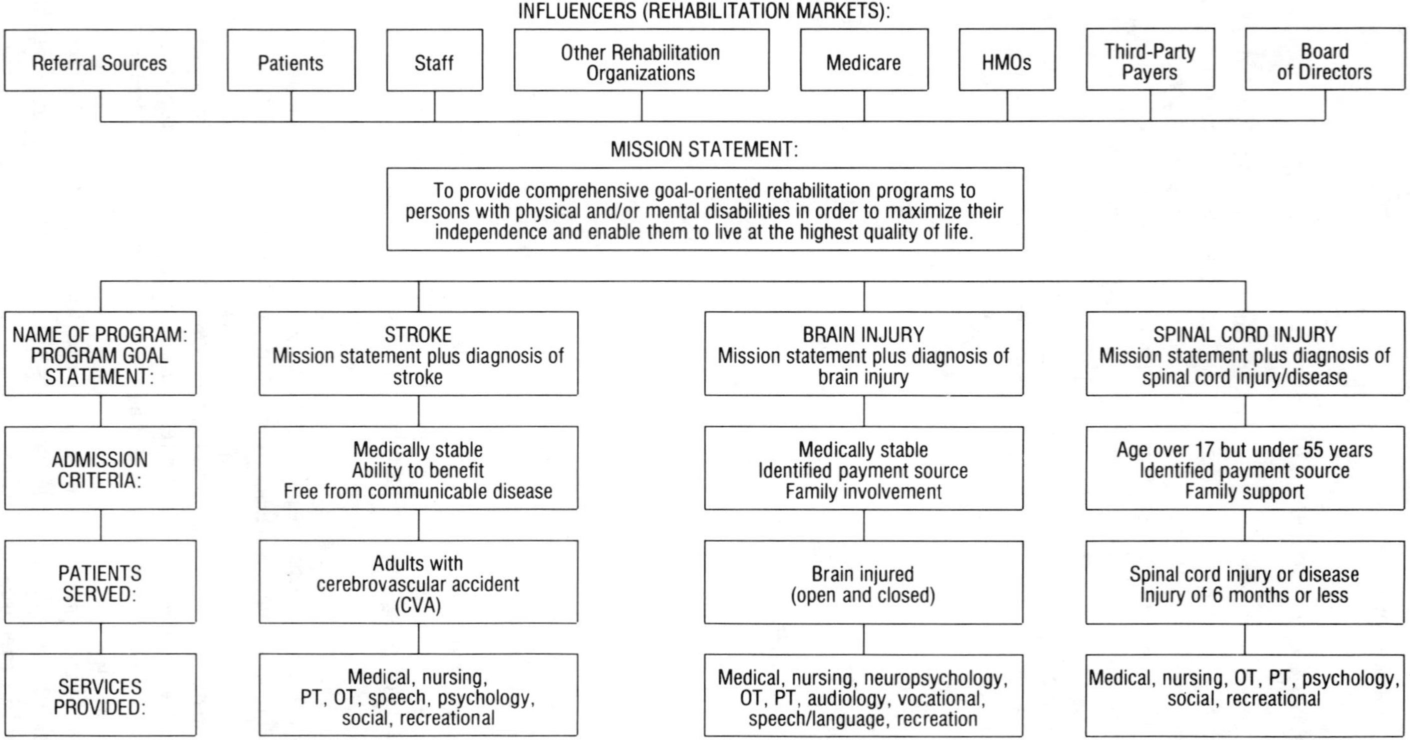

Source: Reprinted from *Quality Rehabilitation: Results-Oriented Patient Care*, coauthored and edited by Brent England, Rita M. Glass, and Carole H. Patterson, American Hospital Publishing, Chicago, 1989.

Program Objectives

Program goals should be written for each outpatient rehabilitation program, and specific services should be designed to ensure that the specific program goals are measurable according to their achievements. Three types of program objectives are addressed by CARF: outcome, progress, and efficiency. *Outcome objectives* reflect the benefits that people receive from program services. *Progress objectives* indicate the degree of patient movement toward discharge via levels of their achievements from the program and into aftercare. *Efficiency objectives* refer to the amount of patient and staff resources that are expended in the pursuit of outcome and progress objectives (time and cost measures).

Objectives are usually measured at the beginning of a program, during the program, at discharge, and again at follow-up, either by questionnaire or visits, to determine that improvement in objective measures has been made over time through the rehabilitation program and that its residual effect continues after treatment ends. Effectiveness and efficiency measures should improve during the rehabilitation process, and improvement should continue after discharge from the outpatient program. Effectiveness objectives (progress and outcome) are usually measured by applying rating scales to functional independence measures such as transfers, ambulation, bathing, and bowel and bladder function. For example, a patient coming in at level 4 in bathing and dressing (on a seven-point scale) may move to level 5 in bathing and level 6 in dressing at the end of the outpatient program, and demonstrate an overall mean-score improvement.

Efficiency measures are also included in a program's objectives. Attendance, length of stay, and cost per patient are typical efficiency measures tracked in program evaluation.

At the present time, the Uniform Data Set's (UDS) seven-point scale, commonly known as the Functional Independence Measure (FIM), is the most widely used and supported measurement instrument in the rehabilitation field. The FIM is a minimum set of information designed to determine the effectiveness of rehabilitation services. It is a measure of disability and is intended to measure the improvement of a person's functional impairment during a treatment program. The functional elements are provided by trained professionals who are involved in each patient's care. It assesses 18 basic functions including self-care, sphincter management, mobility, locomotion, communication, and social cognition of a seven-level scale. These functions are rated when a patient is initially evaluated and again at discharge and follow-up. Measures are then recorded to get FIM scores and average FIM scores, thus demonstrating an objective evaluation of patient outcomes relevant to treatment goals.

Once efficiency and effectiveness objectives have been measured using FIM or another rating scale of choice, actual outcomes are compared to expected outcomes. Objectives are given relative weights, totaling 100, as shown in table 6-1, to demonstrate their importance in the specific

Table 6-1. Program Objectives for Stroke Rehabilitation Program

Primary Objectives	Measures	Applied to	Time of Measure	Data Source	Obtained by	Expectancies			Relative Weight
						Minimal	Goal	Optimal	
To maximize independence in bowel and bladder function	Percentage of patients moving up one level on bowel and bladder functional scale	All stroke patients with problems in controlling bowel and bladder functions	Quarterly	Patient record	Clerk	70%	80%	95%	30
To maximize attendance	Percentage of patients attending scheduled sessions	All stroke patients in inpatient medical rehabilitation program	Quarterly	Scheduling and chart records	Clerk	70%	80%	95%	20
To maximize referral sources	Number of referral sources	All stroke patients referred to inpatient medical rehabilitation program	Quarterly	Referral record	Clerk	.5 per quarter	1 per quarter	2 per quarter	15

Primary Objectives	Measures	Applied to	Time of Measure	Data Source	Obtained by	Expectancies			Relative Weight
						Minimal	Goal	Optimal	
To maximize motor functions	Percentage of patients moving up one level on motor scale	All stroke patients in inpatient medical rehabilitation program with motor problems	Quarterly	Patient record	Clerk	70%	85%	95%	15
To minimize program length (LOS)	Percentage of patients completing the program at or under the average LOS	All stroke patients in medical rehabilitation program	Discharge	Patient record	Clerk	70%	85%	95%	10
To maximize socialization	Percentage of patients moving up one level on socialization scale	All stroke patients in medical rehabilitation program	Quarterly	Patient record	Clerk	70%	85%	95%	10

Source: Reprinted from *Quality Rehabilitation: Results-Oriented Patient Care*, coauthored and edited by Brent England, Rita M. Glass, and Carole H. Patterson, American Hospital Publishing, Chicago, 1989.

rehab program. The more important objectives are given higher weights. In a stroke program, for example, bowel and bladder training may be given a relative weight of 30 percent; attendance in therapy, 20 percent; motor functions, 15 percent; and socialization, 10 percent.

Aside from objectives, client descriptors and supplemental measures are collected. *Client descriptors* are defined by CARF as elements that describe the patient, for example, age, prescribed rehabilitation treatment, and sex. *Supplemental measures* are data elements that describe the program, such as number of patients on Medicare, average length of stay (ALOS) in the program, and percentage of patients with family support. Supplemental measures add an important dimension to demographic information and prove extremely helpful when data are analyzed and interpreted in management reports.

Management Reports

Management reports provide a mechanism for measuring patient progress data and evaluating the program. These are the statistical and narrative analyses of an outpatient rehabilitation program's service delivery and form the foundation for management action. Reports on patient progress should be carefully analyzed and shared, as appropriate, on a regular basis with governing boards, staff, the public, the press, purchasers of services, and other markets.

Statistical sections include summaries of program performance compared with expected levels of achievement, client descriptors, supplemental measures, and other supporting data trends that are compared over time (usually quarterly), and then annually.

The narrative section contains a brief statement of the program's goals and accomplishments, a commentary on the evaluation methodology, extrapolation of statistics (what has been concluded from the data), and recommendations for a course of action.

Action plans are developed from analyzing management reports. Courses of action may include watching trends for a certain period to determine whether a pattern emerges that requires changing who is served; tightening or loosening admission criteria; or changing the amount, type, location, and time of services. Once a plan of action is developed, the impact of the plan on the resources of the hospital should be evaluated. No action plan can be implemented without administrative and governing board support.

Once the design elements, program objectives, and management reports have been in use for a period of time and are ready for review, the outpatient facility is ready to submit to the CARF accreditation process.

The CARF Accreditation Process

The major elements of a program that will be studied by CARF accreditation teams during the accreditation process include the following:

- How program aspects are rendered.
- Who renders care/staff qualifications.
- Quality of program in results, efficiencies, and patient outcomes.
- Financial status. Evaluators will determine if an organization has an appropriate budget for the level of care it provides, is financially solvent, and charges appropriately for treatment.
- The physical facility and its safety features.

The following are the steps in the CARF accreditation process:

1. The organization applies to CARF for accreditation of its outpatient rehabilitation program. A CARF survey can be requested after a facility/program has evaluated its ability to meet all the appropriate standards for a successful accreditation. The Commission on Accreditation of Rehabilitation Facilities standards manuals as well as its self-study questionnaire are the basic resources to use for an overview of preparedness for a successful survey. The application must include the specific aspects of the rehabilitation program that are to be evaluated, such as spinal injury, brain injury, hand therapy, and other specific treatment services. A formal request for survey, listing the programs to be reviewed, is made to CARF. These formal applications requesting a survey may be obtained from CARF. The completed application is then processed by CARF.
2. The Commission on Accreditation of Rehabilitation Facilities develops the survey team for each specific facility, which includes team members with expertise in the rehabilitation areas to be surveyed.
3. The facility is notified of the date of the survey and the names of the surveyors.
4. A two-day survey is conducted, consisting of an initial conference between the surveyors and key personnel, the survey itself, and an exit conference.
   - During the initial conference, the survey team will explain the survey process to the key personnel involved.
   - During the survey itself, the CARF surveyors will interview administration and staff, conduct a visual inspection of the facility, check the credentials of treatment staff, and check documentation and recordkeeping. The CARF evaluators will examine the physical facility for structural soundness as well as safety features and documented safety plans, especially for fire. They will also evaluate

the accessibility of the facility for the patients served. The governance of the facility will be examined, and the competence and backgrounds of the governing board will be evaluated. As for documentation, CARF is concerned with the provision of care and takes the position that "if it is not documented, it is not done."
- During the exit conference, the surveyors will share their findings with the organization's key personnel.

5. The written survey report will be prepared and sent to the facility's administration, detailing the findings and recommendations. The written report is usually prepared within 90 days. It will include suggestions or areas of concern, if any, and recommendations for correcting major deficiencies. Recommendations will focus on correcting major areas of noncompliance.

Levels of CARF Accreditation

There are three levels of CARF accreditation awards. These levels are assigned according to the results of the survey. The highest level is accreditation for three years. The next level is accreditation for one year. A one-year accreditation means that the facility showed some basic deficiencies that require resolution and should be resolved before that next year's review. The last level is abeyance. *Abeyance* means that the survey team will return within a set period to see if major deficiencies/recommendations have been corrected. It denotes findings of multiple areas of noncompliance/deficiency. This means that immediate actions should be taken by the facility/program before any level of accreditation is awarded. Following the facility's plan of action submitted to CARF for these corrective actions and within a specified time frame, CARF, if requested, will again survey the facility/program as to its compliance to correct these deficiencies. If the new survey indicates substantial successful compliance, an accreditation level is awarded.

Quality of Care and Accreditation

Both accreditation organizations discussed in this chapter (CARF and the Joint Commission) require in their standards manuals that the outpatient rehabilitation organization engage in QA activities that are outcome-oriented and measured by specific, objective criteria and their data as part of the accreditation process. The Commission on Accreditation of Rehabilitation Facilities focuses its quality review standards on a program that includes the collection of data that describe measures of efficiency and effectiveness and that is described here and in its standards manuals as "program evaluation."[8] The Joint Commission focuses its quality review standards on the monitoring and evaluation process for the review of both the quality and appropriateness of patient care services related to the structures and processes of care giving.

The Joint Commission has called the process *quality assurance,*[9,10] and its standards currently are focusing on *quality assessment and improvement* in 1991. The two concepts of program evaluation and quality assurance may be integrated. For example, an acute care, hospital-based, comprehensive physical and psychiatric rehabilitation unit at Good Samaritan Hospital in Zanesville, Ohio, has illustrated how to use both program evaluation and quality assurance as outlined in the standards of both CARF and the Joint Commission to demonstrate its quality-of-care levels to anyone who is interested in their outcomes, including patients and their families.[11,12]

Both accreditation organizations require, as part of their accreditation standards, that outpatient rehabilitation organizations monitor patient outcomes achieved by the patient care process. The Commission on Accreditation of Rehabilitation Facilities requires program evaluation that aggregates data collected relative to individual patients as well as total program outcomes stated in measures of functional independence. The Joint Commission requires the ongoing, planned, and systematic monitoring of important aspects of patient care against indicators of excellent patient care in addition to tracking patient outcomes.

The very act of striving to achieve accreditation standards drives the outpatient rehabilitation organization's clinical staff members toward the delivery of high-quality patient care. One of the indirect benefits of achieving accreditation is that the outpatient rehabilitation organization's board, medical, clinical, and managerial staff are required to become full participants in the QA activities prescribed by the standards. This forces the staff to define those specific day-to-day activities that enhance and promote quality. As a result, it further focuses the outpatient rehabilitation staff on the review, evaluation, revision, and delivery of high-quality care and on continually improving the quality of patient care services, activities, processes, and outcomes.

Both CARF and the Joint Commission have standards and programs for outpatient rehabilitation care and recognize that care delivered in such settings can be measured and compared against each accreditation organization's published standards. The outpatient rehabilitation organization can enhance its patient care activities by making the decision to seek accreditation from either one or both accreditation organizations. The outcome of achieving accreditation from either organization is the same; that is, the outpatient rehabilitation organization earns the right to promote the quality of its services to patients and their families, the community at large, governmental and other third-party insurance agencies, business coalitions, and perhaps even its competition in the health care marketplace.

Conclusion

The long-range strategic plans of many outpatient rehabilitation organizations often address seeking accreditation in order to prove their competence. The achievement of accreditation also permits outpatient organizations the opportunity to enhance their actual status, capitalize on the untapped potential for proving their abilities, and create new niches for themselves in the rehabilitation marketplace. In a highly competitive marketplace, accreditation often provides a marketing edge.

Oftentimes, consumers have no real access to information about the quality of services provided by an organization except through promotional literature and, more commonly, through word-of-mouth reports about the organization's reputation. Accreditation provides the opportunity to ensure external measurement of quality and to project that image to referral sources and potential patients. Accreditation status with one of the nationally recognized private, voluntary accreditation organizations, such as CARF or the Joint Commission, permits the outpatient rehabilitation organization to promote its care and services as being recognized by the accrediting body. Use of such information in publicly accessible documents and marketing tools allows the outpatient rehabilitation organization to say, in all truth, that it indeed provides a measurable level of quality and can, in effect, help assure consumers of high-quality care and services delivered in the most effective and efficient manner.

For a full explanation of the requirements of CARF and the Joint Commission, the reader is referred to *Quality Rehabilitation: Results-Oriented Patient Care*[13] and to the standards manuals and publications of both organizations.

References

1. Joint Commission on Accreditation of Healthcare Organizations. *Accreditation Manual for Hospitals,* 1991 edition. Oakbrook Terrace, IL: Joint Commission, 1990, pp. 181–96.
2. Joint Commission on Accreditation of Healthcare Organizations. *Ambulatory Health Care Standards Manual,* 1990 edition. Chicago: Joint Commission, 1989.
3. Joint Commission on Accreditation of Healthcare Organizations. *Accreditation Manual for Hospitals,* pp. 49–53.
4. Joint Commission on Accreditation of Healthcare Organizations. *Accreditation Manual for Hospitals,* pp. 181–96, 218.
5. Joint Commission on Accreditation of Healthcare Organizations. *Ambulatory Health Care Standards Manual,* pp. 4–5.
6. Joint Commission on Accreditation of Healthcare Organizations, *Ambulatory Health Care Standards Manual,* pp. ix–xx.
7. Joint Commission on Accreditation of Healthcare Organizations, *Ambulatory Health Care Standards Manual,* pp. 75–87.

8. Commission on Accreditation of Rehabilitation Facilities. *Standards Manual for Organizations Serving People with Disabilities.* Tucson, AZ: CARF, 1988, pp. 137–44.

9. Joint Commission on Accreditation of Healthcare Organizations. *Accreditation Manual for Hospitals.* Chapters on Quality Assurance and Physical Rehabilitation Services, pp. 181–96, 215–22.

10. Joint Commission on Accreditation of Healthcare Organizations. *Monitoring and Evaluation: Physical Rehabilitation Services.* Chicago: Joint Commission, 1988.

11. Gray, C. Quality assurance in a rehabilitation facility: a decentralized approach. *QRB: Quality Review Bulletin* 14(1):9–14, 1988.

12. England, B., Glass, R., and Patterson, C., editors. *Quality Rehabilitation: Results-Oriented Patient Care.* Chicago: American Hospital Publishing, 1989.

13. England and others.

Chapter 7

Reimbursement and Financial Management

Donald H. Ratner and Jerry Strum

Introduction

Generally, the demand for rehabilitation services is expected to increase 50 to 100 percent over current levels within the current decade. The need for inpatient rehabilitation beds is expected to grow significantly by the year 2000. However, the payment system for health care increasingly favors outpatient programs and services rather than acute care. This is true for other fields as well as rehabilitation. Generally, the payment structures of diagnostic-related groups (DRGs) for the Medicare prospective payment system (PPS) favor fewer acute inpatient services and more outpatient services. In addition, because of the significant dollar savings that can be realized when a person is being rehabilitated while living at home instead of in a nursing home or in an acute inpatient unit, it also appears that hospitals will be seeing significant pressures from commercial insurers and other payers to reduce inpatient rehabilitation utilization and move toward outpatient services. A shift toward the provision of a continuum of care that includes outpatient rehabilitation services after discharge from inpatient care, covering things such as transitional living and other outpatient services, is already beginning.

Outpatient rehabilitation treatment can be provided in a number of different types of settings. In general, outpatient rehabilitation is geared to assisting individuals who have reached a level of relatively independent functioning and may still have the potential for further functional gain. Outpatient treatment can be given within a hospital environment, freestanding facilities, physician office space, or other multiuse facilities.

Specific portions of this chapter were reprinted from *Substance Abuse Services: A Planning and Management Guide,* coedited by Joseph Westermeyer and Ronald S. Krug (Chicago: American Hospital Publishing, 1991).

Many different types of outpatient treatment can occur in each of these settings. Some are simple, individual-type services; others cover more comprehensive, all-inclusive treatment. Because of the payment regulations that cover them, physical therapy and speech pathology are two of the more common outpatient services. To these services need to be added a number of different types of programs, including pain, brain injury, spinal injury, cardiac rehabilitation, hand therapy, sports medicine, work hardening, and industrial medicine programs. More comprehensive programs would include day hospitals generally requiring more extensive nursing care and full-day treatment, transitional living programs, and comprehensive outpatient rehabilitation facilities (CORFs).

This chapter will not make a case for moving to outpatient rehabilitation care but, instead, will focus on the financial factors that will help planners determine whether outpatient rehabilitation services are an appropriate choice for an individual facility. The chapter begins by addressing financial feasibility. (Whereas chapters 2 and 3 addressed the major marketing and business planning issues, this chapter will narrow the focus of planning to the financial foundation needed to develop and maintain an outpatient rehabilitation program.)

Although outpatient rehabilitation services are covered by a variety of different payers, including Blue Cross and commercial insurers, there is a significant variation in the type and amount of coverage both among these payers and in different locations. It is important to understand how each payer in its particular location views outpatient rehabilitation services generally in its payment structures, what services each covers, and how much each will pay. This chapter addresses some of the major issues for these payers and discusses Medicare in depth.

The topics to be covered include:

- Financial feasibility
- Medicare, including general requirements
- Medicare coverage for CORFs
- Medicaid
- Workers' compensation
- Blue Cross
- Commercial insurance
- Health maintenance organizations (HMOs)
- General data collection and billing issues

Financial Feasibility

Before moving full-steam ahead with an outpatient rehabilitation program, it is important to determine whether the program is financially feasible. What are the start-up expenses? What is the current reimbursement picture? These questions can only be answered by conducting a thorough financial feasibility study.

The financial feasibility study must be based on thorough market research, a topic that was addressed in chapter 2 but is reiterated here to stress its relationship to financial issues. If you intend to explore starting a new outpatient rehabilitation service, you will be well advised to develop a classical business plan in order to evaluate whether the services you intend to place in the outpatient center will be successful. (Business plans were discussed in chapter 3.) The business plan will address the type and scope of the proposed outpatient rehabilitation program.

A good financial feasibility study involves estimating the costs associated with beginning the new outpatient rehabilitation service *and* developing a forecasted statement of operations for a minimum of the first three years. The feasibility study also includes forecasting the number of personnel, type and amount of space needed, and the amount of capital required to develop the service. The forecasted statement of operations consists of three sections: revenue, operating expenses, and nonoperating expenses.

Start-up expenses for the project should be carefully developed in a capital budget. These are generally divided into operating expenses, such as personnel expenses, marketing expenses anticipated prior to opening the new service, and equipment and supplies needed for day-to-day operation, and nonoperating expenses, such as real estate acquisition and the capital needed for cash flow.

Revenue

The revenue section of the forecasted statement of operations is based on estimating the number of patients who will be treated in the outpatient program. The revenue forecast should be based on detailed assumptions of reimbursement at all phases of care beginning at the point when patients receive an evaluation for admission to the program, as well as on data regarding frequency of participation (daily, biweekly, and so forth) and anticipated length of stay. Length of stay will vary according to each patient's primary diagnosis. Therefore, it will be necessary to forecast the patient volume by the most common primary diagnosis and average length of treatment needed to help each patient achieve maximum function.

In order to determine potential revenue, the financial feasibility study should include an estimate of the volume of patients who will participate in the program from both internal and external sources. If the outpatient service is being developed by a larger hospital facility, it is reasonable to expect that a certain number of outpatients will result from referrals from within the hospital's existing inpatient services.

The best way to evaluate the potential for referrals from internal sources is to look at the medical records of patients discharged from the hospital during the past year. This information can be used to estimate how many patients would have been treated in an outpatient rehabilitation program during the past year if the program had been operational during that period. This review should not be limited to patients treated in an existing acute rehabilitation program, but should also include a 100 percent sample of patients with injuries or disease processes that would have indicated a need for outpatient rehabilitation care. If a 100 percent sample is not feasible, the research should include a stratified random sample.

This type of research will also help identify the services the outpatient program should offer and the types of patients it will treat, by primary diagnosis. A list of ICD-9-CM codes related to the primary diagnoses should be developed. Medical records on patients discharged with the relevant diagnosis should be pulled and carefully reviewed. Research should focus primarily on the disposition of the patient at discharge and whether the new service would have captured the patient in an outpatient rehabilitation treatment program at the time of discharge.

Each of the data elements abstracted from the medical records will be of value in the feasibility assessment. The review should include the patient's primary residence, his or her disposition at discharge, his or her primary payment source at discharge, and the physician(s) involved in the patient's treatment course. Capture of data elements related to a patient's residence helps to determine if the proposed outpatient service will be accessible to the patient after he or she is discharged from the inpatient program.

Data on the primary payment source help to determine the principal payment sources to be used in developing the revenue section of the forecast. These data also identify the insurance carriers that will need to be contacted and informed about the proposed new service. This ensures that third-party payment procedures and policies are clarified from the beginning. This list will also serve as an archive for carriers that should receive marketing information once the service is operational.

Similarly, primary physicians who appear on the abstracts should be contacted while the feasibility research is being conducted. Involving physicians in the research will help determine whether the service would complement or compete with each physician's practice, indicate what level of involvement the physicians could expect in their patients' progress through the new outpatient treatment program, and suggest the volume of patients each physician might refer to the new program annually.

The next level of research involves looking outside the hospital to the external environment. If an outpatient rehabilitation program could reasonably expect to receive referrals from other community hospitals, the discharge coordinators of those hospitals should be interviewed. The interview process should focus on whether the proposed service would serve as an additional referral resource to the discharge coordinator or would duplicate an existing service already being used by each discharge coordinator. Interviews will be very effective in identifying existing or proposed competitive services that should be researched further. Additionally, interviews with discharge coordinators frequently uncover the names of other physicians who are likely to use the proposed service. These physicians should be interviewed in the same context that a hospital staff physician would be interviewed.

Thorough research of competitive facilities is essential. This includes examining existing outpatient rehabilitation services or facilities that are similar to those proposed, as well as services offered by physicians that might be either similar or potentially competitive. All these factors are important in accurately estimating the outpatient rehabilitation program's potential revenue.

Operating Expenses

Operating expenses include salaries and other personnel expenses, rents, utilities, and so forth. Once the internal and external market research is completed, assumptions can be made about the anticipated patient volume in the new service, the payment source, and the anticipated length of stay. These data will drive the operating expense section of the feasibility study in terms of space, equipment, and professional staff needed to operate the program.

It is also important to estimate the type and scope of support services that are needed or can be obtained from the larger hospital organization. Support services may include business office management, marketing, housekeeping, maintenance, medical records, human resources, billing and accounting, data processing, and auditing.

Personnel expenses are those related to recruitment of personnel prior to beginning the service, in addition to salaries and wages for those personnel involved in a training program prior to beginning the service.

The feasibility study should include a careful analysis of any regulatory requirements associated with beginning the outpatient service, as well as estimates of costs associated with regulatory compliance. Regulatory requirements should be identified in the feasibility package along with a narrative of how compliance is reflected in either start-up expenses or ongoing expenses. Regulatory requirements include state licensure, certificate-of-need (CON) review and approval if applicable, Medicare certification, Medicaid certification, and a review of workers' compensation laws. Regulatory requirements may also include retrofitting or renovating existing structures to meet local safety and building codes. If these *hidden* expenses are not researched, they could financially compromise a new program.

Detailed equipment lists should be developed and the costs associated with acquisition of equipment should be included in a capital budget. The budget should reflect what equipment will be needed during the first year of operation and must either be purchased or rented, and what equipment can be depreciated.

Nonoperating Expenses

Nonoperating expenses are those associated with real estate acquisition, cash flow capital, interest expenses, and regulatory compliance.

Real estate acquisition costs reflect all costs associated with securing the real estate necessary to begin the service.

Assumptions should be made about accounts receivable related to the first year of operation, and adequate capital should be budgeted to cover any negative cash flow until the program reaches the break-even point as forecasted in the statement of operations.

Medicare: General Requirements

Because Medicare is an important payer of rehabilitation services, the feasibility study research should reflect that the Medicare intermediary was contacted and the revenue forecasts in the feasibility reflect current limitations and restrictions on outpatient treatment.

Since the beginning of the Medicare program in 1965, specific outpatient services were generally covered by Medicare Part B payment, when these services were provided by hospitals in an outpatient department. Yet these same services were not necessarily covered when provided by a separate or freestanding outpatient rehabilitation facility. Separate outpatient facilities were only paid under Medicare Part B when providing physical therapy and speech therapy. Thus, this system favored the use of hospital-based inpatient services and in effect discriminated against Medicare users who could have benefited from outpatient services in another setting or location.

Such was the situation until 1981. Starting in July 1981, the CORF amendment of the Omnibus Reconciliation Act of 1980 provided for a certification for an entity called a comprehensive outpatient rehabilitation facility (CORF). A CORF is a certification and a designation, not a licensure, and basically recognizes that the same services that were always provided in hospital outpatient departments can now be provided in another location. The new legislation authorized coverage for a broad range of items and services when they are provided by a physician or other qualified personnel to a beneficiary who is an outpatient of the CORF. Services such as occupational therapy, prosthetics and orthotics, nursing, and so forth, which were not paid for by Medicare when provided in an outpatient speech therapy or physical therapy facility, could now be covered and paid for by Medicare. After July 1, 1987, Medicare began covering other rehabilitative services provided in separate, non-CORF outpatient facilities. Although this legislation did not revolutionize the outpatient rehabilitation field, it did make it possible to provide and be paid for comprehensive rehabilitation services in areas geographically distinct from the hospital itself.

In order for outpatient rehabilitation facilities (including CORFs) to participate in the Medicare program, a number of conditions for participation and requirements for service must be met. Outpatient rehabilitation facilities are defined as nonresidential public or private entities that, at minimum:

1. Are exclusively engaged in providing diagnostic, therapeutic, and restorative services under a physician's direction for the rehabilitation of injured, disabled, or ill outpatients at single, fixed locations.
2. Must provide at least:
   - Physician services on either a full- or part-time basis
   - Physical therapy
   - Social or psychological services
3. Must maintain clinical records on all patients.
4. Must have the policies that govern their services established by a group of professional personnel that includes at least one physician who assumes responsibility for the implementation of these policies.
5. Must guarantee that every patient served is under the care of a physician.
6. Must meet applicable state or local standards for licensing.
7. Must have utilization review plans in effect that are in accordance with federal regulations.
8. Must ensure that overall plans and budgets meet established legal requirements.
9. Must have a separate and distinct space.
10. Must, in general, adhere to any other conditions the Secretary of Health and Human Services may impose that relate to the health and safety of their patients. This may even include conditions concerning the qualifications of personnel in their facilities.

Comprehensive outpatient rehabilitation facilities, which are discussed in detail later in this chapter, have the same requirements as those in the preceding list, but also have some different requirements. Planners cannot assume that the requirements for an outpatient rehabilitation facility are the same as those for a CORF.

It is important to recognize two basic factors regarding Medicare: what outpatient rehabilitation services are covered, and how the payment structure generally works.

What Outpatient Services Are Covered

Rehabilitation services in a hospital outpatient department are included among those that are reimbursed as *incident to* the services of physicians and that are paid for by Medicare at 80 percent of allowable costs. Outpatient physical therapy and speech pathology services are also covered on a cost-related basis (80 percent) when furnished by a clinic, rehabilitation agency, or public health agency (for example, a separate outpatient facility).

As part of the Omnibus Budget Reconciliation Act of 1986, Part B coverage was extended for occupational therapy services both in outpatient settings and to independently practicing therapists. The coverage for occupational therapy services of private practitioners is at 80 percent of reasonable charges with an annual limit in incurred expenses eligible for coverage. Medicare regulations should be consulted to determine the limit. Occupational therapy services in other outpatient settings are paid at 80 percent of costs.

There is a dollar limit for the amount of psychological services that will be covered. This applies to therapeutic psychological services, not covering initial diagnostic testing. Researchers should consult Medicare regulations to determine the dollar limits.

There are some other limitations on what services can be covered, especially for CORFs. These will be discussed in the section in this chapter on CORFs.

Payment Structure: Cost Reporting

To obtain payment from Medicare, facilities must prepare cost reports and other forms and submit them, usually to the regional Medicare office or intermediary.

On an interim basis, Form 1450 (UB-82) is used for billing for all outpatient services. Medicare pays on an interim basis based on the bills submitted. A year-end settlement results from a filed cost report.

Hospital-based outpatient facilities use cost report Form 2552, with special schedules denoted for hospital-based CORFs. Freestanding CORFs and freestanding physical therapy and speech clinics use cost report Form 2088. At the close of a fiscal year, CORFs and other outpatient rehabilitation facilities reach a reimbursement settlement with the Health Care Financing Administration (HCFA) by filing a Medicare cost report. The cost report forms are used by:

- Rehabilitation agencies, clinics, and public health agencies certified as outpatient physical therapy (OPT) providers on or after July 1, 1968
- Comprehensive outpatient rehabilitation facilities (CORFs) for the first cost reporting period that began on or after July 1, 1981, and for which a facility is certified as a CORF.

The cost report is arranged into cost centers. There are four classifications: (1) general service cost centers, which are not billed to patients; (2) reimbursable service cost centers, which are billed to patients; (3) nonreimbursable cost centers (patient care); and (4) nonreimbursable cost centers (other) (see figure 7-1).

The cost report forms are designed to determine how much of the total cost of operating the program and providing the services should be allocated to Medicare patients. The cost report takes all the costs of the program or clinic and determines which ones are not allowable. Using the remaining allowable costs, the cost report then allocates cost from the overhead cost centers such as housekeeping, depreciation, maintenance, and so forth, to the revenue-producing cost centers. The revenue-producing cost centers are those for which charges to patients are made for services rendered. The overhead is allocated to these revenue-producing cost centers through the use of a cost allocation method known as a *step-down*.

Once the overhead costs are all allocated to the revenue-producing cost centers, the amounts are then split between Medicare utilization and non-Medicare utilization, using the ratio of Medicare charges for each area to the total charges for each area. This methodology thus prorates the cost of running the program to Medicare based on its utilization of the program. Medicare then pays the calculated reasonable cost at a rate of 80 percent.

The cost apportionment may use cost findings based on one of three methods: (1) gross charges, (2) weighted units of service, or (3) number of visits. The gross charges method is based on a concept known as the ratio of cost to charges. This takes total gross charges and calculates a ratio based on the relative weight of the Medicare charges to total charges. This ratio is then applied to the costs defined as *allowable costs* in the regulations. It is developed for each individual rehabilitation service.

The weighted units of service method is the ratio of health insurance program (Medicare) individual-weighted units of service to total-weighted units of service (all patients) applied to the total allowable costs. This ratio also is developed for each individual rehabilitation service.

The number of visits method is the ratio of health insurance program patient visits to total patient visits (all patients) applied to total allowable costs. This ratio is developed for each individual rehabilitation service. This method may be used only if the intermediary/carrier determines that the data needed for the other methods are not available.

It is important to understand a subtle distinction about what is reimbursed between the two groups of providers—CORFs and other rehabilitation treatment providers. For outpatient physical therapy and outpatient speech pathology providers (including those that are hospital based), the provider is reimbursed on the lower of reasonable cost or customary charges, or reasonable cost minus amounts that may be billed to Medicare

Figure 7-1. Medicare Cost Centers

General Service Cost Centers

1. Capital Costs: Buildings and Fixtures
2. Capital Costs: Movable Equipment
3. Employee Health and Welfare
4. Administrative and General
5. Maintenance and Repairs
6. Operation of Plant
7. Laundry and Linen Service
8. Housekeeping
9. Cafeteria
10. Medical Supplies and Other Expenses
11. Medical Supplies—Library
12. Professional Education and Training

Note: The direct expenses including salaries and ''other'' for the above cost centers are accumulated, closed out, and then apportioned down to the Reimbursable Service Cost Centers on a ''step-down basis'' using a statistical basis.

Reimbursable Cost Centers include:

1. Skilled Nursing Expenses
2. Physical Therapy
3. Speech Pathology
4. Occupational Therapy
5. Respiratory Therapy
6. Medical Social Services
7. Psychological Services
8. Prosthetics and Orthotic Services
9. Drugs and Biologicals
10. Medical Supplies
11. Durable Medical Equipment Sold
12. Durable Medical Equipment Rented

Nonreimbursable Costs include:

1. Sheltered Workshops
2. Recreational Programs
3. Resident Day Camps
4. Preschool Programs
5. Diagnostic Clinics
6. Home Employment Programs
7. Equipment Loan Service
8. Physicians' Private Offices
9. Fund-raising
10. Coffee Shops and Canteen
11. Research
12. Investment Property
13. Advertising
14. Franchise

Source: Strum, J. Reimbursement and financial management. Presentation, American Hospital Association Meeting, Outpatient Rehabilitation Program: Options in Planning, Marketing, and Operations, Chicago, June 6–7, 1990.

beneficiaries for providing services. On the other hand, CORFs are not subject to the lesser of costs or charges provisions. Instead, CORFs are reimbursed based on the reasonable cost that remains after subtracting any applicable deductibles and is the lesser of:

- Eighty percent of the remaining reasonable cost
- The remaining reasonable cost minus billed coinsurance

Although the preceding is a simplistic explanation of the fairly complicated cost-reporting mechanism, it should suffice to explain generally how Medicare cost reports work for outpatient rehabilitation services.

Medicare and Comprehensive Outpatient Rehabilitation Facilities

Comprehensive outpatient rehabilitation facilities are engaged primarily in providing diagnostic, therapeutic, and restorative services to injured, disabled, or sick outpatients under medical direction. They are expected to provide on-site services with only one home evaluation visit allowed.

Planners must thoroughly explore the specific requirements for CORFs to identify whether they are feasible for the market and meet the hospital's objectives for the outpatient rehabilitation program. It is critical to conduct the market research required to determine if Medicare is going to be your major payer for your type of patients. For example, developing a CORF for a market made up of young, employer-insured, urban professionals is unlikely to be feasible. Financial feasibility is obviously the other closely related major factor. Determining costs and revenues under Medicare is not easy, but a sound knowledge of Medicare policies and reimbursement procedures is a necessary strategy. Figures 7-2 and 7-3 show the pros and cons of CORF development.

When considering CORF development, a number of questions must be answered:

- What is the market share for CORF patients in the service area?
- Is a CORF financially feasible? Can it make money, or is it a loss leader?
- What would be the problems in finding a location for a CORF?
- Can a CORF be easily staffed?
- Can a CORF provide a high-quality program for the patients served?

In developing the forecasted operating budget, you will need to estimate potential utilization or forecast patient volume by expected payment source.

Figure 7-2. Pros of a CORF: General and Hospital-Specific

Pros of a CORF: General

A. Should increase reimbursement for additional treatment services.
B. Helps program credibility to third-party payers, health care providers, and so forth.
C. Can be readily marketed.
D. Indicates a commitment to comply with federal regulations for a formalized organized approach to comprehensive patient programming.
E. Only three required services:
   1. M.D.
   2. Physical therapy
   3. Social services or psychology
F. Permits joint venturing with physicians to reduce present or future competition.
G. Reimbursed on a *reasonable* cost basis.

Pros of a CORF: Hospital-Specific

A. Enhances marketing of inpatient rehabilitation programs because inpatients can be easily transferred to an outpatient program.
B. Serves as a direct treatment source from in-house patient programs.
C. Allows for the identification of diversified and coordinated services.
D. Promotes continuity of care from the inpatient program to outpatient programming.
E. Permits association with an institution that has an inferred commitment from the medical staff to refer patients to CORFs.
F. Permits fluctuation of staff from other service areas when patient demand/census varies.
G. Coordinated use of rehabilitation medical director of inpatient program.
H. Reimbursement on a reasonable cost basis is a prospectively determined amount based on a DRG.
I. Now permits contractual services outside the facility, such as physical therapy, occupational therapy, speech pathology.

Source: Swope, M. Pros and cons of a CORF. Presentation, American Hospital Association Meeting, Outpatient Rehabilitation Program: Options in Planning, Marketing, and Operations, Chicago, June 6–7, 1990.

Figure 7-3. Cons of a CORF

A. Restricts services to one physical plant unless the facility has dual certification.
B. Regulations restrict staffing, space use, and equipment to be used only in the specific CORF operation.
C. Allows only for designated and not commingled space (inpatient-outpatient CORF).
D. 100% review of claims with potential for denial based on a number of factors.
E. Increases cumbersome medical review criteria which impede operations and increase cost.
F. Delays in reimbursement payments still a problem. Protracted payment turnaround from Medicare contractors which may create cash flow problems.
G. Increases documentation and utilization review requirements with variable demands being placed by Medicare reviewers, which may depend on local interpretation.
H. Problems in meeting staffing needs, especially a fluctuating patient population.
I. Number of specialists required may be difficult to recruit, especially with an increased number of rehabilitation facilities and limited number of trained specialists to manage and develop rehabilitation programs.

Source: Swope, M. Pros and cons of a CORF. Presentation, American Hospital Association Meeting, Outpatient Rehabilitation Program: Options in Planning, Marketing, and Operations, Chicago, June 6–7, 1990.

One common, potential trap is to assume that the length of stay on an acute rehabilitation unit will be shortened for all CORF patients, although it is possible that some Medicare patients may be able to be placed in a CORF and thus have their length of stay in the acute program shortened. However, planners should carefully review the medical records of the hospital inpatients, because there are two categories of patients who may not be able to participate in a CORF program: those without home support systems, and the frail elderly. Generally speaking, Medicare patients who can successfully transfer out of an inpatient program into a CORF program have in-home support systems such as a spouse or relative who can facilitate getting the patient back and forth to the outpatient service for treatment. If the patient does not have an in-home support system, it is unlikely he or she will be able to participate. Additionally, experience has shown that very frail, elderly patients (such as those 70 years of age or older) have limited ability to participate in a comprehensive outpatient rehabilitation program, even with in-home support systems. The business plan estimates should factor out these categories of patients.

As stated previously, CORFs are reimbursed on a reasonable cost basis except that they are not subject to the lesser of costs or charges provisions. They are paid 80 percent of allowable costs by Medicare and can bill the patient for the Part B deductible and the 20 percent coinsurance amount.

In addition to the previously mentioned general Medicare requirements, CORFs also have to meet further conditions in order to participate in the program. These can be found in Sub-Part B of 42 C.F.R. Part 488 of the Regulations, and are summarized here. Comprehensive outpatient rehabilitation facilities are required to follow specific guidelines related to governance and administration:

1. Each needs to have a separate governing body.
2. Each provider is required to furnish information about the identity of any person who may have ownership or controlling interest in the facility.
3. The governing body must appoint an administrator to be responsible for the overall management and enforcement of its policies.
4. An institutional budget plan must be prepared under the direction of the governing body providing for an annual operating budget, a three-year capital expenditure plan if expenditures in excess of $100,000 are anticipated, and an annual review and updating by the governing body.
5. Written care policies are required relating to:
   - Arrangement for services rendered by employees
   - Personnel responsibilities during medical emergencies
   - The handling of drugs

- Procedures for patient admission care and discharge
- Clinical recordkeeping
- Treatment plans
- Requirements for physician care
- Other related items

The treatment program itself must provide the following:

1. The patients must be initially assessed and evaluated by a physician and must receive all their services on the CORF site, with the exception of the single home evaluation visit.
2. All patients have to be assessed by every qualified professional who will be involved in their care, prior to implementation of the plan of treatment. They must also be reassessed after they undergo any significant changes in their functional status.
3. The CORF physician is responsible for establishing a treatment plan, assisting with the creation of policies related to patient care, and participating in treatment and progress evaluations along with utilization reviews.
4. Every CORF is required to establish a treatment plan for each patient before treatment begins. It must specify the services that are to be provided and the goals for treatment, and must undergo physician review at least every 60 days.
5. Like other outpatient rehabilitation facilities, CORFs must maintain clinical records. It is important that they present an adequate picture of the care being given to and the progress being made by each patient. The patient's record must be maintained for at least five years after discharge.

In addition, CORFs are required to undergo utilization review (UR), which entails writing a UR plan that is reviewed at least once per quarter by the UR committee.

They are required to have a separate and distinct space that is not used for other programs or non-CORF rehabilitation services. Additionally, CORFs have to provide the kind of physical environment needed to protect the health and safety of their patients, personnel, and the public at large. They must have established fire safety and disaster procedures.

Additional requirements and issues will require special exploration when determining the feasibility of CORF development. These include requirements that must be met in order to receive reimbursement as a CORF under Medicare. These requirements include provisions regarding the covered services, location, personnel qualifications, referrals for treatment, treatment plans, and data collection. Also, planners must determine how a CORF would fit into existing health maintenance organization and independent practice association contracts or the potential for contracting.

Covered Services

Medicare will pay CORFs only for covered services. Services provided by CORFs are covered only if they are reasonable and necessary for the diagnosis or treatment of an illness or injury to improve the function of a malformed body member. Other services can be provided but may not be reimbursed by Medicare. The regulations generally require that services provided in a CORF may be covered if a hospital patient would receive coverage as an inpatient. By definition, there must be a potential for restoration or improvement of lost or impaired functions. In other words, if the patient receives repetitive services that do not require the skilled services of nurses or therapists, such as maintenance programs or general conditioning or ambulation, these services are not covered under Medicare Part B reimbursement.

Services that are covered and paid for by Medicare include medical/physician services; physical, occupational, speech, and respiratory therapy; nursing services; social and psychological services; some drugs and devices; and home evaluations (one home visit).

Medical/Physician Services (CORF Physician Services)

Physician services that are reimbursable under a CORF include consultation with and medical supervision of nonphysician staff and administration, establishment and review of treatment plans, and other administrative activities. Certain medical services do not directly constitute CORF physician services but can be reimbursed by Medicare using a separate billing form (Physician Billing Form 1500). These are generally diagnostic- and therapeutic-type services, which are billed specifically as physician services and are reimbursed by Medicare Part B on a reasonable charge basis. These services are subject to the same 60 percent charge limitation normally applied to physicians' services furnished in outpatient settings.

Physical, Occupational, Speech, and Respiratory Therapy

Physical therapy is covered if its services are designed to improve the functioning levels of patients. However, as previously stated, maintenance therapy, which entails repetitive services required to maintain a certain level of functioning, is not covered. It should be noted that if a patient has reached his or her restoration potential, the *establishment* of a maintenance program is covered by Medicare, but not the maintenance therapy itself.

Occupational therapy is covered. Speech therapy is generally covered with the limitation that the physicians, and not the speech pathologist, must create the plan of treatment. Respiratory therapy is covered.

Nursing Services

Nursing services are covered if they are provided by or under the supervision of registered nurses. Included are any nursing services specified under the treatment plan or any other nursing programs that are necessary to obtain rehabilitation goals.

Social and Psychological Services

Social and psychological services are covered if they are stipulated in the treatment plans and contribute to improvement in the patient's condition.

Certain psychological services are covered by Medicare, including the assessment, diagnosis, and treatment of the beneficiary's mental and emotional problems that relate to rehabilitation; psychological evaluation of patient response to and rate of progress under the treatment plan; and the assessment of the individual, family, and home situations that affect patient rehabilitation treatment.

There is a dollar limitation on the amount of psychological services that are covered by Medicare. The CORF psychiatric limitation is part of the limitation on physicians' outpatient psychiatric services. Under the regulations, a patient is subject to a limit under Medicare Part B program reimbursement per year for outpatient physician services and CORF services combined for treatment of a mental, psychoneurotic, or personality disorder. This limit applies to therapeutic services and does not apply to initial psychiatric or psychological testing. However, additional payment may be authorized. As part of the CORF cost report settlement, the intermediary evaluates the accumulated payments for outpatient psychiatric physicians' services and CORF reimbursement. If the accumulated payments total the limit, additional payment may be authorized for the difference between the limit and the accumulated payments. Administrators should consult Medicare regulations to determine the limits that would apply to Medicare beneficiaries.

Drugs and Devices

Medicare also covers prosthetic and orthotics devices; drugs; supplies; appliances and equipment; and durable medical equipment.

Home Evaluations

Medicare will also pay for home evaluations, but only for one visit. The purpose is to allow treatment plans to be tailored to take into consideration the patient's home environment and its potential impact on rehabilitation goals. However, Medicare does not generally pay for alterations to the home to facilitate rehabilitation, nor is a home evaluation covered unless there is clear indication that the home environment may adversely affect the goals of the treatment plan. Only one professional will be paid for doing the home evaluation.

Location of Services

Except for the one home evaluation, services must be furnished on the premises of a CORF, and the program reimbursement is made only to the participating CORF and not to a private individual.

Comprehensive outpatient services can be located away from the main hospital campus, which may offer increased accessibility to persons with disabilities. However, you may also want to consider a hospital-based CORF, if your facility has surplus space and patients experience no overwhelming problems in getting to the outpatient services.

Personnel Qualifications

The regulations for CORFs require that services must be furnished or supervised by qualified personnel in accordance with the regulations in 42 C.F.R. Part 488.70. This section of the regulations sets forth the qualifications that must be met for facility physicians or the CORF medical director, a licensed practical nurse (and vocational nurse), an occupational therapist (and occupational therapist assistant), an orthotist, a physical therapist (and physical therapist assistant), a prosthetist, a psychologist, a registered nurse, a rehabilitation counselor, a respiratory therapist, a respiratory therapy technician, a social worker, and a speech-language pathologist. (These requirements were implemented by rules and regulations published in the *Federal Register,* 48 F.R. 56293, Dec. 15, 1982. Redesignated and amended at 50 F.R. 33034, Aug. 16, 1985; and 51 F.R. 41352, Nov. 14, 1986.)

A facility physician must be in the facility for a sufficient time to:

1. Provide, in accordance with accepted principles of medical practice, medical direction, medical care services, and consultation
2. Establish the plan of treatment in cases where a plan has not been established by the referring physician
3. Assist in establishing and implementing the facility's patient care policies
4. Participate in reviews of treatment, patient case review conferences, comprehensive patient assessments and reassessments, and utilization review.

In addition, the facility must provide for emergency physician services during all operating hours.

Referrals for Treatment

To become a patient of a CORF, the patient must be under the care of a referring physician who certifies that the beneficiary needs skilled rehabilitation services. The referring physician must advise the CORF of the beneficiary's medical history, current diagnosis and medical findings, desired rehabilitation goals, and any contraindications to specific activity or intensity of rehabilitation services.

Treatment Plans

All CORF services must be furnished under a written plan of treatment established by a physician. The physician may be either a physician associated with a CORF or a referring physician and must provide a detailed plan of treatment that meets the following requirements:

- The plan must contain the diagnosis, type, amount, frequency, and duration of services to be performed, as well as the anticipated rehabilitation goals.
- The plan must be sufficiently detailed to permit an independent evaluation of the patient's need for the indicated services and of the likelihood that he or she will derive meaningful benefit from them.
- The plan must be reviewed by the CORF physician at least once every 60 days. Following review, the physician should certify that the plan of treatment is being followed and that the patient is making progress in attaining the established rehabilitation goals. When the patient has reached a point where no further progress is being made toward one or more of the goals, Medicare coverage ends.

Data Collection

A number of data requirements must be met if a facility is to be reimbursed under CORF regulations. In order for CORFs to be paid by Medicare, a physician must *certify* that the services were required, that the patient needed skilled rehabilitation services, that a plan for furnishing these services was established and reviewed by a physician, that services were furnished while the patient was under physician care, and that the plan was reviewed at least every 60 days by a facility physician with the physician certifying that the plan was followed and progress was made. This certification must be sent in with the billing form. Once the bill and certification have been submitted, the intermediary subjects all bills to a thorough medical review.

Many CORF providers have experienced long delays in getting paid by Medicare. This has been due to a number of reasons, including the following:

- A detailed review of all bills is mandated by the 100 percent review requirement. This obviously slows down the payment process.
- Because most audits by payers are based on patient records, the information must be available on the patient charts, or there is a high probability that payment will be disallowed or delayed.
- The review process frequently takes a long time because of backlogs at the intermediary.
- Intermediaries do not always ask for the same information for each set of claims.
- There is frequently poor response time on inquiries to intermediaries.

There has been movement on the government's part to remedy the situation, and we are beginning to see improvement and an increase in the speed in the payment of CORF bills. However, this information on billing delays needs to be factored into the facility's business plan and cash flow projections, because it could have a significant adverse impact on operations.

Limited Referrals from PPOs and IPAs

Persons planning an outpatient rehabilitation service should be aware that approval for treatment of preferred provider organization (PPO) and independent practice association (IPA) patients in the service may be limited as a result of a CORF facility.

Preferred provider organizations and IPAs make profits by limiting participation in outpatient services to members who either discount their billings for the services or share in a residual of the net profit on an annual basis. Both have shown a reluctance to approve placement in CORFs outside their membership organizations. When the business plan for a CORF is developed, the market analysis section should reflect that an appropriate level of research has been completed with respect to PPO and IPA penetration within the planned market area to permit factoring out these potential patients.

Medicaid

Medicaid is a public health insurance program that funds treatment for the medically indigent, financed under Title XIX of the Social Security Act. The program is funded jointly by federal and state governments and is administered by each state. This latter factor often results in variations in reimbursement levels and in the process of reimbursing providers for services. Medicaid payment is made directly from the state medical assistance agency to service providers and is based on bills and specific forms submitted by the provider or patient (or both) to the agency.

Medicaid contracts are generally location-specific, and providers of rehabilitation services may be able to establish an agreement with the Medicaid program in a given state for reimbursement.

Medicaid reimbursement is often lower than the costs incurred in providing rehabilitation services. Of course, this varies from state to state. Planners must evaluate the Medicaid reimbursement policies within their own states along with expected reimbursement from other sources to determine if losses can be offset. If Medicaid is the dominant payer within a given market, providers must examine the services that will be reimbursed under current policies and estimate reimbursement rates. Reimbursement rates are usually determined by dividing the expected Medicaid budget for an upcoming fiscal period by the expected units of service for the period.

Workers' Compensation

Workers' compensation plans are state-based insurance programs that provide for coverage of medical treatment and compensation to employees for work-related injuries or diseases. Generally, workers' compensation laws are only concerned with workers who have suffered work-related injuries and need rehabilitation treatment to return to work.

Workers' compensation laws vary widely from state to state. Some states permit the patient to choose his or her physician, whereas others specify the physician that the patient must be treated by. This distinction is important to evaluate, because a patient may be limited in his or her choice of a particular outpatient rehabilitation program. Some states operate their own state-supported outpatient programs for injured workers. Providers located in these states will have little or no opportunity to penetrate the workers' compensation market. Still other states have case management staff, who determine where a patient will receive treatment and at what level. Therefore, hospital-based physicians may have limited opportunity to refer a patient to a hospital-based program.

Some states have fee schedules, which place a limit on the amounts paid for a particular treatment or therapy. Finally, some states have extraordinarily long periods of time before the provider is compensated for services. This would influence cash flow targets in a financial feasibility analysis.

Planners and financial managers must become thoroughly familiar with state workers' compensation laws and reimbursement practices.

They must know which services are covered under workers' compensation and which are not.

Blue Cross

Blue Cross is another major payer for hospital-based outpatient rehabilitation services. Like Medicare, Blue Cross has requirements for payment based on the type of services, and policies for obtaining reimbursement.

If the outpatient service will involve treatment of patients covered by Blue Cross, the research should include a thorough review of payment practices by Blue Cross in the particular state where the program is located. If a good number of patients and a case mix including Blue Cross patients is anticipated, the financial feasibility research should reflect that an interview with Blue Cross representatives was conducted and that the findings are adequately accounted for in the statement of operations.

Generally, the services covered by Blue Cross are based on the particular contracts and limitations within the contracts. For example, an employer group health plan with Blue Cross may exclude psychological services and occupational therapy from reimbursement.

Blue Cross generally reimburses usual and customary charges, subject to copayments and cost findings. These provisions are relatively easy to uncover by contacting Blue Cross or the Blue Cross intermediary for a particular state. Interviews with Blue Cross staff will also uncover any unique billing considerations that will need to be considered, such as special forms, special fee schedules, and so forth.

Blue Cross conducts concurrent utilization review, generally on a two-week basis, but may review some cases only on a 30-day basis. Reports outlining the patient's treatment plan by a single modality or group of modalities may be required.

Commercial Insurance

When the initial financial feasibility research was conducted, abstracts should have been made of commercial insurance carriers that have historically reimbursed for the types of rehabilitation services proposed. These abstracts can be prepared from interviews conducted with major commercial carriers. Interviews with representatives of commercial insurance carriers will uncover any billing and coverage issues unique to a particular commercial insurance carrier and any special restrictions on reimbursement for outpatient programs.

These carriers should also be contacted to determine if they require special forms for billing outpatient rehabilitation services. Many private insurance carriers accept the UB-82 form required by Medicare; however, some may accept a per diem billing attached to their own more simple form without the individual detail required on a UB-82. Some also make it possible for reimbursement to be issued directly to the patient after the patient has paid for treatment. This helps ensure quick payment.

Most commercial insurance carriers fully cover outpatient rehabilitation services, subject to some copayment provisions or deductibles by the patient or other insurer. However, some other commercial insurers have length-of-stay restrictions and frequency-of-treatment restrictions.

Many commercial insurance carriers use utilization review to impose restrictions and, after a certain length of time, may under their own case management refer the patient to day treatment programs, then to home health care. If a particular commercial insurance carrier has an effective case management system and the proposed service is perceived as having a long length of stay, referrals to the service through case managers will be limited. The outpatient rehabilitation service should be designed to offer cost-effective alternatives to inpatient treatment and any other existing treatment, or the service will not be used by commercial carriers.

Health Maintenance Organizations

Health maintenance organizations (HMOs) are prepaid health care organizations that both fund and provide the services included in the benefit package purchased by employers. They were originally conceived as "cooperative" payment plans to provide all health care services for a given population. Early plans were developed in the western states in the 1930s. However, the real popularity of HMOs as health care insurance options began in the 1970s as a potential cost-containment vehicle for rising health care costs.

Health maintenance organizations take several different forms, depending on the makeup of the medical staff of direct providers in the organization. For example, independent practice associations use independent practitioners practicing alone or in small groups to provide prepaid health care under criteria established by the corporation, partnership, or other legal entity. Group model HMOs use one designated independent multispecialty group for physician care, and network HMOs use more than one large group for physician services.

The primary purpose of HMOs is to provide a broad range of services that prevent or reduce the need for expensive procedures, technology, or specialists. As a result, HMOs try to limit the amount of inpatient care delivered in order to keep costs as low as possible. They also ask the hospitals in their contracted network to give large per diem discounts for rehabilitation services.

Health maintenance organizations' benefits for outpatient rehabilitation treatment vary according to the type of plan and employee group.

Planners in areas with heavy HMO penetration must ensure that their rehabilitation services will be reimbursable under an HMO contract and evaluate whether to "package" specific outpatient rehabilitation services for HMO members. Alternatively, providers that are in areas with high HMO penetration but that do not have contracts with HMOs might target other markets that are underserved or unserved.

A review of any current managed care contracts held by the hospital will determine if any unique restrictions for outpatient rehabilitation services will apply to the new service.

General Data Collection and Billing Issues

A major billing and collection problem inherent in the outpatient environment is that there are a large number of relatively small bills, such as services for some therapies or other charges. Because of this, the billing and collection system must be designed to handle high-volume, low-dollar items efficiently. The collection system also should be designed to capture as much cash at the time of service as possible to avoid expensive follow-up costs and potential for large bad-debt write-offs. Finally, the system must be adequate to identify information such as amounts of deductibles, copayments, and total daily charges at times of service.

All these issues need to be addressed in the design of the data collection system. Whether you use a mainframe computer, a minicomputer, a shared system, a personal computer, or a manual system is not the issue. If the outpatient facility is connected with a hospital or other entity, it may appear easy to tie in to existing systems. It is extremely important to adequately evaluate whether these systems can meet all the data requirements of the outpatient facility and are flexible enough to meet the needs of the facility's management.

Frequently, hospital-based computer systems are geared more toward inpatient billing and collection and may or may not have adequate information available for an outpatient environment. There is a significant difference between the needs of an inpatient-oriented facility and an outpatient-oriented facility. Outpatient facilities, for example, should be able to get information for billing and collection immediately. Also, the general accounting systems, which keep track of revenues and expenses and are common in inpatient facilities, frequently can provide adequate basic information but may be too cumbersome for a small facility.

Other data needs such as tracking patient visits, scheduling, demographics, productivity management, and staffing, all of which can be crucial in maintaining the profitability of a small outpatient facility, may not even be addressed in the existing hospital information system.

In planning the design of your information system, all the data elements already mentioned should be listed and management should determine what information is needed, and in what format. If the existing system or the system in the larger facility can provide this information in an adequate format and on a timely basis, it can be used. Trying to make an existing system do what it was not designed to do, however, would probably cause more headaches than the ease of using the system is worth. In such a situation, either a different system should be used or one should be specially developed.

There are certain software packages on the market for different elements of the various data collection systems that can be purchased independently. Otherwise, management could design a completely new computerized system on its own, or a simple manual system could be designed and used until such time as volume increases to a point where a computerized system is required. The important element is that the system must be made to work for the facility. Management will find that an improperly conceived system will end up causing major problems in running the business.

Conclusion

There is currently a significant demand for outpatient rehabilitation services, and this demand is expected to increase. In order to be able to satisfactorily meet the demand for services, an outpatient rehabilitation facility must be aware of the rules and regulations governing participation in various outpatient programs, what services are covered, payment regulations, payment issues, and data collection issues. Only when these elements are understood and successfully incorporated into the operation of the facility can the provision of outpatient services and successful operation of the business be accomplished.

Bibliography

Section 1861 (cc) Social Security Act, 42 USC 1395x (cc).

47 F.R. 56281 Comprehensive Outpatient Rehabilitation Facilities: Final Rule, Dec. 15, 1983.

42 C.F.R. Part 488, Conditions of Participation for Comprehensive Outpatient Rehabilitation Facilities.

48 F.R. 8902, Medicare Program Payment for Physician Services Furnished in Hospitals, Skilled Nursing Facilities and Comprehensive Rehabilitation Facilities: Final Rule, Mar. 2, 1983.

Chapter 8

Legal Aspects of Outpatient Rehabilitation Services

L. Edward Bryant, Jr.

Introduction

This chapter deals with the primary legal aspects of developing and managing outpatient rehabilitation services. Because many different people are involved in planning an outpatient rehabilitation program, a consideration of the *legal aspects* must first acknowledge the great diversity of *nonlegal views.*

Involving different aspects or views in planning an outpatient rehabilitation program ensures different viewpoints, and there is often little consistency among key planners. The views of the following persons or entities must be taken into consideration in planning an outpatient rehabilitation program:

- Patients
- Consumer groups
- Public policymakers
- Health care administrators
- Orthopedic surgeons
- Physiatrists
- Various allied health professionals (physical and occupational therapists and so forth)
- The Health Care Financing Administration (HCFA)
- State governments
- Commercial insurers/Blue Cross/Blue Shield
- Representatives of health maintenance organizations (HMOs), preferred provider organizations (PPOs), and independent practitioner associations (IPAs)
- Religious sponsors

- Hospital trustees/directors
- Business-employer alliances
- State health care bureaucrats
- Accrediting organizations
- Competitors
- Financial officers and accountants
- Management consultants
- Investment bankers
- Lawyers for any of the foregoing
- Unknown hangers-on

Each of these sees what is transpiring somewhat differently and will translate the legal significance of the activity differently, using different perspectives and representing different disciplines.

The process of determining the business viability of offering hospital-affiliated outpatient rehabilitation services may sometimes exclude a number of views. The lawyers involved, however, must take into account all those other persons who have different, sometimes unfriendly, views as they attempt to advise those developing outpatient rehabilitation programs. Like other professionals, attorneys can best do their jobs when they also are able to see the situation before them through the eyes of their opponents or their clients' antagonists. Otherwise, the program itself might be developed and marketed, but dire results might occur. For example, a competitor might be able to enjoin the provider from rendering a particular service by taking the provider to court. This could happen because the planners failed to recognize antitrust or certificate-of-need (CON) problems beforehand or failed to consult legal counsel in a timely fashion. Alternatively, the provider of outpatient rehabilitation services may offer the services, only to find out that no one will pay for them or that payers are slow in paying for one reason or another. Exploring the right legal alternatives first when developing an outpatient rehabilitation program will often determine who succeeds and who fails.

This chapter begins by discussing the various legal alternatives for organizing an outpatient rehabilitation program. Then the various corporate structure alternatives for organizing an outpatient rehabilitation program are described, including joint ventures and other legal options. Federal income tax factors or variables are also analyzed, as well as some of the general principles of the Medicare/Medicaid antifraud and abuse rules. The chapter then discusses various types of laws that might affect program planning.

Corporate Structures

Before the advent of multicorporate structures through the many hospital corporate restructurings of the 1970s and 1980s, hospital-based, hospital-sponsored, and hospital-affiliated activities were typically similar in the structuring of the entity. Today, they are not. Instead, through alternative corporate structures health care systems, including hospitals, are able to offer outpatient rehabilitation services in several ways, which can help ensure:

1. Greater flexibility for governance and/or management
2. Better payer positioning for better reimbursement or more competitive prices
3. Lawful avoidance of CON regulation
4. Sheltering of needed assets
5. Formation of capital in ways otherwise subject to confiscatory regulation that will not be offset through health care regulation

The various corporate structure alternatives for operating hospital-sponsored or hospital-affiliated outpatient rehabilitation programs include the following:

- Corporate divisions of hospitals
- Tax-exempt human services corporations
- For-profit taxable corporations
- Tax-exempt joint ventures
- Taxable joint ventures
- Joint taxable corporations
- "Captive" professional corporations

Corporate structures range from the very simple to the fairly complex, and they have only a few characteristics in common. They all point out the absolute need for clearly stated goals and objectives and for a business plan with realistic *pro forma* financial statements before an enterprise is launched.

The Corporate Hospital Division

Many people do not understand what a corporate hospital division is—at least from a legal standpoint. Legally, a division is not an entity at all, but an *operation* of a corporation. A *division* is an identifiable operation within a corporate structure that is capable of being accounted for separately and even managed and planned for separately. It is not unusual, for example, to find four hospitals, two nursing homes, two home health agencies, and a comprehensive outpatient rehabilitation facility (CORF) all being operated as *divisions* of the same corporation. Divisions may lawfully operate under their own names as long as their true status is disclosed, as in Presbyterian-St. Luke's Hospital, *a division of* Rush-Presbyterian-St. Luke's Medical Center.

However, just because an outpatient rehabilitation program is operated as a division of a corporation that also operates a hospital does not mean that the rehab program is a hospital-based outpatient program. That would be strictly an issue of the *intention* of the hospital and its willingness to have the applicable hospital licensure, accreditation, or payment standards apply to the outpatient activity. In fact, many hospitals conduct outpatient activities on a so-called satellite basis, in which they never quite decide whether a patient in the program is a *hospital patient*. This point is a critical distinction to draw. Regardless of where the program is located physically, if an outpatient is assigned a hospital outpatient number, has a medical record that meets all the licensure and accreditation requirements of a hospital outpatient's medical record, and is billed by the hospital for hospital outpatient services, few will disagree that the program is a hospital-based outpatient program or that the patient is a hospital outpatient. Nonetheless, the laws of some states require that the activity not be treated as a hospital outpatient activity unless special licensure requirements are met for each site.

On the other hand, if the activity is merely being conducted by the corporation that also operates a hospital, the patients are not identified as hospital outpatients, hospital outpatient medical records are not kept for the patients, and none of the indicia of hospital outpatients' status are met, then the activity may be totally unlicensed and may "fall through the cracks" from a regulatory point of view. Hospitals are well advised not to enter into programs without a complete analysis of the legal standards applicable to all patients in such programs and of whether these standards are obligatory or discretionary.

An additional important point needs to be made regarding treatment of the outpatient rehabilitation program as a hospital division. Hospital-based outpatient services are sometimes reimbursed or paid for differently than are other ambulatory services, usually through the authorization to add appropriately allocated hospital overhead to the fees or cost reports of the ambulatory care provider. The decision to treat the ambulatory program as a hospital outpatient program cannot be either assumed or taken lightly.

The Tax-Exempt Human Services Corporation

Exempt human services means exemption from federal taxation under §501 of the Internal Revenue Code, usually under Code §501(c)(3). Status as an exempt human services corporation can only be attained by an organization which is both organized and operated exclusively for charitable, educational, scientific (or religious) purposes, and otherwise meeting the stringent provisions of that code section.

Probably the most frequent use of this stand-alone corporate format would be for home health agencies, which, under the laws of most (but not all) states, can receive a license to conduct that business. As long as the organizational documents and the actual operations of the entity show that it will engage in charitable activities (educational, scientific, or religious grounds are utilized less frequently), the organization is entitled to exemption from federal taxation.

When the activity is hospital affiliated and it is deemed important for the operation to be owned or controlled by a hospital or one of its corporate affiliates, the exempt human services corporation may be the logical corporate format.

In order for the not-for-profit corporation to obtain federal tax-exempt status, it must show either (a) that it is, through its organization and its operations, charitable, educational, or scientific (usually medical research), or (b) that its operations are substantially related to another tax-exempt organization, such as an affiliated tax-exempt hospital. If one of the tactical purposes of locating the activity in a separate corporation from the tax-exempt hospital, however, is to avoid a form of regulation (CON, rate setting, and so forth) that would be applicable to the hospital, declaring that the outpatient human services corporation exists to support the hospital may have the legal effect of obtaining tax-exempt status but losing the argument for avoiding health industry regulation.

Lawyers would generally prefer not to advise utilizing a corporate format that might be enjoinable even though the regulatory agencies are overworked, understaffed, and underbudgeted for compliance activities. In other words, don't use a legally questionable format just because someone else has thus far avoided legal problems while doing so. In the past 10 years, the health care world has seen a proliferation of freestanding not-for-profit and tax-exempt corporations that have been utilized in unlicensed form to conduct the affairs of licensed professionals on an outpatient basis within integrated health care systems. Many such organizations have little or no legal organizational basis and would be hard to defend legally, but they exist nonetheless because either the rules are unclear or the rules are often not enforced when they are clear. Oftentimes the violations are not detected because the regulators or competitors simply assume that the hospital is conducting the enterprise.

Exempt, not-for-profit human services corporations can be a viable form of delivering hospital-affiliated outpatient rehabilitation care. However, depending on the facts, they can be in the "grayest of gray areas" legally. Therefore, they should be examined very carefully by legal counsel very familiar with not-for-profit corporate structurings to determine whether there are clear and measurable advantages when compared with their possible legal risks.

Nowhere is this illustrated better than with the CORF. The CORF has no licensure as such, and it only exists in order to receive payment under the Medicare program for outpatient rehabilitation services. It is possible to show that a CORF located in a not-for-profit corporation is capable of being both organized and operated as a charity. However, the absence of the state-issued license is a factor to be considered in such cases, and this helps explain why most CORFs seem to be operated simply as divisions of corporations that also operate not-for-profit hospitals or other recognized and licensed providers. Another reason, of course, is that Medicare-certified CORFs rarely make much revenue in excess of expense and are, therefore, not worth the organizational expense of a separate entity.

There are also nontax and nonregulatory reasons for using a separate not-for-profit corporation for outpatient rehabilitation services, including CORFs. Some of these reasons include the goals of having more accountable management, a smaller or more focused board of directors, and the intention to not saddle the CORF's operations with the managerial baggage of a large hospital. If a separate corporation is used, however, various important corporate design issues must also be taken into consideration.

The legal issues that need to be addressed before selecting the tax-exempt human services corporation structure include the following:

- Whether the functions being considered are licensed by the state
- Whether Medicare coverage is important financially
- Whether a CON is necessary or legally avoidable
- Whether the corporate practice of a profession is involved
- Whether referral payments or other inducements to refer patients will be utilized in any way

The For-Profit Taxable Corporation Owned by a Tax-Exempt Hospital

The single most distinctive organizational element of the for-profit taxable corporation in the context of the tax-exempt hospital is that, unlike the affiliated not-for-profit organizations (which are in effect not "owned" by anyone other than the public), the taxable corporation is actually owned by either (a) another organization, (b) individuals, or (c) a combination of an organization and individuals. When a for-profit taxable corporation is formed, it issues stock in return for the contribution of equity capital. That stock must be registered in the name of an individual or entity (or a nominee for one of them) on the books of the corporation, so that it is known to whom dividends or dissolution proceeds are payable and who votes for directors, as well as for other similar legal reasons. Those individuals and entities all have federal taxpayer numbers, and transactions with them and dividends paid to them must by law be reported under those numbers.

Another distinction is that the value of the stock of the for-profit taxable corporation, which is owned by a tax-exempt organization, is included on the balance sheet of the owning tax-exempt organization as an *identifiable asset,* whether valuated at book value or market value. Put another way, a taxable corporation owned by a not-for-profit corporation is, in some ways, the same as a bank account owned by that same not-for-profit corporation. The value of the stock is available, if necessary, to pay the creditors of the shareholding organization. If the not-for-profit shareholding corporation is required by law to be audited annually (as are hospitals participating in Medicare), there is no legal way to "hide" the value of the stock.

By statute, a controlling shareholder or group of shareholders may ordinarily force a dissolution of the taxable corporation, prompting a distribution of its net corporate assets to the shareholder or shareholders. The dissolution process is much different for a not-for-profit organization, which must distribute net assets after payment of debts to other not-for-profit organizations, typically the not-for-profit hospital or other not-for-profit entity within the health care system.

Selling health care services to the public in itself is not a tax-exempt activity. Unless a corporation demonstrates that it has been organized and is being operated exclusively for charitable, educational, or scientific purposes, it will not be entitled to tax-exempt status. Many organizations that apply for tax-exempt status do not obtain it.

A single for-profit taxable corporation with multiple shareholders, rather than a partnership or unincorporated joint venture, is probably the simplest way of operating such a joint enterprise, particularly if the hospital will be owning a majority of the interests and wishes to remain sheltered as much as possible from malpractice exposure and other types of liabilities. There is an additional problem with the use of for-profit taxable corporations affiliated with tax-exempt hospitals, however. That problem is inurement. Code §501(c)(3) prohibits tax-exempt organizations from doing anything that would permit their net revenues to inure to the benefit of private individuals. Hypothetically, the tax-exempt organization that permits any inurement to occur risks having its exempt status revoked. If, for example, a tax-exempt organization owns 100 percent of the stock of a taxable corporation, inurement regarding the ownership of that stock cannot occur because no private individual is involved. On the other hand, if the tax-exempt organization sells half of the stock to a nonexempt individual or organization, it must thereafter be especially careful on all future capitalizations of the taxable corporation, lest it end up contributing proportionately more in value than the taxable shareholder in question. At any given time, the taxable corporation could be liquidated and/or dissolved, and the taxable shareholder could end up receiving proportionately more for the stock than was contributed to the corporation's equity. This would be an inurement in violation of Code §501(c)(3).

Another problem for the tax-exempt hospital or health care system owning a for-profit taxable corporation is that of unrelated business income taxation (UBIT) under Code §§511–514. Under Code §512(b)(13), when a tax-exempt hospital owning 80 percent or more of a taxable corporation loans money or leases real estate to its taxable subsidiary, the Code taxes the same to the exempt shareholder as if it were a taxable corporation. This is because the subsidiary deducts its interest and rental expenses, and it is not seen as fair that they receive *both* a deduction *and* an exemption. Problems with UBIT require sophisticated tax planning, but they are not a reason for refusing to consider having taxable subsidiaries.

For-profit taxable corporations are capable of the same kind of tax planning that all other taxable corporations are permitted to engage in, even when owned by tax-exempt organizations (with a few exceptions, such as the UBIT rules under Code §512(b)(13) previously described). At any rate, the enterprise has to be very successful before substantial taxes will be paid.

The Tax-Exempt Joint Venture

The tax-exempt joint venture is a legal aberration or an exception to the general tax rule. This is because the general tax rule is that when a tax-exempt organization participates as a partner in any enterprise, the partnership income, if any, will be taxable to it. This rule is based on the premise that joint activities of tax-exempt organizations are not encouraged outside Code §501(e), permitting tax-exempt cooperatives to assist otherwise unrelated tax-exempt hospitals. More likely than not, health industry partnerships will often involve other parties who are taxable. The income from the activity is then taxable as a general rule because it is deemed not related directly and substantially to the tax-exempt purpose of the exempt organization.

Notwithstanding this general rule, however, tax-exempt parties have for some time been able to receive favorable private letter rulings from the Internal Revenue Service (IRS). This includes rulings that in certain cases, partnership income is in fact related substantially to the tax-exempt purpose of the exempt organization and would therefore not be taxable as UBIT. Examples include medical office buildings located next to hospitals to attract new medical staff members and partnerships involving high-tech medical diagnostic or therapeutic equipment related to medical conditions which the hospital treats. Arguably, the passive income from a limited partnership interest is likewise tax-exempt because of its passivity, even without a private letter ruling, but there would appear to be no reliable authority for that position. (Private letter rulings are by statute applicable only to the parties to the ruling and cannot be cited as binding authority in any other case.)

As a result of the ongoing consolidation within the inpatient health care industry nationwide, there is a tremendous surge of jointly ventured hospital or hospital-related activities, including laboratories, medical equipment, and other health care functions, such as those related to outpatient rehabilitation. Some of these are conducted in unincorporated joint ventures (which, legally, are general partnerships) between two tax-exempt hospitals. Even in the absence of a private letter ruling from the IRS, it is possible that, in a dispute, the tax-exempt hospitals might win their case based on the premise that the income from hospital-related outpatient activities for the benefit of both of their hospital operations should be tax-exempt to both of them. There are no guarantees, however, and legal counsel will be very cautious in advising clients in this area.

It would often make better sense to obtain IRS private letter rulings to be safe. Of course, if the jointly ventured operation is projected to be a money loser, loss leader, or break-even operation, under present law this point is moot because no income tax would be payable.

The Taxable Joint Venture

An unincorporated joint venture is a general partnership by definition. The legal presumption under the Code is that its income will be taxable to all venturers in the absence of a private letter ruling to the contrary. When the joint venturers are not all or mostly tax-exempt entities, the chances of obtaining a private letter ruling exempting the income (other than for those cases where the venture is clearly related to a limited partnership) are problematic. It may make the most business sense, therefore, to use the taxable unincorporated joint venture structure for partnerships that include taxable partners in which the exempt entity insists on an active role. Many tax-exempt health care systems today utilize their taxable corporations as the partners in some enterprises with other taxable entities and unrelated tax-exempt entities, declining even to attempt to achieve tax-exempt income from their investment in the joint venture. When doing this, these hospitals concede taxable status for that particular operation or program.

If a hospital-affiliated outpatient rehabilitation program is to be operated in conjunction with licensed health care professionals or other taxable parties, and if the corporate practice of the licensed health care profession is not an issue, most parties involved will generally find that a taxable joint venture affords them the most flexibility, taxes notwithstanding. Thus, many durable medical equipment enterprises (including those developing and selling orthotics and prosthetic devices) will utilize a taxable joint venture format. Likewise, pain centers and sports fitness centers are often most successful when using this format, with the professional services themselves being billed separately by the licensed professionals through a negotiated arrangement. This is also a successful format for managing (as opposed to operating) the practice of an outpatient health care professional (such as one or more physical therapists), so long as the management fee is structured in a way that avoids the implication that the unlicensed management corporation is itself practicing physical therapy or splitting fees with a professional.

Where states have statutes governing licensed health care professionals that prohibit fee splitting in connection with their practices, it is important to structure fee arrangements in connection with management contracts that will successfully overcome any likely legal scrutiny. Again, the best structure is often a taxable joint venture.

A taxable joint venture is an unincorporated entity, with the result that the taxes on the net income from the joint venture, if any, are paid not by the joint venture itself, but by the joint venturers. This format has the advantage of totally avoiding federal taxation at the venture level and passing the tax results to the investors. This in turn affords a great deal of flexibility for tax planning for most parties to the joint venture and avoids the double taxation (corporation and shareholder levels) that results from corporate dividends.

The taxable joint venture also permits buying in and out of the enterprise to include new parties or allow others to withdraw from the enterprise, all of which should be spelled out specifically in the joint venture agreement.

Conversely, this structure may be a disadvantage to the hospital because of the ease with which a general partner or joint venturer can ordinarily terminate the venture and retrieve his or her proportional share of the assets. Great care should be taken in negotiations and in drafting joint venture agreements to avoid this problem, which is often solved with a reasonable noncompetition covenant.

The Joint Taxable Corporation

The joint taxable corporation is owned by multiple shareholders. Some shareholders may be taxable individuals or organizations, and some may be tax-exempt organization shareholders. A joint taxable corporation also allows for a mix of majority and minority shareholders. A joint taxable corporation might be developed when an entity is required to serve in a role that avoids personal liability for the shareholders, but where most of the benefits of the relationship might come through other structured relationships in the course of business, such as provider contracts or a related unincorporated joint venture. Joint taxable corporations are often created to manage a professional enterprise or serve as a broker for managed health care, neither of which functions is necessarily highly capitalized.

From a tax planning point of view, this is a less valuable format than the taxable joint venture because the joint taxable corporation presents another level of taxation and will not qualify for the pass-through tax treatment afforded to unincorporated partnerships, joint ventures, or "subchapter S" corporations as long as any of the shareholders is a corporation.

The purchase of a minority interest is made on great faith that the minority shareholder(s) will be treated well and that the profits, if any, will somehow eventually redound proportionately to the benefit of the minority shareholder. If this is doubtful and the minority interests seem unlikely to be profitable, the hospital affiliate is well advised to buy or retain at least 51 percent of the stock in all events. A 50 percent interest can always be deadlocked by the other 50 percent.

Joint taxable corporations should be approached very carefully in order to avoid making an uncontrollable investment and to avoid both (a) inurement in favor of nonexempt shareholders and (b) UBIT to the tax-exempt shareholder. Remember that when someone else wants control of a joint venture, he or she generally has a good reason for wanting that control.

Captive Professional Corporation

The term *captive professional corporation,* though used frequently, is troublesome. It is probably more wisely termed the *friendly professional corporation.* Generally, professional service corporations are intended by the legislature to be owned by professionals and no one else. Their enabling statutes so provide. In many cases, the interests of physicians or other licensed health care professionals and hospitals are ancillary to and not inconsistent with regard to a proposed enterprise, such as an outpatient rehabilitation facility, which could be mutually beneficial to both groups. Where their interests are similar, and unless the arrangement is expressly forbidden by law, it is appropriate for a hospital or hospital affiliate to enter into a friendly professional corporation agreement with a professional service corporation or other legal structure owned and controlled by physicians or other licensed professionals. As an example, a hospital or hospital-affiliated corporation might agree to manage the outpatient rehabilitation practice of one or more licensed professionals having a specified relationship or agreement with the hospital. Thus, the hospital's medical director or vice-president might be willing to purchase stock in a professional service corporation and to operate it strictly in accordance with state law, while agreeing at the same time in writing only to transfer the stock to other specified licensed professionals in the event of retirement, loss of license, and so forth. However, the decision should be based on whether the relationship or agreement between the hospital and the physician or licensed professional is legally in order, under the laws of the applicable state. If it is, negotiating an arrangement through which licensed individuals form a professional corporation and operate it in accordance with their own interests would not be in violation of the letter or spirit of the applicable Professional Service Corporation Act. Purchasing management (as opposed to governance) from another source is a generally acceptable practice throughout the health care industry and professions.

It is important to ensure in the contractual documents of the professional service corporation that the licensed professionals who own and govern it are likely to be friendly to the hospital or its affiliates by specifying clearly the rights and responsibilities of each.

Many licensed professionals are willing to enter into negotiated arrangements with affiliates of hospitals where they perceive that their own professional service corporations receive financial or operational advantages as a result. Those advantages may include lower rent in a strategically located medical office building, an exclusive agreement to operate an outpatient rehabilitation facility for the hospital, or any number of other, additional arrangements that are both ethical and lawful.

Federal Income Tax Factors

There is no black and white when it comes to the federal income tax treatment of hospital-affiliated outpatient rehabilitation programs. How a program will be taxed, or if it will be taxed, depends on a number of very important variables or factors, specifically, the following:

1. The nature of the function being conducted
2. Whether or not the function is an integral part of the operations of a tax-exempt hospital or another exempt organization
3. Whether there is a charitable, educational, or scientific element that dominates the function
4. Whether, in addition to the proposed function, there is substantial income unrelated to any exempt function
5. Whether any or all of the venturers or partners are taxable
6. Whether, for those that are taxable, tax planning is a matter of importance
7. Whether any of the corporate transaction issues might apply (such as tax-loss carryovers, corporate liquidations, and so forth)

A key piece of advice: It always makes better sense first to structure an outpatient rehabilitation program in the way that will make the most business sense and will get the best operational results and *then* to see what the tax implications will be, rather than to try to structure a business *simply* for a tax reason.

Medicare/Medicaid Antifraud Provisions

One of the most troublesome legal problems confronting the health industry today is the exposure many parties have to the Medicare and Medicaid antifraud and abuse statutes. The problem is a classic example of frustrating regulation in the health industry.

In 1972 and again in 1977, Congress passed and strengthened the antifraud and abuse provisions of the Medicare and Medicaid statutes. These provisions make it a federal felony to give or receive, either directly or indirectly, any payment, remuneration, or other consideration of value in return for the referral of patients who would be reimbursed in whole or in part under Medicare or Medicaid. In 1972 and 1977, the overwhelming majority of payment for Medicare and Medicaid services to health care providers was based on reimbursement of their reasonable costs (except for physicians, who were paid their usual and customary charges). Under such circumstances, it made good sense to prohibit arrangements by which providers or middlemen were being paid to involve people in the Medicare programs, because that had the effect of simply incurring more costs for the federal and state governments.

In 1983, most of the Medicare inpatient hospitalization programs went to prospective payment. Since then, many other aspects of the Medicare and Medicaid programs have evolved away from true cost reimbursement, with the result that referral fees cannot profitably be built into the costs of providers as they were formerly by some, and with the further result that referral fees generally will not increase the amounts paid by the Medicare or Medicaid programs (assuming that only necessary care is rendered).

Unfortunately, it is not clear enough under these criminal statutes what intent needs to be present in order for a referrer or beneficiary of a referral to be capable of being convicted. The components of the violation other than intent are fairly clear and are so broad as to cover virtually any conduct. Generally, as long as the referral payments given are made even in *part* for the referral of Medicare or Medicaid patients, a violation of these statutes can be found to exist by the courts.

It must be emphasized that the sanctions under these statutes are criminal, involving fines and imprisonment or both, as well as civil, involving exclusion from the Medicare program and payments back to Medicare. It must also be emphasized that not all such statutes are clear to the layperson. It is a constitutional principle of law that all criminal statutes must be clear enough on their face to be understandable by the persons to whom they apply; if not, they may be voided for vagueness by the courts. Of course, no health care provider wishes to be the test case for whether the antifraud and abuse statutes are vague. It is best to seek legal advice before swimming in unknown waters.

Some states have enacted legislation generally prohibiting the referral of medical or health care patients for a fee. This type of constraint can apply strictly to Medicaid patients, regardless of payment for some form of services. Unfortunately, although apparently well intentioned and aimed at prohibiting ethics violations and rising costs in health care, these laws do not realistically address the fact that health care providers and professionals are being forced to compete in ways hardly thought possible a few years ago. The message is: Compete, but not like other businesses.

It is because of laws like these that lawyers are important parties to planning outpatient rehabilitation services. Planners and sponsors of outpatient rehabilitation services need to know about these laws and to get written advice from their attorneys on how to operate in order not to violate them.

State Laws

From the incipiency of our republic, health care has been thought of legally as essentially a local function. Reserving nonfederal matters to the states through the Tenth Amendment ensures that state laws will provide an almost infinite combination of rules and constraints in health care. As a result, there are 50 possible differing standards regarding the legal aspects of hospital-sponsored outpatient rehabilitation facilities. For the physical therapist practicing only in Springfield, Illinois, this may not be of great significance, but to the same professional practicing in East St. Louis, Illinois, the differences between Missouri and Illinois law may be of great importance, because his or her patients may come from both states. Moreover, for that multistate chain of facilities offering any of the different types of outpatient rehabilitation services at its various locations, the variety of state laws must always be taken into consideration in anticipating and solving legal problems.

When planning an outpatient rehabilitation program, it is valuable to know what kinds of related or seemingly interchangeable activities might be legally prohibited. The primary state law impediments/factors to offering outpatient rehabilitation services are as follows:

- There are prohibitions concerning the unlicensed corporation of a licensed profession.
- There are prohibitions on professional fee splitting.
- Being Medicare-certified as a CORF is no guarantee of receiving licensing, despite some illusions to the contrary.
- Medical societies in most states are generally very successful in obtaining special legislation or administrative rulings helpful to physicians when they believe their interests require the same. These rulings may affect how or whether hospitals can set up a program.

The unlicensed corporate practice of a licensed health care profession could be a legal problem. Essentially, most states have permitted licensed professionals to practice their profession in a corporate form, but only with certain stringent statutory qualifications. For example, under the Illinois Professional Service Corporation Act and the Illinois Medical Corporation Act, all shareholders and most officers and directors must be members of the same licensed profession if the professionals wish to practice their profession in corporate form. This means that a professional service corporation in Illinois cannot have a physician shareholder and a physical therapist shareholder at the same time. It also means that a regular business corporation would be a legally inappropriate and enjoinable way for a hospital to try to conduct the affairs of an outpatient rehabilitation services organization. It is important to understand that a standard business corporation ordinarily may *not* engage in the practice of a licensed profession.

Another way in which state law affects health care practices is through anti–fee-splitting legislation. These laws generally restrict the way certain forms of businesses operate and share fees among different professional individuals. For example, the anti–fee-splitting provisions of the Illinois Medical Practice Act proscribes activities by which physicians are precluded on penalty of loss of license from simply splitting the proceeds of profits of their medical practice with nonphysicians such as physical therapists, or for that matter with other physicians who have not earned the split fee. This is an important legal issue. No physician will want to enter into an arrangement that could cause the loss of his or her medical license. Ordinarily, the party splitting the fees with the licensed professional is not penalized the way the licensed professional is. However, having a business arrangement fall apart because of a material illegality is hardly a way to ensure the operation of a successful business.

To understand the interaction between federal and state law, it is critical to understand that CORF Medicare certification means very little under state law. As an example, a CORF might be entitled to Medicare certification, but at the same time be enjoinable in court by virtue of practicing a licensed profession in unlicensed corporate form or by virtue of violating the fee-splitting or other state law prohibitions applicable to the professionals involved. Comprehensive outpatient rehabilitation facilities have unique federal law statutes enabling them under the Medicare laws to receive payment for outpatient rehabilitation services that are comprehensive and generally meet the conditions of participation (see chapter 7). Essentially, a CORF may receive both a *facility* fee and a *professional* fee (computed as a single fee).

The long and the short of all this is that the unlicensed corporate practice relates to the corporate status; the fee-splitting laws relate to the financial relationships; and the CORF certification, for example, relates strictly to the question of Medicare reimbursement for the activity involved. All these relationships and legal definitions must be in sync in order for an outpatient rehabilitation business to be successful.

A last reminder relative to state law impediments: When state medical societies see circumstances developing that appear to be contrary to the interests of their members, they are often able to pass legislation that remedies the problem. There is nothing unlawful or improper about this. It simply means that physicians as a lobbying force have a very good track record in most states. Rather than anticipating such legislation, however, it would seem sufficient at this point to indicate that this is merely a possibility that needs to be factored into the political feasibility issues in designing an outpatient rehabilitation program.

Conclusion

As the beginning of this chapter tried to illustrate, there are many parties to planning and implementing an outpatient rehabilitation program. That is why there are so many legal aspects to making a program work, particularly in the health care industry. There are regulators of every description, competitors, and other outside parties who are always available to help make or break the enterprise.

The legal aspects of outpatient rehabilitation care are many. However, the alternative business structure formats start to narrow dramatically as the business aspects of the enterprise are crystallized. The objective is to eliminate as quickly and as rationally as possible those structural alternatives that are legally infeasible and otherwise not consistent with the proposed business. From a practical point of view, the narrowing of the alternatives will depend not just on the experience and integrity of the managerial and clinical parties, but also on the identity and leadership of the initiating parties.

Those being asked to invest capital into the enterprise should insist on commonsense controls rather than assume that other parties have their interests at heart. If the initiating party is the hospital or its affiliate, it needs to measure early in the negotiations exactly what it brings to the table and whether those components are essential or substitutable. Its negotiations should reflect the conclusions on those points.

There is no substitute for a good business plan, and there is no substitute for experienced management and clinical personnel in making that plan work. The most successful of the outpatient rehabilitation services enterprises are those where real leadership has been asserted, risk has been assumed, common sense has prevailed, and the well-thought-out business plan is based on the feasible legal alternatives available and is scrutinized by an experienced attorney before it is finalized.

Part Two

Innovative Programs in Outpatient Rehabilitation

Chapter 9

St. Joseph Hospital Rehabilitation and Fitness Center

Suzan D. Boyd and Becky Coven

Introduction

St. Joseph Hospital and Health Care Center is a 497-bed, not-for-profit, community, teaching hospital, located in Chicago, Illinois. It serves a diverse catchment area ranging from affluent to working-class income groups and from young working professionals to the largest over-65 population in Chicago. The hospital is owned and operated by the Daughters of Charity National Health System, the largest Catholic not-for-profit health care system in the United States. St. Joseph Hospital is affiliated with Northwestern University Medical School and trains medical residents in various specialties.

This chapter discusses development of the hospital's rehabilitation and fitness center, the program's implementation, its marketing and promotion, problems in implementation, and its evaluation. The chapter concludes with some perspectives on future directions for outpatient rehabilitation.

Background and Development

When the idea of the rehabilitation and fitness center was conceived, the department of rehabilitation services was in the Division of Ambulatory and Ancillary Services and included the following programs:

- Physical therapy
- Occupational therapy
- Speech–language therapy
- Cognitive rehabilitation

- Audiology
- Electronystagmography (ENG)
- Home health physical therapy
- DRG-exempt rehabilitation unit (an eight-bed unit managed by the Division of Nursing)
- Rehabilitation and fitness center
- Corporate health programs (industrial health)
- Skilled nursing facility rehabilitation

The hospital did not identify rehabilitation services as a key initiative in its strategic plan in 1982. However, the potential profitability and merit of such a venture resulted in revision of the strategic plan to include expansion of rehabilitation services. The idea for a freestanding outpatient rehabilitation center was conceived in December 1982, the proposal was approved in March 1983, and the center opened in October 1983.

Internal factors justifying expansion into outpatient rehabilitation services were:

- *Unmet patient demand:* In 1982, St. Joseph Hospital was 90 percent occupied. Rehabilitation services was unable to provide therapy twice a day when necessary. The advent of diagnostic-related groups (DRGs) necessitated development of a DRG-exempt unit requiring three therapy hours per day and twice-a-day treatments when indicated for nonexempt patients in order to facilitate healthy discharge.
- *Unmet and underdeveloped outpatient demand:* Priority allocation of staff and space was given to inpatient needs, and schedules and space were allowed for only limited outpatient use. Treatments for outpatients were scheduled between 8:00 a.m. and 9:00 a.m. and late in the afternoon following completion of the inpatient treatment schedule. Even if more staff had been available to provide outpatient therapy throughout the day, space limitations would have interfered due to high inpatient utilization. These factors resulted in an inability to accept all outpatient referrals.
- *Loss of revenue:* Revenues were significantly diminished by the hospital's inability to meet inpatient and outpatient demand. In addition, hospital loss of revenue might be assumed, following DRG implementation. If inpatients did not receive enough therapy to facilitate discharge, they had to stay in the more costly inpatient program.
- *Physician interest:* As the concept of a freestanding outpatient rehabilitation center developed, physicians thought it would meet their needs and were very supportive. The orthopedic surgeons were particularly interested.
- *Outpatient focus:* The focus of rehabilitation services in the Division of Ambulatory and Ancillary Services was a significant factor in the hospital's initiating development of an outpatient rehabilitation center,

because the division was responsible for strategic initiatives in satellite and new venture developments. The realization that inpatient and outpatient rehabilitation were two distinct products was key in the acceptance of the proposal by the chief executive officer (CEO) and the hospital board.

External factors justifying expansion were:

- *Outpatient health care trends:* In 1983, as it is today, the trend in health care was to place increased emphasis on using outpatient facilities and services whenever possible. At that time, third-party payer reimbursement was being restructured to develop payment incentives that would ensure provision of services at the least expensive level of care. Surgery was going through its initial major shift from a primarily inpatient setting to an outpatient service.
- *Lack of competition:* Market surveys indicated there were no freestanding outpatient rehabilitation centers in the area and that by being first in the market, St. Joseph Hospital could offer top-quality rehabilitation services at low cost and gather a large percent of the untapped outpatient market.
- *Advent of DRGs:* Medicare DRGs were in the process of being implemented. This made it imperative that St. Joseph Hospital make high-quality and cost-effective outpatient rehabilitation accessible. Also, the Medicare population around the hospital was increasing and was predicted to grow.
- *Demographics:* In addition to the projected increase in the elderly population, demand for sports medicine and the growing need for chronic rehabilitation substantiated the need for outpatient service capabilities.

After reviewing the internal and external factors, demand for services was predicted based on linear regression. Long-range demand for outpatient services was difficult to quantify based on historical utilization because utilization patterns were changing. We were uncertain about the source or volume of new referrals. Thus, our projections reflected a conservative but viable growth trend for outpatient rehabilitation.

Program Implementation

A number of factors made implementation of a new outpatient program a challenge. These included corporate structure and location.

The corporate structure at St. Joseph Hospital did not allow for placement of the center in a separate corporation, which might have reduced overhead expenses. However, because the center would be in a separate building, it would not be allocated full-hospital overhead expenses for departments such as environmental services, maintenance, and plant operations.

Location of the facility was crucial to its success. The decision was made to locate the program close to the referral sources. In order to maintain proximity to physician referral sources and ensure continued identification with the hospital, space was taken in the hospital's professional office building, one block from the hospital.

The building houses over 100 physicians and is situated on a major thoroughfare for pedestrian traffic, automobile traffic, and public transportation. It has an ambulance entrance and customer parking across the street. Construction costs for the rehabilitation and fitness center were minimized because the office building was being renovated and provided a building construction standard design for each suite. Total construction costs were below building standard, because the gym area did not require walls and partitions.

Disadvantages to the location were the high rental cost per square foot and the inability to have all the square footage in one suite. Two suites directly across the hall from each other were thus chosen. One suite was developed to include a reception area, a staff office, occupational therapy, and a multipurpose treatment room; the second was devoted totally to treatment booths, hydrotherapy, and a gym. The total area was approximately 2,000 square feet.

Once basic development considerations had been addressed, other operational requirements and issues were defined. The major operational issues were staffing (including supervision, recruiting, salaries, and hours of operation) and financial (including equipment costs, pricing strategies, and billing).

Staffing Issues

Staffing issues in rehabilitation are critical, due to the shortage of rehabilitation therapists and the high costs related to hiring new personnel. Initial staffing goals were:

- To make the most effective use of current professional staff by transferring as many as possible to outpatient facilities, thus ensuring maximum productivity for both inpatient and outpatient services
- To provide enough staff to service our current outpatient caseload and allow for minimal initial growth

Meeting these goals would result in high outpatient productivity, minimal excess treatment capacity, and low start-up costs. Staff would be added as growth occurred.

Management responsibility for the center remained in rehabilitation services under the administrative director. On-site supervision was provided by the center's director, a physical therapist who worked 20 percent of the time in direct provision of patient care and 80 percent in management.

During start-up, rehabilitation services transferred two inpatient positions to the outpatient center (including the on-site director) and added 1.5 physical therapists, resulting in a total of 3.5 physical therapy positions. One position was filled by a rotator from the inpatient area who would spend three months at the rehabilitation and fitness center.

Initially, occupational therapy and speech outpatient demand was low and could be covered as needed by inpatient departments. Although speech outpatients were more easily treated in the hospital, speech therapy was provided at the rehabilitation and fitness center for patients who also had physical or occupational therapy so that patient care would not be fragmented.

Initial staff recruitment in October 1983 was not difficult. The new off-site facility provided the opportunity to work with general ambulatory and orthopedic patients. This group of patients attracted greater professional interest than the older, more acute inpatient caseload.

Staff salaries were to be the same as inpatient staff salaries. However, due to difficulty in recruiting staff for the 11:00 a.m. to 7:30 p.m. shift, the center instituted a $.90 per hour shift differential, equivalent to the hospital night nursing shift differential for that position.

The rehabilitation and fitness center selected hours of operation from a survey completed by the current outpatient caseload. That survey indicated that the hours should be from 7:30 a.m. to 7:30 p.m., Monday through Friday, and from 9:00 a.m. to 1:00 p.m. on Saturdays. At start-up, one physical therapist worked from 11:00 a.m. to 7:30 p.m., and the director worked 8:00 a.m. to 4:30 p.m. but agreed to adjust her hours depending on demand. The other full-time physical therapist worked from 7:30 a.m. to 4:00 p.m. and the part-time therapist worked afternoons. All therapists (except the director) rotated Saturdays.

Financial Issues

Once staffing issues were resolved, financial considerations were addressed. The expenditure of funds related to start-up were divided into capital and noncapital costs. The capital equipment determined to be essential was based on clinical needs of the current caseload. Total capital costs were $82,000. This figure included $38,000 donated to purchase a Kin-Com (computerized exercise equipment). Costs for noncapital supplies were based on approximately one month's expenses for patient care and nonpatient care items based on the current caseload.

Pricing strategies were addressed in four ways:

1. An outpatient charge survey was conducted at nearby hospitals.
2. Current costs and charges were reviewed for accuracy.
3. Current patient mix was reviewed, volume for specific types of treatments was determined, and high-volume charges were identified.
4. Potential profitability of the center was determined given varying percents of discounts based on inpatient charges.

Services were priced at 10 to 15 percent below hospital charges. Ten percent reductions were initiated for the most frequently ordered procedures, and 15 percent reductions for less frequently utilized procedures.

It was determined that in operating the new center, billing systems should be developed that would be responsible to patient needs but that emphasized cash collection. Negotiations with the finance department resulted in the rehabilitation and fitness center developing a manual system that would readily interface with the hospital's computer information system. Thus, registration is on-site at the center, along with cash collection.

The commitment to make the center's services financially viable required that the therapists give their patients a bill at the time of service. This procedure, in which therapists were directly accountable for fee-for-service, was different from inpatient procedures, and its success required acknowledgment and resolution of negative feelings toward this direct accountability. Failure to handle this transition consistently can interfere with initial cash flow, as it did at the rehabilitation and fitness center. Cash collections can be facilitated by careful instruction by the director and the hospital billing staff being available to provide in-services on the latest insurance and financial information.

Final billing is a function of the hospital finance department. Patient bills are sent out monthly, based on charges written manually on a charge sheet by the therapist and entered subsequently into the hospital computer. These forms are in duplicate so that one can be given to the patient at the time of service and one can be kept in the patient's file. In this way, patients can immediately see the services for which they are being charged. This reduces confusion that frequently occurs if patients receive only a bill from the hospital once a month rather than at the time of service. Reduced confusion results in increased revenue because patients tend to understand the services for which they are being asked to pay.

Marketing and Promotion

After the major operational issues had been addressed, it was necessary to focus on how the rehabilitation and fitness center would be marketed to referral sources. The major marketing goal was to solidify services with our base business, that is, St. Joseph Hospital and Health

Care Center attending staff; and the marketing effort was initially limited to the medical staff. This is also because the management of the rehabilitation and fitness center did not want to make a tactical error by choosing to aggressively market services without the ability to handle referrals effectively. (The center's operating philosophy is to be able to see new referrals within one week and ideally within three working days.)

Marketing to the medical staff was done via informal and individual physician contact. Frequent telephone discussions of patient progress built positive physician relationships. Because responding to any problems in a timely manner is essential, monitoring patient/physician satisfaction became a frequent activity. The quality of care and patient feedback to their physicians cemented the rehabilitation and fitness center's growing reputation.

A six-minute slide-tape presentation was developed to introduce the center to the hospital attending staff and was shown at a quarterly medical staff meeting. The presentation was well received by the physicians and elicited strong interest in the center.

Marketing to St. Joseph Hospital's medical staff continues to be informal and occasionally through articles in hospital publications. These articles have related successful patient case studies focusing on new patient programs such as temporomandibular joint syndrome.

As the rehabilitation and fitness center grew and staffing increased, the decision was made to market outside the St. Joseph Hospital medical staff. In an effort to address the health maintenance organization/preferred provider organization (HMO/PPO) market, the rehabilitation and fitness center administrator met with alternative delivery system groups to discuss center services. Efforts were not fruitful because, for the most part, medical directors or individual HMO/PPO physicians decide where to send outpatient rehabilitation patients for service. In addition, this was attempted in early 1984 when HMO/PPO growth in Chicago was just beginning. Now that St. Joseph Hospital and Health Care Center has multiple HMO/PPO agreements, the rehabilitation and fitness center is receiving an increasing number of referrals.

In October 1984, the center targeted a group of 2,100 orthopedic surgeons, rheumatologists, neurologists, neurosurgeons, family practice physicians, and other potential referral sources in the Chicago area by sending out a "Dear Doctor" letter with a business reply card. However, only one response was received, and this physician wanted information on how she could set up her own center.

The only other attempt at marketing outside the medical staff was a display ad that ran in alternate months in two journals targeted to Chicago and Illinois physicians. The goal, to increase awareness and name recognition, has evidently been accomplished: referrals from outside the medical staff have doubled.

In 1986, transportation to and from the center at minimal cost to the patient was added to center services, as was free parking. Physicians and patients have seen these as very positive patient service programs. In addition, these services add to the positive word-of-mouth marketing that is so critical to the success of any program.

Further efforts at more traditional marketing did not seem indicated because growth far exceeded 1982 projections in the initial business proposal. Outpatient rehabilitation growth for the first nine months of operation was 108 percent above what had been predicted and 66 percent above treatments performed the previous year. The second year of operation resulted in a 41 percent increase in referrals. Treatments at the rehabilitation and fitness center exceeded projections by 59 percent. In the first six months of fiscal year 1986–1987, growth again exceeded these initial projections by 28 percent.

Problems in Implementation

Among the challenges to implementation of the rehabilitation and fitness center were staffing and other problems, including referrals.

Staffing Problems

As the rehabilitation and fitness center moved into 1984, both staffing and program development issues emerged. Staff recruitment became a critical problem as Chicago and much of the nation began to experience severe shortages in rehabilitation staff. In conjunction with the human resources staff, a recruitment/retention program was developed that has been successful in attracting more rehabilitation therapists to St. Joseph Hospital. The program included:

1. College loan payback
2. One hundred percent payment for special continuing education courses such as spinal mobilization
3. One hundred percent payment for national association dues
4. At least $300 each year for continuing education courses
5. Financial assistance for students in exchange for one year of service

These benefits were designed to differentiate St. Joseph Hospital from other Chicago hospitals. Consistent review and revision of the benefits program helps maintain a competitive advantage. In addition, emphasis on extensive money for continuing education allows the hospital to invest in the therapists' professional growth and influence the quality of patient care.

Productivity is another issue (see chapter 3). During the first four years of the rehabilitation and fitness center's operation, actual outpatient treatments exceeded those budgeted each year. In 1983, the first year of operation, the center performed 20 percent more treatments than were budgeted; in 1984, this increased to 90 percent; in 1985, the center performed 89 percent more treatments than were budgeted; in 1986, the center performed 59 percent more treatments than were budgeted; and in 1987, 21 percent more treatments were performed than were budgeted.

Initially, development of the center allowed for outpatient referrals to increase by an average minimum of 20 percent per month. The substantial growth of outpatient business has occurred in conjunction with the center's ability to justify increased staffing by assuring maximum staff productivity. At St. Joseph Hospital, monitoring productivity is part of the daily procedure and is built into patient charges. This is beneficial, as it is easy to compute productivity and assures that therapists are charging their patients. Productivity standards include both direct and indirect time, and thus, it is not unreasonable to request an 85 to 100 percent productivity target. The average for the rehabilitation and fitness center usually exceeds 100 percent every month.

Other Problems: Referrals, Growth, and Space

Although the rehabilitation and fitness center has shown steady, successful growth, there have been and continue to be other unforeseen problems that need constant attention.

One problem that has been present since opening is that a large percentage of the center's volume is attributable to four orthopedic surgeons. This group initially referred 70 percent of their patients. Center staff have worked to elicit referrals from other sources and are now attracting referrals from a broader base of orthopedists and primary care physicians.

A second problem has been difficulty in expansion of outpatient occupational therapy. The potential for growth is present. However, issues related to adequate staffing, physician utilization, and program development need to be resolved.

The last major problem is continued need for increased space. Recent expansion and a move to a new consolidated suite has increased treatment space. However, space for staff is at a premium due to continuing growth of the physical therapy staff.

Evaluation

The rehabilitation and fitness center has benefited the hospital in four major areas:

1. The inpatient rehabilitation department is able to meet inpatient demand more consistently. With a 14 percent decrease in hospital admissions, inpatient rehabilitation had experienced only a 3 percent

decrease in treatments. Hospital Medicare length of stay has dropped and maximum treatment time can be given to inpatients. Staff are able to provide the required three hours of daily treatment for patients in our DRG-exempt rehabilitation unit.

2. The rehabilitation and fitness center has enhanced the hospital's image as a progressive, community, teaching hospital. It has attracted a group of young, nonacutely ill patients who previously were not familiar with the hospital. When the center opened, Medicare accounted for 35 percent of the volume. Currently, Medicare volume is 29 percent, with Blue Cross/Blue Shield and commercial insurance accounting for approximately 50 percent; the rest are private pay.
3. The success of the center provided the impetus for the opening of a work hardening site. In addition to outside referrals, the new work hardening site handles hospital employees and returns them to work quickly and in a more functional state.
4. In the first nine months of operation, the center broke even. During the first full year of operation, the center yielded a positive margin and has continued to do so. The concomitant growth in volume and revenue, with excellent productivity and monitoring of expenses, has resulted in profitability exceeding expectations.

Future Directions

Future strategies for the rehabilitation and fitness center will include:

- Increasing staff productivity through the use of computers for clinical documentation
- Coordinating efforts with the hospital medical staff development office to recruit physicians demonstrating active use of outpatient rehabilitation services
- Modifying clinical management practices to accommodate more stringent third-party payer requirements

The St. Joseph Hospital Rehabilitation and Fitness Center continues to provide a productive and profitable experience for the administrators who spent many hours planning the center and the therapists who provide high-quality patient care. In addition, patients and physicians consistently report a high degree of satisfaction with the center.

Chapter 10

Industrial Medicine Lehigh Valley

Lawrence Goren, M.D.

Introduction

Industrial Medicine Lehigh Valley is part of a freestanding outpatient rehabilitation and sports medicine facility that opened in January 1989 in Bethlehem, Pennsylvania. The other part of the facility is Sports Medicine Lehigh Valley. The facility serves a middle-class and upper-middle-class suburban area. The area is projected to have continuing growth in light and medium industry (including several industrial parks), which serve as sources of patients for the industrial medicine side. Several universities with athletic programs serve as sources of patients for the sports medicine side.

Industrial Medicine/Sports Medicine Lehigh Valley is owned and operated by two entrepreneurial-minded physicians. Lawrence Goren, M.D., a former emergency room physician, is in charge of Industrial Medicine Lehigh Valley (hereafter known as IMLV). Emil J. DiIorio, M.D., an orthopedic surgeon, runs Sports Medicine Lehigh Valley (SMLV). The founding physicians' entrepreneurial spirit, willingness to innovate, commitment to service, and insistence on excellence pervade every aspect of the enterprise.

This chapter discusses the facility and program development, implementation, program elements, pricing, marketing and promotion, problems in implementation, evaluation, and future directions of IMLV.

Development

In 1986, Dr. Goren was an emergency room physician at St. Luke's Hospital in Muhlenberg, Pennsylvania. Dr. Goren had felt for some time that many of the injured patients he was treating needed outpatient care after their release, including outpatient rehabilitation. He also felt there was a need for an occupational health program that would get injured workers back to work and prevent future injuries. He decided to start an industrial medicine practice based at St. Luke's. The demand for occupational health services was huge, and within 1½ years he was seeing 1,000 patients a month. The hospital could not accommodate this volume of patients, either for treatment or for rehabilitation. Further, Dr. Goren's patients found the standard inpatient rehabilitation facilities at St. Luke's to be depressing and unstimulating, the hours did not meet their needs, and there was no opportunity for the kind of one-to-one attention that Dr. Goren wanted.

During this same time, Dr. DiIorio had started a sports medicine practice out of his orthopedic surgery practice, from which he was seeing about 40 patients a day. Dr. Goren began referring an additional 30 to 40 industrial injury patients per day to Dr. DiIorio. The results were excellent, and the two doctors came up with the innovative concept of developing a program that would apply sports medicine techniques to rehabilitating injured workers, a fairly new concept at the time.

The doctors decided to merge their expertise to provide both treatment and rehabilitation on an outpatient basis to injured workers and athletes. Their mission, in addition to healing patients' injuries, was to "light patients' fire" to maintain their health and fitness. They believed that workers (whom they referred to as "industrial athletes"), as well as athletes, needed to maintain their competitive edge in order to achieve maximum productivity, remain in good health, and avoid future injuries. The doctors' own burgeoning practices and the excellent results they had achieved with the injured workers whom Dr. Goren had referred to Dr. DiIorio convinced them of the demand for such an innovative program. The doctors asked St. Luke's to provide space for their new program, but the hospital's strategic plan called for other priorities.

The doctors then decided to form a partnership and build their own facility. They envisioned a building that would house two types of medical practice—industrial medicine and sports medicine—each with its own rehabilitation center. They decided not to seek a joint venture arrangement or affiliation with a hospital because they wanted to be able to move quickly and independently, free from the "institutional inertia" that could prevent them from responding rapidly and effectively to the needs of patients and payers. They decided to remain independent and obtain their own funding.

No formal market research or market needs analysis was conducted. Both doctors knew from the success of their own practices that a market existed for the kind of facility they envisioned. Their own practices would provide an influx of patients, and their Lehigh Valley location would provide continuing access to injuries.

Implementation

With their partnership formed and their decision made to build their own facility, the doctors' next step was to obtain the necessary funding. It was not difficult to persuade a local bank (whose executive staff included some former patients) to lend them the money needed to get started. They estimated that they would need about $300,000 in working capital and about $400,000 for equipment. The major expense, of course, would be designing and building the new facility. All told, including the building, their start-up costs were about $2.2 million.

The main factors in implementation were selecting the site location and design and staffing and the hours of service.

Selecting the Site Location and Design

The doctors had several key criteria for choosing a site:

- *It had to be easily accessible:* This was perhaps the most important criterion. The chosen site was near a major thoroughfare that runs through the Lehigh Valley.
- *It had to have parking available:* The site selected had ample free parking–more than 150 spaces.
- *It had to be convenient to likely sources of patients:* As discussed earlier, the site chosen was in a prosperous, growing industrial area with several nearby universities.

Once the site was chosen, the doctors spent a lot of time, attention, and money on the facility's design and construction. They made site visits to other centers to assess their strong and weak points. They hired an architect and a builder who had extensive experience with medical office buildings. In a brainstorming session, the doctors free-associated with the builder and architect about their goals and what the building should embody. Their criteria included the following:

- The building had to be open and airy, with lots of glass. The ambience had to be upbeat and stimulating, and there had to be abundant views of the outdoors so that patients could focus on pleasant sights.
- The facility had to have the right kind of "flow-through" because the doctors would be combining two different practices and treatment areas. The doctors wanted a bridge leading from each of the two treatment areas to a central strengthening area, where the patients would be merged. Thus the patients would mix together as their treatment progressed. This merging of athletes and workers would foster healthy competition and would be stimulating and motivating.

- Because the facility would house the doctors' offices and practices as well as the two rehab centers, the building's design had to make it easy for the doctors to interact freely with and observe patients as they went through rehab.

The architect prepared several plans, and the doctors chose the design that came closest to what they envisioned. Their involvement continued as the building was being constructed. They made daily visits to the site and requested almost daily changes.

The result was an impressive 45,000-square-foot facility with two stories. The first floor, encompassing 25,000 square feet, is devoted to rehabilitation. In its center is a 3,300-square-foot weight room that is glass-enclosed so that injured workers and athletes have a constant motivating view of weight lifters building strength and fitness. The second floor consists of offices, a 70-seat conference room, and a 2,300-square-foot soundproofed work simulation area. This area is used for demonstrations and for special programs that are developed for corporate clients.

Staffing and Hours of Service

Because IMLV serves about 200 patients per day (SMLV serves about 400) and the hours of operation are long, the staffing needs are extensive. Further, as patient volume increases, the staff will continue to grow. As of December 1989, the staff at IMLV included:

- 6 full-time physical therapists
- 1 part-time physical therapist
- 6 full-time physical therapy assistants
- 2 part-time physical therapy assistants
- 1 hand therapist
- 2 occupational therapists
- 4 registered nurses

For the athletic program, there are:

- 2.5 athletic trainers
- 1.5 aquatic specialists
- 1 strength and fitness coach

The staff also includes 10 clerical employees, 1 full-time housekeeper, and 2 part-time housekeepers. The housekeeping staff handles the facility's laundry.

Industrial Medicine/Sports Medicine Lehigh Valley has been able to recruit and retain excellent staff members for several reasons:

- By mutual agreement, the physicians and the therapists worked out an agreement whereby the therapists have their own subcorporation and thus are working for themselves as well as for the physicians. An incentive plan pays bonuses to therapists based on their patient load. This system, which maintains high patient volume while also providing high-quality care that will bring in more patients, directly benefits the therapists as well as the doctors.
- The therapists are coequal members with the physicians on the treatment team—their professional expertise and autonomy is recognized.
- Ample educational opportunities are provided, including (1) payment of continuing education costs; (2) weekly grand rounds, for which outside physicians are brought in and therapists make presentations; and (3) involvement in the development of special programs in such areas as ergonomics—the study of how people perform work-related movements, through which therapists can receive hands-on experience and knowledge in new fields.
- The facility is an attractive, pleasant place in which to work.
- The facility is successful and highly regarded, and its patient volume and programs are expanding.

The hours of service are 8:00 a.m. to 8:00 p.m. Monday through Friday, and 8:00 a.m. to 5:00 p.m. on Saturday. During the week, the doors remain open until 10:00 p.m. so that patients can use the equipment and so the evening programs can be accommodated.

Program Elements

A major goal in planning the program was the focus on the individualized treatment of each patient. All patient care is individualized; there are no protocols at IMLV.

Each patient is seen initially by a physician, either Dr. Goren or a referring physician, who sends a "prescription" describing the nature and scope of the injury to the physical therapist (PT). The PT evaluates the patient, and then the patient, the physician, and the PT meet to decide on the program the patient will pursue. Thus the patient-education aspect of IMLV's program begins on the first day the patient is seen. The physician monitors the patient's progress by observing him or her in therapy two or three times a week. Outside referring physicians are encouraged to do this as well. Thus the physician's involvement is ongoing, not just at follow-up appointments or at case conferences. Because IMLV emphasizes individualized care and intensive service, the staff is available to patients at all times, not just at scheduled appointments.

Everyone with an injury gets therapy-based modalities, including hot packs, ice massage, electrical stimulation, and ultrasound. The program also includes stretching, both with a therapist and on one's own. There is also a wide range of strengthening equipment. Figure 10-1 is an equipment list for IM/SMLV.

The commitment to education, good health, and injury prevention continues after regular service hours through the evening programs that are offered free of charge to patients and the community at large in the conference room. Examples of programs that IM/SMLV has offered include:

- Skiing
- Jogging
- Running
- The dangers of steroids
- Preventing back injury
- Strength and fitness

Pricing

The doctors' entrepreneurial spirit, confidence, and commitment to high quality extended to their pricing strategy. Believing that "you get what you pay for," they surveyed the prevailing charges in their area, raised them by 10 to 20 percent, and then added more services/program values: more time in rehab, more individualized attention. Their strategy was to provide more services up front and more aggressively, so that even though the initial cost was higher, payers would save money in the long run because patients got better faster and did not get hurt again. Services are priced by modality, and there are no discounts. The physicians believe that cut-rate deals, with accompanying cut-rate service, do not save health care dollars over the long run.

Marketing and Promotion

Industrial Medicine/Sports Medicine Lehigh Valley does no traditional marketing and promotion and never has. There are no glossy brochures, no sales and marketing staff, not even any business cards. From the start, IM/SMLV wanted to stand out as being different, so the physicians and the therapists did their own marketing, face to face.

For IMLV, Dr. Goren targeted companies with over 50 employees that were likely to have major problems with injuries. Team members visited the appropriate person (usually the personnel manager or the health and safety director), explained the services that IMLV offered, and emphasized that IMLV would provide individualized care and would satisfy the company's unique needs with a specially developed package

Figure 10-1. Equipment List for Industrial Medicine/Sports Medicine Lehigh Valley

Type of Equipment	Number
Modalities	
Dyna Sound Ultrasound Units	3
Sonopulse Ultrasound Unit	1
Medcosonalotor Ultrasound Unit	1
Dyna Wave High Volt Galvanic Stimulation	3
Dynalator Combination High Volt Ultrasound	1
Neurotech Muscle Stimulator	1
Portable Programmable Unit for Neurotech	1
3-M Myocare Plus Muscle Stimulator	3
Programmer for Myocare Plus	2
Electro-Accuscope	1
Hydrocollator Hot Pack Unit	2
Hydrocollator Cold Pack Unit	2
Fluidotherapy	1
Whirlpools	4
Work Hardening	
Valpar 1, 4, 8, and 9	
WEST 2A, 7	
B.T.E. WS-20 Work Simulator	1
CAD-TEX	1
Blankenship Boxes and Sled	
Exercise	
Biodex Multijoint Testing and Rehabilitation Units	2
Biodex Cuff Weights (20 lb.)	1
Biodex Free Weights (dumbbells 5–100 lbs.; Olympic weights to 650 lbs.)	
Body Masters Variable Resistance Equipment	
Chest Press	2
Leg Extension	2
Leg Curl	2
Back Extension	2
Torso Rotation	2
Lat Pull Down	2
Tricep Press	2
Arm Curl	2
Multi Hip	2
Calf Raise	1
Pullover	1
Rowing	1
Leg Press	1
Abdominal Shoulder Press	1
Aerobics	
Treadmill	2
Versa Climber	1
Rowing Ergometer	3
Bicycle Ergometer	5
Fitron	1
Uppercycle Arm Ergometer	2

of services. This in itself set IMLV apart; it is rare for a physician to call on potential customers. Industrial Medicine Lehigh Valley challenged companies to try them once. When companies did, IMLV provided top-notch service that ensured that companies would use them again and spread the word about the facility. Sports Medicine Lehigh Valley followed this strategy with university athletic directors. Thus the marketing strategy is based on networking and on providing excellent service and results. The networking is ongoing, as is the commitment to excellence.

The evening educational programs were developed out of a genuine belief that IM/SMLV had a debt to the community; they are tied to the doctors' commitment to educate people so that they can maintain good health and avoid injury. Happily, they have proved to be excellent marketing tools as well.

Dr. DiIorio writes a weekly column on sports medicine that appears in the sports section of the local Sunday paper. This, too, has proved to be an excellent marketing tool.

Problems in Implementation

The problems encountered by IMLV in its first year of operation have been the same as those faced by any rapidly growing business and include the following:

- Finding top-notch staff members as the business grows and the demand for services increases
- Helping staff members to use their time as efficiently and effectively as possible
- Maintaining high quality and a service ethic in the face of rapid expansion and increasing demand

So far, IMLV has been able to meet its staffing needs, which increase along with patient volume, without relaxing standards, and it is determined to continue to do so. Factors such as the program's success, the attractiveness and good design of the physical plant, and the excellent working and financial relationship the therapists have with the physicians have helped to attract and keep good people.

Evaluation

Industrial Medicine Lehigh Valley has proved that its innovative approach of applying sports medicine techniques to the rehabilitation of injured workers and its commitment to high quality and individualized service can be both effective and profitable. Industrial Medicine Lehigh Valley has more than justified its founders' confidence and commitment.

Within less than a year of operation, IMLV served and continues to serve about 200 patients per day. The majority (about 80 percent) are internal referrals from Dr. Goren's industrial medicine practice; the balance are referred by outside physicians and facilities. Workers' compensation is the payer for 80 percent of IMLV's patients. The rest are covered by private insurance. The facility does not serve Medicare or health maintenance organization patients. The breakdown of injuries is as follows:

- 25 percent have back or spine injuries.
- 25 percent have knee or shoulder injuries.
- 25 percent have ankle or hand injuries.
- 25 percent have neck, elbow, or work hardening injuries.

The breakdown by age is:

- 50 percent are aged 25 to 45 years.
- 35 percent are aged 45 to 60 years.
- 15 percent are over age 60 years.

Industrial Medicine Lehigh Valley, after just under a year of operation, is extremely profitable. Its gross revenues are about $225,000 per month, of which about 65 percent is profit.

Future Directions

Long-term plans for IM/SMLV include putting together a network of facilities, all within 50 to 100 miles of the parent facility. The best way to accomplish this, the doctors believe, is by networking, a belief that is consistent with their marketing strategy. Industrial Medicine/Sports Medicine Lehigh Valley is well known within its networking radius of about 100 miles and enjoys an excellent reputation. The doctors have had numerous offers for joint ventures, and they have not yet decided where and how they will expand.

Future plans also call for diversification into such fields as ergonomics, and the doctors are considering developing an ergonomics team. All along, IMLV has provided special programs and services to meet the unique needs of its corporate customers. Examples include a stretching program for employees of Alpo Pet Foods and a back program for United

Parcel Service (for which the doctors videotaped workers in IMLV's work simulation room). Industrial Medicine Lehigh Valley plans to expand these kinds of special services. Possibilities include a training program for plant physicians and a safety symposium for plant supervisors. Ultimately, IMLV would like to develop an industrial safety division to advise companies on safety and injury prevention.

Chapter 11

The Work Hardening Program at the Institute of Physical Medicine and Rehabilitation

Lynn Floyd-Decker and Cindy Couri Behrends

Introduction

The Institute of Physical Medicine and Rehabilitation (IPMR) is a communitywide, not-for-profit corporation chartered by the state of Illinois in 1950 to provide comprehensive rehabilitation services. It is fully supported by fees received for treatment and services. It receives no government or community funding for program support or expansion. The Institute of Physical Medicine and Rehabilitation has received continuous three-year accreditations, the highest accreditation awarded by the Commission on Accreditation of Rehabilitation Facilities (CARF) since inception of that national accrediting body.

The Institute of Physical Medicine and Rehabilitation provides services in three area hospitals (one operating a 26-bed rehabilitation unit), two school districts, several nursing homes, a comprehensive outpatient rehabilitation facility (CORF), a geriatric day-care facility, and the Return to Work Center, based in Peoria, Illinois. It has a staff of more than 180 full- and part-time personnel, including assistive device technicians, exercise physiologists, medical social workers, occupational therapy personnel, physiatrists, physical therapy personnel, psychologists and psychotherapists, rehabilitation nurses, speech pathologists, transportation orderlies, vocational evaluators, and a complete administrative staff.

The Return to Work Center has three components:

- *Vocational evaluation:* This process evaluates an injured person who has undergone rehabilitation and matches them with a new or redefined job.
- *Case management:* This tracks the progress of the injured person from injury through return to work.

- *Work hardening:* This is a therapeutic approach that uses graded conditioning tasks to progressively improve the injured person's biomechanical, neuromuscular, cardiovascular, and psychosocial functions in conjunction with real or simulated work activities, so that the person can return to work.

Because these three programs are so closely related, they are all included in this discussion of return-to-work strategies. However, our focus is primarily on the development and implementation of the work hardening program. This chapter explains the program's development, various elements (evaluation and treatment), staffing, financial issues, and marketing and promotion.

Program Development

In the early 1980s, IPMR established a unique utilization review protocol, which encouraged clinicians to refer patients to a review committee. The purpose of this review committee, which included staff therapists as well as physicians, was to monitor and improve the quality of services provided, both on a case-by-case basis and for the institute as a whole.

In reviewing individual cases, the review committee became aware of a number of important factors that indicated the need for additional return-to-work services:

- Certain patients who had completed rehabilitation and whose therapists had recommended termination were being referred to the institute again, because no alternative services were available.
- Some patients who had incurred injury to one part of the body, and who had received treatment for that injury and then been returned to work, were subsequently reentering the medical system with new injuries to other parts of the body. For example, when a worker who had injured his hand returned to work, he unconsciously adopted an unnatural posture and compensatory techniques to avoid using the hand and, as a result, developed a low back strain.
- We were seeing many instances of the "revolving door syndrome," in which a patient would incur an injury, receive conservative treatment for that injury, return to work, and reinjure the same part of the body. We believed that this situation often occurred because the *cause* of the original injury—poor body mechanics, poor job layout—had not been addressed; only the symptoms had been treated.
- In other cases, patients were returned to work when it was believed they were ready. But because there was no objective system to compare the patient's physical capabilities to actual job demands, the return to work was often not successful.

The vocational evaluation component existed at this time at IPMR, but the review committee's growing awareness of the factors in the preceding list made it clear that something else was needed. Vocational evaluators were performing physical capacities evaluations, but they lacked required expertise in anatomy. Health clubs and exercise centers were investigated as possible referral sources, but were rejected because they did not meet the actual needs of the patients.

In 1984, the center added the case management component to coordinate services for individual patients and facilitate communication among patients, physicians, employers, insurance companies, attorneys, and therapy providers.

Case management is provided by rehabilitation nurse specialists, who review and interpret medical records, assess the injured worker's (the client's) attitude and motivation to return to work, and provide support for the client and his or her family. Case managers can also contact employers to assess job requirements and the possibility of modified job descriptions for injured workers who might be capable, after rehabilitation, of performing a substantial portion of their former jobs, but not all of the tasks.

The early intervention provided by this new program expedited many workers' return to a productive work life and resulted in medical cost containment for the payer by helping to close cases more effectively and earlier. Still, however, it was not enough.

The concept of work hardening was just beginning to surface in rehabilitation literature, and one of our staff members attended a seminar given by Leonard Matheson, the creator of the concept. After further investigation of the concept and its potential application to our needs, we submitted a proposal to add such a program to IPMR's existing services.

Because the proposal could be implemented without renting additional space, board approval was not required. The IPMR administrator approved the proposal to add the work hardening component to the institute's services in 1985. It was combined with vocational evaluation and case management to form the Return to Work Center.

Funding came from IPMR's operating budget, but the hope was that we would eventually be financially self-supporting.

Because the work hardening program would share equipment and interact with the center's other two components, it was decided that it would share their existing space. This space consisted of 1,200 square feet in IPMR's rented office building, which also provided office space for 15 other organizations.

We now use three times that space, having been given approval to expand when our client waiting lists reached nine weeks. One-third of the space is used for administrative purposes, and two-thirds for therapeutic activities. We can accommodate 16 people per session, two sessions per day, in the current space. Because of continued growth, a new freestanding facility of 5,500 square feet is currently being erected, with completion expected by January 1992.

During our first year, we spent $15,000 for both equipment and continuing education for the staff. Because significant theoretical and practical information about implementing such a program did not exist, much of what we did in the first year was based on trial and error.

In selecting equipment, however, we believe strongly that we made the right decisions. The work hardening concept includes an important attitudinal component that relies on "real" work experience. Because it is difficult for most workers to see an analogy between their job requirements and exercise, we decided not to furnish the center with the kind of equipment usually found in health clubs. One measure of the psychological effect is that when injured persons walk into our 3,500-square-foot center, they often look around in bewilderment and ask if they are in the right place. This is the beginning of their transition from viewing themselves as patients to viewing themselves as workers. This has proved to be very important in influencing their self-images.

Rather than providing exercise equipment for workers who need to practice lifting, we chose containers such as bags and crates of various sizes and shapes. Because most of our clients work in jobs that involve manual labor and physical strength, we also have such things as a handjack, an industrial cart, a ladder, a wheelbarrow, a shovel, a sledgehammer, a 50-gallon drum, and very specific job-related items such as a keg of beer or a mailbag.

We purchased stationary bicycles, a treadmill, and free weights, which constituted the bulk of our initial equipment outlay. We also use standardized testing equipment, which we had before we began the program.

Because of our increased client base, we have recently installed isometric testing machinery that measures back movements in several planes. This equipment was purchased for $70,000. However, our conviction remains strong that it is neither necessary nor desirable to outfit a work hardening center with expensive equipment at start-up.

In 1988, we added job placement to the center's services. It assists clients in developing resumes, filling out job applications, practicing interviewing skills, and conducting a job search to identify leads and prospective employers. We use a computerized transferable skills report and labor market survey to find the best jobs available in the local area for each individual.

Program Elements

Work hardening treatment is an all-day, five-day-a-week program aimed at preventing reinjuries, increasing the worker's productivity, and determining the worker's probable maximum level of function on the job (as defined by the Department of Labor's physical demands listing). In the IPMR work hardening program, there are no "patients," only "clients," all of whom are *workers*. This is a critical point because many patients referred to the program had become dependent on the health care system. They expected things to be done to or for them; they viewed themselves as sick, injured people. But to be employable, one must view oneself as a worker. Therefore, in developing our program, the concepts involved in traditional therapy were not only minimized, they were rejected.

There are two major components to the work hardening program: physical capacities evaluation and work hardening treatment. The primary purpose of the physical capacities evaluation is threefold:

- To determine the client's current level of function (based on the Department of Labor's physical demands definitions)
- To determine the physical requirements of the client's current or proposed employment
- To determine whether the client is providing maximum voluntary effort during the evaluation

The program averages four to five evaluations per week at a cost of $350 to $450 per evaluation. The physical capacities evaluation takes approximately five to seven hours and includes review of critical job demands, medical and personal history, behavioral performance, musculoskeletal assessment, and functional and general aspects.

Critical job demands are those aspects of the job with which the client's pathology may interfere, or which would substantially increase the client's risk of reinjury by their performance. They are unique for each client and are determined by comparing the physical demands of the job to the client's pathology. To ensure a clear picture of the physical demands, the worker's description of his or her job is compared to the *Dictionary of Occupational Titles* and verified by the employer. If further clarification is needed, an on-site job analysis is performed.

During this evaluation, when obtaining a personal history, it is often noted that the client has no idea whether his or her former position is available because the client has not talked with his or her employer in months. Initially, when we started contacting employers, we were often the first communication they had from the medical field since the employee's injury, and we were met with a certain amount of skepticism.

Some employers had preconceived ideas with regard to an injured employee; they were disgruntled with workers' compensation and medical costs and felt inconvenienced by equal employment laws. We found that some employers were not receptive to changing practices that had created or aggravated injuries in the past.

We explained that services could only be provided if they were preauthorized by the employer and/or their insurance company. We acknowledged that in some cases the traditional medical model needed a more aggressive phase, and for that reason, our program was established. We explained that the purpose of the program was to provide a full-day conditioning program concentrating on job-specific tasks to prepare the employee to return to work and reduce the risk of reinjury. As a result, employers became more receptive and were pleased to know that the employee was in a work hardening program on a full-day basis and not just sitting around all day.

Consistency of performance, worker traits, and pain behaviors comprise the behavioral performance component. Consistency is determined by comparing client effort during two different activities that utilize similar body movements and by comparing the client's effort during easy versus more strenuous tasks. Worker traits are attributes essential in the workplace such as punctuality, cooperation, and follow-through of instructions. The frequency and intensity of demonstrated pain behaviors are compared from one activity to another and to their pathology. These results help to quantify and lend insight into the client's image of himself or herself as a worker.

The musculoskeletal assessment component of the evaluation assesses strength, flexibility, and mobility, providing a baseline with which to compare the results of the functional component.

During the functional aspects component, the client is instructed and evaluated on various lifts, carrying, and pushing–pulling as well as job-specific tasks. Specific test procedures have been developed for each activity to ensure that objective data can be produced by any therapist and to provide test–retest reliability. Each activity is started with "no load" and weight is added based on the client's tolerance. Maximum performance is determined when the client feels he or she has reached his or her limit, the therapist decides the client should stop (for example, because of poor body mechanics), and/or any restrictions or limitations previously requested by the client's physician have been reached.

The general aspects component of the evaluation may include determining the reported location, type and ratings of pain, vital statistics, and activities of daily living (including sleeping posture).

Results of the evaluation provide a comparison of the client's present level of function to his or her job requirements, with an assessment of the client's effort and major limiting factors noted. A written report is then submitted with evaluations and recommendations that could include the following:

- The client is functioning at job level and can safely return to work.
- The client has a minor problem, and one or two sessions of an instructional program called a kinetic workshop is sufficient. (The kinetic

workshop is a three-hour session to instruct the client in proper body mechanics and posturing, flexibility exercises, and job-specific problem solving.)

- The discrepancy between the client's level of function and job requirements is so significant that vocational retraining should be considered.
- There were significant inconsistencies in the evaluation, indicating that maximum effort had not been provided by the client during testing, so the client would not be a candidate for work hardening.
- Remediation seems plausible, and the client should be enrolled in work hardening treatment.

On the first day of treatment, clients are informed of expectations, goals, and the consequences of noncompliance. They sign a contract in which they agree to meet the program's expectations in terms of such issues as attendance and so forth. They are given assignment sheets and specific activities and are expected to take the initiative in setting up, performing, and recording in writing the performance of each activity.

Therapists are there to supervise the method of performance, answer questions, and help clients understand the increased discomfort the body sustains during reconditioning. The staff is *not* there to nurture the client in the traditional sense; we focus on increased productivity rather than symptom relief.

Specific methods of treatment for each individual are determined by the therapy team based on the client's performance during the physical capacities evaluation, according to the client's previous or proposed employment, his or her diagnosis, and the physician's current restrictions. As much as possible, the functions and tasks required by the client's particular employment are simulated. In addition, warm-up flexibility, endurance, and strengthening exercises are utilized.

Much emphasis is placed on client education. We believe very strongly in the concept, "If I treat you today, I've helped you today. If I teach you today, I've helped you for a lifetime." Individual instructions are provided in proper body mechanics (with special emphasis on lifting with the lumbar spine in lordosis), posturing, pacing, energy conservation, safety, job-specific adaptations, relaxation techniques, sleeping positions, and biofeedback.

Over time, clients' major concerns and questions have been translated into group lectures. These topics include physiology of pain; anatomy and physiology of muscles, strains, and sprains; stress management; sexual dysfunction; structure of the back; common pain; and anti-inflammatory medications and their side effects.

Staff conferences with all team members are held weekly to review each client's progress and update his or her assigned activities to facilitate the client's reaching target levels of function.

The major components that make our program successful include an integration of disciplines, documentation of measurable progress submitted in a timely fashion, a work-oriented environment, and strict client attendance rules.

Staffing

Initially, an occupational therapist and a part-time physical therapist were transferred from traditional therapy settings to establish this new program. Although their initial evaluations were similar to traditional occupational or physical therapy evaluations, it soon became apparent that if this program were to succeed, there had to be a change in focus from traditional therapy to the work hardening program. It was extremely difficult for the physical therapist to work half-time in the acute care setting and half-time in work hardening, because the philosophies are quite different. The approach taken by the therapist in an acute care setting is initial symptom relief with the long-term goal of curative treatment. However, the focus in work hardening is to determine the client's physical capabilities and increase these to a functional, employable level.

In addition to the vocational evaluators that were already on board and the rehabilitation nurses, there are now two full-time therapists/administrators (who spend about 20 to 30 percent of their time on administration and the rest on treatment), a physical therapist assistant, two certified occupational therapist assistants, a part-time psychologist, and two secretaries.

Because most of the cases we handle involve litigation, and because we are the endpoint of the client's treatment and are best able to assess what the injured person is capable of, we spend a good deal of time giving depositions and participating in court actions. In estimating adequate staff levels for a new program, time for such activities should be included in initial projections.

The staff is cross-trained so that each person is able to perform most components of the evaluation. This is essential to provide a rotation of responsibilities, prevent staff burnout, and ensure a global approach. Personalities must be considered in the selection of staff to prevent "turf" battles.

Financial Issues

The great majority—89 percent—of the program's services are paid for by workers' compensation insurance, which provides for quick turnaround and few disputes. The rest are paid for by medical insurers and the Illinois Department of Rehabilitation Services.

In Illinois, workers' compensation is financed by private insurers and regulated by the state. In other states, the state funds the program and, in these cases, arranging for approvals and payments can be more complicated. Thus, in setting up such a program, it is important to determine how workers' compensation operates within that particular state.

No services are performed until the therapist contacts the appropriate claims representative from the insurance company or employer, explains the proposed services, and receives approval for the recommended services and the recommended duration of treatment. In some cases, approval is received for only a portion of the recommended duration, and thus service can be rendered for only that period.

When the program first started, the time we spent on this administrative task was considerably longer than it is now. Most insurers were not familiar with work hardening, so each time we called for an approval, we had to explain the entire concept and program in great detail. Now, however, the claims representatives are some of our best sources of referrals, and although the amount of a case's paperwork has remained static, the overall time involved in this procedure has been reduced dramatically.

We based our charges on existing charges for work hardening services in our area. At this level of patient fee, the program was operating in the black within six months of start-up, and it continues to be a profit center. Treatment is now $85 per half-day and $140 per full day.

Marketing and Promotion

When the program first started, letters of introduction were sent to all physicians in the county. In addition, a slide presentation was prepared to tell the story of the program. When new insurance companies or physicians' offices were contacted to request an authorization or a prescription, a slide presentation was offered. This was first presented in-house to the IPMR physicians and therapy staff. Since then, it has been presented to safety directors in industry, plaintiff and defense attorneys, insurance organizations, rehabilitation specialists, rehabilitation nurses, and civic groups such as the Kiwanis Club. During the first year of operation, it was presented five times. In our third year, it was presented 35 times.

We have not been very successful in interesting our local news media in the program, but we have found that our growth depends more on word of mouth and a solid reputation than on media interest. In those two areas, our success has been enormous.

Reaction from the medical profession has been very positive, and we receive referrals from 82 physicians. In addition, we now receive referrals from insurance companies, rehabilitation specialists, and attorneys—the very people whose skepticism we had to overcome when we started the program. We also receive referrals from former clients.

Evaluation

After four years of operation, the only serious problem we have is keeping up with ever-increasing demand. We continue to grow at the rate of about 150 clients per year. After expanding our space to reduce waiting time to enter the program, we are inching back up; currently, there is about a three-week wait. We hope that the increased space offered by the planned new building will again reduce that time to zero.

Our patient mix has remained relatively stable—between the ages of 30 and 49 years, 75 percent male, the majority (65 percent) with back-related injuries.

We have reduced the average time in work hardening from 7.1 weeks at start-up to 4.8 weeks, with a related treatment cost reduction of $1,380. More than 240 employers have been served with employees in the program.

We offer a refresher course to former clients in the evenings, two times a year, so that they can review work hardening principles. There is no charge for this course.

The soundness of the work hardening approach is illustrated by our observation that encouraging mutual support among workers, rather than relying on traditional therapist nurturing, does much to promote clients' progress toward returning to work. Those who have been in the program for a few weeks usually encourage and reassure those just beginning. And peer pressure is often a motivating factor in improving performance.

Of the clients who have participated in the program thus far, 50 percent have returned directly to work, 10 percent have been released to seek employment, 22 percent have been referred for further medical treatment, 13.5 percent have been discharged for noncompliance, 3 percent have settled their cases with the Industrial Commission, and 1.5 percent have been discharged due to physician sympathy toward the client.

Most clients discharged for noncompliance are released because of unexcused absenteeism. The contract signed by each client who enters the program states that he or she will be discharged after two unexcused absences. Clients also receive a warning reminder after the first unexcused absence. We view these discharges as positive. Work hardening is *work*, and the client receives a "salary" in the form of workers' compensation payments. The alternatives are sitting at home all day and going back to work. When a client is discharged for noncompliance, workers' compensation benefits are often withdrawn soon after. Because these clients tend to be severe symptom magnifiers, the discharge and subsequent withdrawal of benefits is often just the jolt of reality that is required. The process also weeds out the small percentage of compensation recipients who are looking for a free ride, rather than doing their part in their own rehabilitation.

The same holds true for those clients discharged after settling their arbitration cases with the Industrial Commission. Although these workers are involved in arbitration regarding their injuries, the employer or insurer continues to make payments to them. At the employer's or insurer's discretion, these workers may be referred to work hardening, and those who do not like having to "go to work" every day often settle their cases quickly.

Our Return to Work Center has reinforced a holistic client approach and continues to challenge the health care practitioner's ability to return the injured worker to gainful employment through a "one-way/don't-turn-back" door.

Bibliography

American Occupational Therapy Association. *Planning and implementation of vocational readiness in occupational therapy.* Presentation, St. Louis, June 1–2 and June 28–30, 1985.

Andersson, G. B. J., Worsing, R. A., Jr., and others. Work capacity expands. Presentation, Work Capacities, Inc., Kansas City, MO, Sept. 26–27, 1986.

Apts, D. *American Back School.* Presentation, Hilton Head, SC, May 22–25, 1985.

Blakenship, K. *Work capacity evaluation.* Presentation, American Therapeutics, Nashville, TN, Aug. 1–3, 1985.

Gimbel, G., Tramposh, A., and Blowers, R. W. *Ergonomics in the workplace: practical applications.* Presentation, Work Capacities, Inc., Chicago, Aug. 28–29, 1987.

Isernhagen, S. *Specialties in Occupational Medicine.* Presentation, Polinsky Medical Rehabilitation Center, Superior, WI, Aug. 1–2, 1986.

Johnson, E. W. The back. First annual Rex O. McMorris, M.D., memorial lecture series, Institute of Physical Medicine & Rehabilitation, Peoria, IL, Oct. 17, 1985.

Lett, C. F. *Functionally fit for work basic systems course.* Presentation, Work Capacities, Inc., Pittsburgh, Dec. 1–3, 1987.

Matheson, L. *Work capacity evaluation.* Presentation, St. Louis, July 18–19, 1985.

O'Donnell, R. J. *Objectifying the lumbar spine.* Presentation, Health Education Institute, Chicago, Aug. 1, 1987.

Rancho Los Amigos Engineering Center. *Neuromuscular electrical stimulation.* Presentation, Rancho Los Amigos Engineering Center, Downey, CA, Mar. 20–21, 1981.

Tramposh, A. K. Work capacities. Third annual Rex O. McMorris, M.D., memorial lecture series, Institute of Physical Medicine & Rehabilitation, Peoria, IL, Sept. 10, 1987.

Wadell, G. A new clinical model for the treatment of low-back pain. *Spine* (European edition) 2(7):632–44, 1987.

Work hardening: occupational therapy in industrial rehabilitation. *American Journal of Occupational Therapy* 39(5):314–21, May 1985.

Zlutnick, S. Pain and behavioral intervention. Second annual Rex O. McMorris, M.D., memorial lecture series, Institute of Physical Medicine & Rehabilitation, Peoria, IL, Oct. 2, 1986.

Chapter 12

A Vocational Services Program for Brain-Injured Patients at Sister Kenny Institute

Carol M. Norris

Introduction

Sister Kenny Institute was founded in 1942 by Sister Elizabeth Kenny, an Australian nurse who was a pioneer in polio treatment. It is a not-for-profit rehabilitation hospital located in Minneapolis, Minnesota, and serves as the rehabilitation division of Abbott Northwestern Hospital. Although Sister Kenny Institute is known nationwide for its range of programs for persons with disabilities due to injury or disease, this case study will focus on the facility's vocational services program for people with brain injuries.

Program Development

The number of patients sustaining head trauma admitted to Sister Kenny Institute increased from 30 inpatients in 1982 to 41 in 1983. In response to the growing need for inpatient head trauma services, as well as additional community-based outpatient services, Sister Kenny Institute introduced an outpatient head trauma adjustment program (OHTAP).

The initial focus of this program was the enhancement of the vocational potential and psychosocial adjustment of adults with head trauma. Later, people with many different kinds of brain injury were included, and emphasis shifted to vocational rehabilitation and placement.

Problems with the program quickly became obvious. Standardized work sample testing proved to be too abstract to be used as the sole vocational evaluation strategy for individuals with brain injuries. In addition, existing work adjustment programs did not address the specific characteristics of persons with brain injuries. These programs were generally located in sheltered workshops, where other participants were primarily mentally retarded, mentally ill, or developmentally disabled. It was observed that individuals with brain injuries tended to resist joint programming with clients who were diagnosed with these disabilities. We knew that something different was needed, but we were not sure what it was.

In 1983, we became aware that the Rehabilitation Services Administration of the U.S. Department of Education was offering grants for innovative programs for persons with disabilities. Working largely on the basis of our experience of what did *not* work, we submitted a proposal. The goals outlined for the program in the proposal were as follows:

- To develop and implement a transitional employment program for adults who had sustained mild to moderate head trauma
- To develop and implement a prescreening and vocational evaluation program for adults with head trauma to assess their potential for competitive work
- To develop outreach and case-finding services that were extended to secondary and postsecondary schools, hospitals, community-based facilities, the Minnesota Division of Vocational Rehabilitation, and insurance carriers, and to identify potential participants with head trauma for the transitional employment program
- To establish a project advisory committee, composed of area employers, purchasers of service, service providers, and representatives from Sister Kenny Institute's Projects with Industry placement program (PWI)
- To provide competitive job placement services for adults with mild to moderate head trauma who had successfully completed the transitional employment program
- To develop and initiate long-term follow-up and support services to maintain successful job placement of competitively employed individuals with head trauma
- To develop and implement a training workshop to educate vocational professionals on the vocational impact of head injuries

A major benefit of this program was that patients would have continuing programming when their outpatient therapies were completed. Once they had reached a plateau in their outpatient therapies, they would be referred for vocational planning and become involved in a completely different system, one that extended services into the vocational arena. Patients who may have previously sat at home and watched television all day would become involved in vocational programs based on specific individual goals to be achieved.

In 1984, we received a three-year grant in the amount of $104,219 a year for the development of such a program as part of the Sister Kenny vocational services department.

Program Elements

We wanted to avoid diluting the program's effectiveness by making it too broad, based on diagnosis (head trauma). Therefore, rather than focus on all the impairments in a specific diagnostic category, we solicited individuals having any kind of brain injury that led to cognitive impairment. Our clients are people who have suffered a brain injury that has reduced their ability to perform the tasks they performed before the injury occurred, but who still have marketable skills.

The program consists of clinical vocational evaluation, counseling, situational assessment, and job placement. When a client is first referred to the program, a neuropsychosocial evaluation is performed before any other assessments are made. The purpose of the neuropsychosocial examination is to determine the nature and extent of each client's cognitive impairments so that accommodations can be made in both evaluation and job placement.

Through trial and error, we learned the importance of doing this procedure first. If a client undergoes vocational testing and performs work samples before neuropsychosocial testing is done, any poor performance may be due to factors other than the simple inability to perform. For example, if the brain injury has resulted in an impairment in understanding spoken language and the instructions for the evaluation are spoken rather than written, the client may perform poorly because he or she did not understand the instructions. If this client had received the instructions in writing, he or she might have performed better on the evaluation.

The neuropsychosocial examination is followed by a vocational evaluation to determine the client's current aptitude, skills, and interests. In this evaluation, we use commercially available, standardized work samples manufactured by VALPAR. Each sample duplicates some part of a job. For example, one work sample tests the individual's ability to do rapid manual manipulations on a moving part—duplicating assembly-line work. All VALPAR work samples include scores for variables such as speed and accuracy that have been established based on nationwide norms and against which the individual can be graded.

The next step is to perform a situational assessment. The client is placed in some kind of "real-work" job situation within Sister Kenny Institute that would normally be filled by a volunteer. The purpose of this step is to determine not only the client's actual job capabilities, but also the level of his or her psychosocial adjustments, for example, ability to work with others, ability to maintain a schedule, and so forth.

Perhaps the most important aspect of situational assessment is its ability to provide a clear picture of exactly how much accommodation for the client's cognitive impairment will be required on the job. To some extent, we try to rig the job situation to gain this kind of specific information.

For example, one of our clients was a woman with bookkeeping skills. Her brain injury had made it difficult for her to concentrate; distraction was a major problem. She was placed in a hospital department that needed help with bookkeeping, and the quality of her work was assessed. But we also assessed the extent to which distraction caused her difficulties by arranging for various levels and types of distraction around her as she worked. In this case, we were able to say to her potential employer, "This client must work in an area that is away from major traffic corridors and common areas. She is more distracted by auditory stimulation than visual, so placing her near a window is not a problem." In this way, we were able to take one additional step toward ensuring her success on the job.

When we have learned as much as we can about how the client will perform a specific task, we begin the job placement process. Through Projects with Industry (the federal grant that supports our placement program), we have access to approximately 400 employers in the Twin Cities area. Throughout this process we are seeking a good job match, one where the client can meet the employer's performance standards and the employer can support the employee in the use of compensatory strategies to maintain job performance.

Ongoing counseling is provided for both client and employer to ensure a good fit between the two. If a client is not working out in a job setting, we remove the client and begin a reevaluation process based on the problems encountered in the job.

The number of clients in the program is small because of the selective nature of competitive employment. It is financially feasible to provide these specialized services to a small population because of the vocational services department's primary focus on providing services in other areas.

Placement service is provided through the PWI program, which is funded through the Rehabilitation Services Administration. This service places 230 people into competitive employment annually. In 1987, 43 of them were from the brain injury program; in 1988, 38; in 1989, 57; and in 1990, 25.

We also provide a support group for clients who are working. Originally, this group was run by a consulting psychologist. However, we soon learned that the group functioned quite well on its own and required only a vocational counselor to act as a facilitator, which is how it functions now.

The purpose of the group is to allow clients to support and help each other in the day-to-day difficulties they encounter on the job. Brain injuries frequently have no impact on an individual's intelligence, values, world view, philosophy, ambitions, or desires; rather, their impact is primarily on ability to perform. A university professor who is now working as a file clerk because her ability to perform her former job has been impaired by injury faces many more difficulties than vocational counseling addresses. This group gives clients the opportunity to share their frustrations and successes with others who are facing similar adjustments.

As part of the vocational services department, we were subject to an administrative and organizational culture with which we were already familiar. Because we were working under grant funding, we had no difficulty obtaining approvals for staffing, budget, and program development.

The expectation of the vocational services department was that we would be self-supporting by the end of the three-year grant period, which was a goal we met.

Location

The brain injury program uses the same space and equipment the vocational services department uses. Space includes two large areas, one for the clerical training program and one for vocational evaluation; and offices. The vocational services department was originally housed on the first floor of the hospital building.

In 1986, the hospital was experiencing a lack of space. We saw this as an opportunity to move away from a hospital setting and into one with an atmosphere having more to do with work than medical care. We leased a space in downtown Minneapolis, about 2 miles from the hospital campus. This location, which is in the heart of the business community, is readily accessible to our brain-injured clients. Most important, the location illustrates our philosophy that rehabilitation is not complete until an individual is able to return to competitive employment.

The program is situated in an office building in which our offices are surrounded by those of other employers. No special accommodations were made, except for the installation of an automatic door opener. The building is on a major bus line, has an accessible parking ramp, has on-street parking available adjacent to the building, and offers direct access to a major freeway.

Staffing

Most of the grant funds were used to cover the expense of staff salaries, consultants, and staff training.

The original program staff included a part-time project director (who was the department director), a full-time coordinator, two part-time counselors, a part-time job placement specialist, a part-time vocational evaluator, and a secretary. All these people were full-time employees of the vocational services department. We also used the services of a research and education director, who helped with program evaluations; a psychologist; and a statistician. These people were employed on an as-needed basis.

The project director concentrated specifically on budgetary and financial matters. The project coordinator actually developed the program. The vocational counselors, job placement specialist, and vocational evaluator were involved in direct-service provision, assessing functional abilities, identifying compensatory strategies, moving participants into competitive employment, and providing postplacement follow-up and support.

The research and education director and statistician were involved in outcome documentation and statistical analysis required for grant reporting. The psychologist provided descriptions of functional cognitive deficits and helped formulate a plan for teaching compensatory strategies.

This model was different from prevailing programs, many of which are staffed by occupational therapists and psychologists in their vocational training programs, especially when their clients have cognitive deficits and are involved in cognitive retraining programs. With this particular program, we felt that vocational counselors could easily understand the cognitive deficits and their functional deficits given their background in understanding a broad range of disabilities. These new counselors were provided with many opportunities to develop an understanding of the disability of cognitive deficits. They attended conferences, acquired textbooks, subscribed to journals, and particularly studied material from the National Head Injury Foundation.

The expertise these vocational counselors brought to this program was their understanding of adjustment issues; their training to view employers as customers and understand their needs; and their ability to work with community networks. Initially, the vocational rehabilitation staff collaborated with traditional medical therapists (for example, occupational therapy, nursing, neuropsychology, cognitive retraining specialists) in order to increase the team's understanding of this disability.

By the end of the third year of operation, we had made some staff changes. The jobs of the program director and program coordinator were combined into one full-time position. The part-time vocational evaluator become a full-time employee. We began to use a neuropsychologist in place of the psychologist, and we eliminated the statistician's role, which was largely required by the conditions of the grant.

It is important to note that most of the individuals who staffed the original program are still part of the current staff, despite the conventional wisdom that people who work with brain-injured individuals will burn out quickly. We believe that our staff has remained—and remained productive—at least partly because this is a newly developing and interesting field and we provide for as much continuing education in this area as each staff person desires.

Financial Issues

The vocational services department is different from other hospital departments in that all its services are preauthorized and paid 100 percent. The Minnesota Department of Rehabilitation Services (DRS) negotiates an operating agreement annually with the department. Once that agreement has been approved, the state DRS pays the negotiated fees.

The Veterans Administration (VA) negotiates fees and pays the same prices as DRS. Minnesota's Department of Workers' Compensation does not negotiate an operating agreement, but does pay 100 percent of preauthorized fees, using the same guidelines as those used by DRS and the VA. Except for those provided by the job placement component of the program, all services are paid for by third parties. Job placement operates under a federal grant, which allows us to provide this service free of charge to all participants deemed qualified by the Department of Rehabilitation Services.

Marketing and Promotion

When this program was developed, there were no competitors in the geographic area providing vocational rehabilitation services to people with brain injuries. In recent years, many other programs have been developed. However, our program continues to be viewed as maintaining specific expertise. We have established a particular niche in the continuum of services in that our program focuses on returning people to competitive employment. Other programs, developed by area competitors, have focused on supported employment, community-based employment, subminimum wage programs, job coaching, independent living services, and residential programs. Periodically, we are confronted with a philosophical limitation in that some referral sources do not want a vocational evaluation. In those instances, we try to educate the referral source regarding the value of a vocational evaluation and the benefits that can accrue to the client.

Because of the specialized nature of the program, we find ourselves marketing it more to referral sources than potential clients. We held a seminar for rehabilitation specialists and health care providers to educate them on brain injuries. This was necessary because patients with inappropriate diagnoses for the program (for example, those with seizures) were being referred to us.

Other marketing techniques—attending conferences, having booths at conferences, and mailings, for example—are handled by the vocational services department.

Evaluation and Future Directions

An unexpected benefit of this program's operation has been the development of additional community services. Four years after we received our grant, an entire spectrum of community services directed specifically to the needs of individuals with cognitive deficits caused by brain injury is available in the Twin Cities. These services not only provide healthy competition for existing programs and continuing motivation to improve services, but they also provide a sufficient range of services so that both low- and high-functioning individuals can find programs suitable to their functioning level.

Considerations for the future include some kind of blending of medical and vocational services within Sister Kenny Institute. The fact that the payers for the two types of service are different (with the exception of workers' compensation) is an obstacle that would need to be overcome before such a move could be made. The benefit to the patient, however, would be great. A patient receiving medical treatment for a brain injury could begin vocational evaluation and job placement without a waiting period in-between. We are continuing to study ways in which to create a joint program.

Chapter 13

The Professional Voice Program™ at Schwab Rehabilitation Center

Kathleen C. Yosko

Introduction

Schwab Rehabilitation Center, a not-for-profit, freestanding rehabilitation hospital in Chicago, Illinois, has been providing specialized treatment for persons with physical and cognitive disabilities for more than 75 years. The nationally known center is one of approximately 125 freestanding rehabilitation hospitals in the country. Located on the west side of Chicago, it is a permanent affiliate of Mount Sinai Hospital Medical Center.

Strategic planning allows both clinical and medical staff to step back from the daily operations of an organization and reflect openly on the marketplace, financial, and patient care considerations that affect the organization's growth—and often its survival. The rehabilitation professionals must first be sensitive to changes that have already begun to mold the "new" acute care environment. Prospective payment, accompanied by a decreasing need for inpatient hospitalization, has had a serious economic impact on the acute care industry. The result is an environment that has led to the downsizing of acute care facilities, accompanied by an increased sense of competition among providers. The competition has been so great at times that many organizations have been forced to collaborate through joint ventures, mergers, and so forth in order to ensure their economic stability.

However, these changes in the acute care industry have appeared to fuel a boom for expanded rehabilitation services. In a sense, rehabilitation, once a sleeper in the 1960s and part of the 1970s, has become "big business." With the continued exemption from prospective payment, investors, along with a wide variety of rehabilitation providers, have decided to enter the rehabilitation market. In 1986, rehabilitation industry revenues were estimated at $4.5 billion. This number exceeded $11 billion in 1990, reports the Keckley Group, a hospital market research firm based in Nashville, Tennessee.

Along with the growth has come an increased sense of competition among rehabilitation providers. Also, the need for discounting care to private insurance companies – as well as health maintenance organizations (HMOs), preferred provider organizations (PPOs), and, in some states, Medicaid – to ensure an adequate referral base, while maintaining revenues over expenses, has perhaps become the challenge of the decade.

Schwab's highly successful Professional Voice Program™ was one result of a thorough assessment of these issues and an aggressive and skillful marketing strategy.

Program Development

The impetus for developing the Professional Voice Program™ came from the communicative disorders department in 1986, which was receiving referrals from a local otolaryngologist to provide voice therapy for several commodities traders. The traders were experiencing repeated bouts of hoarseness as the result of shouting bids on the floor of the Chicago Board of Trade. The hoarseness was hampering the traders' ability to function effectively, because a trader's voice plays an essential role in his or her livelihood.

The traders received two months' outpatient therapy at the communicative disorders department, while they continued to trade. Their voices improved, and the effectiveness of Schwab's voice program spread through discussions among traders. Within a few weeks, the communicative disorders department received several more referrals for evaluations. Along with the requests for service came an appeal to locate the Professional Voice Clinic site more conveniently for service provision. At that time, Schwab had only the main westside facility and its northwest satellite available for treatment space, neither of which was in close proximity to clients seeking therapy, primarily the commodities traders in the Loop, the city's business center.

The idea of a vocal rehabilitation program aimed at a clearly defined market (people who use their voices professionally) was presented at a 1986 strategic planning session devoted to expansion through outpatient programs and attended by board, administrative, and key clinical directors. The Professional Voice Program™ was viewed as being in concert with the overall mission of Schwab Rehabilitation Center. The program objectives were as follows:

- To tailor Schwab's outpatient specialty and rehabilitation services to meet the needs of a high-profile target market

- To dispel the staid image of rehabilitation services by responding with an innovative and dynamic program to the health needs of an upscale, professional community
- To further enable Schwab to position itself in the rehabilitation marketplace by establishing a reputation for excellence and clinical responsiveness
- To provide an additional source of self-pay and commercially insured patients, thus improving the demographic profile of Schwab's patient population
- To position the hospital as a national leader in meeting changing rehabilitation needs and extending valid rehabilitation services into alternative settings

The establishment of the program received support from the hospital's strategic planning group.

The original product or service of the Professional Voice Program™ was to offer traders an opportunity to learn techniques for maximizing the use of their voices while actively trading and to avoid excessive tension on the vocal cords, which can lead to swelling, pain, hoarseness, and even voice loss. Therapists of the Professional Voice Program™ would concentrate therapy on four aspects of voice production: pitch, loudness, rate, and quality. Traders could learn a variety of preventive techniques including increasing breath support and control, which would provoke less stressful vocal cord vibration. By employing these techniques, traders could continue to shout with minimal risk of damaging their voices.

The strategic planning group determined that in order for the program to flourish, the services should be moved to a downtown location so that they would be more convenient to the target market. Before doing so, the marketing department was asked to perform a thorough analysis of the type of speech services available in the city's downtown and near north areas. Information and data for the market analysis were collected through the American Speech and Hearing Association and telephone surveys with speech therapists in the greater Chicago region. The analysis revealed a total of 30 private and not-for-profit speech service providers in the geographic area, which we had determined to be convenient for access to the trading hub of activity. Despite the number of speech service providers in the targeted geographic area, it was felt that competition for professional voice services similar to that which Schwab intended to provide was minimal. None of the three providers currently offering voice services had been successful at developing either a high profile or acceptance in the trader market.

Refueled with this information, the marketing department set about finding a location for test-marketing the Professional Voice Program™. A referring otolaryngologist offered to time-share space in his Loop office with the Professional Voice Program™. Time-sharing of space proved to be a wise choice, which assisted with revenue maximization by keeping overhead expenses at a minimum. Traders seeking therapy tended to desire their treatment from 4 p.m. to 7 p.m. (after the close of business) or very early in the morning, when office hours for the otolaryngologists tended to be light. Therefore, Schwab would pay only for office time that it needed and used.

Staffing

In keeping with Schwab's approach to all rehabilitation services, a staff person who developed the original program concept was selected to act as product-line manager in implementing the program. This person was a speech therapist with both clinical and business skills.

The original staff consisted of existing Schwab therapists. The staffing level was 1½ full-time equivalents, so therapists who were interested in working in the Loop office would work there part-time and at Schwab part-time.

Many of the Schwab staff therapists were interested in working in the program, so further incentives were not needed. Therapists would be working with a well population of motivated professionals, almost 100 percent cash pay. In addition, therapists who worked in the program were able to attend a variety of trade and promotional shows.

Staff members who worked in the Loop office were allowed to adjust their hours to meet the special scheduling requirements of the program's clients. Thus, if a therapist began work in the Loop office at 7:00 a.m. and then returned to Schwab for the rest of the day, his or her work day would end at 3:00 p.m. In this way, we were able to place the most qualified therapists in the program's offices when they were needed without hiring additional full-time therapists or temporaries.

In programs involving a long-term relationship with a corporate client, our goal is to use the same therapist, as much as possible, in the various programs with that client so that a strong relationship can develop between therapist and client.

Financial Issues

It was determined that the Professional Voice Program™ would be maintained as a cost center of Schwab Rehabilitation Center. Careful consideration was then given to the pricing of services, keeping in mind that all clients would be either self-pay or commercially insured. Payment was to be due at time of service to eliminate billing costs and bad-debt expenses.

Marketing and Promotion

The Schwab Rehabilitation Center approach to growth is that it should be deliberate, but steady. The center employs no marketing research firm, but relies on a coherent and aggressive marketing strategy provided by an in-house department that has grown from one to five people in the past three years.

Implementation of the Professional Voice Program™ occurred midway through the budget year, so funds for promotion were limited. We sought maximum exposure for every dollar spent, which meant less paid advertising, which can be expensive and ineffective if not well targeted. Instead, it was determined that the initial marketing plan would include elements of promotion, publicity, and sales calls.

Booth space was purchased at the Futures and Options Expo in the fall of 1986. This positioned Schwab at the center of thousands of potential clients. The Schwab booth achieved added distinction in that it was the only health care provider in attendance. Free voice screenings were given on location. The booth drew so much attention that a Public Broadcasting System reporter saw fit to interview our therapist and place the interview segment on the broadcast of the "Nightly Business Report." A follow-up mailing was sent to all attendees of the Futures and Options Expo and follow-up calls were directed to those who received free screenings.

A mailing of distinctive announcement cards of the Professional Voice Program™ was made to otolaryngologists in the Chicago market, followed up by phone calls and direct marketing visits. Additionally, mailing lists were obtained and direct mailings were sent to traders of the Chicago Board of Trade and the Chicago Mercantile Exchange. A voice seminar was subsequently requested and provided for the Chicago Mercantile Exchange.

To continue to maximize program exposure, adult voice education classes for professionals began to be offered at private Chicago evening schools for adult lifestyle courses.

The results of Schwab's initial marketing efforts became readily apparent. Within a six-month period, enrollment for individual therapy grew from 3 to 40 clients. Additional revenues were also being generated from private trading houses requesting group training sessions within their office complexes. The need for corporate discounts for individual therapy soon became apparent and was implemented.

Evaluation

The rapid growth of the Professional Voice Program™ quickly allowed break-even and growth projections to be met. However, the shared office space soon became problematic because more clients sought service on a timely basis. Marketing and administrative staff maintained that the key to promoting this seedling market niche was site selection. Informal focus groups among enrolled traders confirmed staff inclinations that convenience of location would be a key factor in traders seeking and continuing therapy. A decision was made to find a permanent home for the Professional Voice Program™ in the spring of 1987.

The new home of the Professional Voice Program™ was strategically located at 327 South LaSalle Street in downtown Chicago, across the street from the Board of Trade and the Chicago Board Options Exchange. The office is finely appointed and has a corporate ambience in keeping with the clients served. The office building offers expansion capability and is readily accessible to a secondary market of other high-risk voice users, for example, attorneys, actors and actresses, broadcasters, and management and sales professionals. Marketing efforts are now being directed to these clients in addition to other select corporate clinical services.

Additionally, because of the rapid program expansion and requests for out-of-state and even international consultation, administration elected to have the Professional Voice Program™ trademarked on February 19, 1987.

From Schwab's perspective, the success of the Professional Voice Program™ cannot be measured solely by revenue milestones alone. As mentioned earlier, one of the objectives of the Professional Voice Program™ was to further enhance Schwab's goals of becoming a national marketplace leader in meeting changing rehabilitation needs. The Professional Voice Program™ joins our other programs such as the *Four Phase Head Trauma Program* and the *STEPS Industrial Injury Clinic* in promoting that goal.

The local, national, and international publicity Schwab has received from the Professional Voice Program™ has been phenomenal, giving us access to free institutional advertising that we otherwise perhaps could not afford. Recent story placements have occurred in the following print and broadcast media, to highlight only a few:

- The *National Futures Association Newsletter*
- The Canadian Broadcasting Company's "As It Happens"
- The *London (England) Daily Express*
- The "Voice of America"
- *Wall Street Letter,* a publication of Institutional Investor
- Dr. Barry Kaufman's medical report on the NBC affiliate WMAQ-TV, Chicago
- The Chicago *Sun-Times* Sunday Business section
- National Association of Rehabilitation Facilities' *Medical Management Review*

- *Chicago Medicine*
- The American Hospital Association's "American Medical News" broadcast

The quality of the Professional Voice Program™ is apparent. A recent unsolicited endorsement by a satisfied trader who had undergone successful treatment in the Professional Voice Program™ gained Schwab story placement in a recent documentary "The Trading Game," on Chicago's ABC affiliate, WLS-TV. The documentary featured the stressful lifestyles of traders, including "life on the floor of the exchange." The documentary highlighted the disabilities that befall traders, including chronic voice problems. Additionally, according to an article in the January–February 1987 issue of the American Hospital Association's *Hospital Planning and Marketing* newsletter, the Professional Voice Program™ "not only provides a service that was hardly available before, it takes the service to patients where they work." Finally, in the marketing section of the September 20, 1987, issue of *Hospitals* magazine, the in-house ad that Schwab produced for the program was reprinted and ran with the caption, "Although most rehab services aren't advertised to the general public, Schwab Rehabilitation Center has created a consumer niche with its Professional Voice Program™."

These are all profitable programs. But even if the profit were marginal, we would be tempted to continue them because of the enormous amount of positive, free publicity they have garnered for Schwab. However, the success of the program has led to some difficulties. Our Loop office needs expanding, and we are seeking effective ways to handle a growing caseload.

The windfall of international, national, and local media coverage has served to establish Schwab as a national leader in providing innovative rehabilitation services. The Professional Voice Program™ has received calls from around the country to provide assistance in establishing similar programs. It has served to dispel the staid image of rehabilitation and replace it with a dynamic identity.

The efforts of the Professional Voice Program™ to achieve its objective through creative and strategic marketing have shown that a carefully conceived health services program can achieve national recognition on a shoestring budget. With innovative, adaptive marketing techniques, the Professional Voice Program™ was nurtured into a high-profile service, catering to the needs of an influential target market while enhancing its overall mission and goals.

Future Directions

Along with expanding our Loop location, hours, and perhaps staffing levels, Schwab has developed several innovative new programs as a result of interest in the Professional Voice Program™. The aim of the Foreign and Regional Accent Modification Program is to help foreign speakers of English working in U.S. corporations speak comprehensible English.

A new program to help professional women speak at an effective level of assertiveness in business situations led to a program for adult women stutterers.

By request, we began a service of five different types of corporate seminars on voice, stress reduction, public speaking, articulation, and foreign regional accent modification. Many of these are offered on the basis of corporate contracts.

The Professional Voice Clinic continues to flourish. Since 1986, the program has grown to such an extent that additional staff and space in a more centralized location in downtown Chicago are now being sought to meet the changing needs of patients.

Chapter 14

Geriatric Rehabilitation at Sister Kenny Institute

Nancy E. Rehkamp

Introduction

Sister Kenny Institute, a not-for-profit rehabilitation hospital, is well known for its interdisciplinary care of persons with disabilities brought on by illness or severe injury. The facility is located in Minneapolis, Minnesota, and was founded in 1942 by Sister Elizabeth Kenny, an Australian nurse who pioneered the treatment of polio.

Sister Kenny Institute continues to be a leader in high-quality patient care, state-of-the-art treatment techniques, disability prevention, research and education, and special projects that enable persons with disabilities to reach maximum functioning and independence. The range of services provided at the facility includes inpatient, outpatient, and follow-up care and programs tailored to each patient's needs.

Sister Kenny Institute serves as the rehabilitation division of Abbott Northwestern Hospital, a 750-bed primary tertiary care center. Abbott Northwestern, one of Minnesota's premier health care centers, is known for its work in perinatal care; cardiac services, including heart and heart–lung transplants; behavioral health programs; geriatrics; neurology and neurosurgery; low back care; and oncology.

Program Development

National trends show that the 75- to 84-year-old age group is growing twice as fast as the 65- to 74-year-old segment of the population. The segment of the population over 85 years of age is projected to grow from 1 to 5 percent of the total population by 2050.[1] According to various studies, the elderly currently represent 12 percent of the population and will represent 21 percent by the year 2030.

Because of the large growth in the number of elderly and the ongoing advances in medical care, it is projected that 38 percent of the 15 million elderly people will be functionally dependent by the year 2000.[2] This makes development of cost-effective rehabilitation to maximize the independence of the elderly an urgent concern.

This need for development of geriatric rehabilitation programs has perhaps been more apparent to those of us working in Minneapolis-St. Paul than elsewhere. The introduction of the Medicare prospective payment system (PPS), the dramatic expansion of Medicare health maintenance organizations (HMOs) in Minnesota, the aggressive discharge review criteria implemented by the Minnesota Foundation for Health Care Evaluation, the increased pressures by payers to find more cost-effective alternatives to inpatient care, and the growing elderly population in Minnesota have forced rehabilitation health care professionals in the Twin Cities to critically evaluate existing programs and develop new ones.

The administration at Sister Kenny Institute recognized early in 1984 that a need to develop alternatives to traditional inpatient acute care and inpatient rehabilitation programs existed. This realization occurred shortly after the introduction of the Medicare PPS, at a time when there was a shortage of rehabilitation beds at Sister Kenny Institute. Patients, particularly stroke patients, were looking for ways to continue, as outpatients, the improvements they had made in inpatient rehabilitation. In addition, families of patients were looking for increased support and education from the therapy staff as they took their loved ones home.

Out of all these pressures came the development of the Sister Kenny Institute Day Hospital Program. The staff believed we could ensure the patients' continued progress, continue the therapy and patient teaching that was abbreviated by shortened hospital stays, and respond to the patients' request to go home sooner by developing a hospital stay that did not include the evening, night, and early morning hours. The staff also felt strongly that many patients needed and could benefit from a structured, intensive rehabilitation program, even though they no longer met the criteria for inpatient rehabilitation.

The purposes of the day hospital program are to reduce the risks of long-term institutionalization, improve the transition from hospital to home, reduce the chances of rehospitalization, and help improve the functional and cognitive status of patients. The program differs from conventional outpatient settings in that services are based on a comprehensive assessment of patients' health care needs and goals, and the program includes nursing care and access to all services available to inpatients without requiring patients to stay overnight.

Program Elements

The stated goals of the Sister Kenny Institute Day Hospital Program are fairly simple and are consistent with our inpatient rehabilitation program goals. The goals include the following:

- To increase the options available to the patient and his or her family within the health care delivery system
- To assist the patient in avoiding inappropriate use of health care resources
- To provide a cost-effective alternative for those individuals who are in need of a continuing rehabilitation program
- To provide a structured, supportive environment and a multidisciplinary team to work with the patient to improve his or her physical and/or cognitive skills
- To provide education and support to the patient's care givers

Abbott Northwestern admits over 3,000 Medicare patients each year; however, it was assumed that not more than 2 to 3 percent of those patients might benefit from and choose to enroll in the day hospital program.

The admission criteria for day hospital patients were established early by a team of physicians, nurses, social workers, and therapists. The criteria required that patients:

- Have restorative potential
- Need an intensive rehabilitation program including two or more rehabilitation services
- Have a physical and/or cognitive disability or illness
- Be medically and psychiatrically stable
- Have the desire and motivation to participate in the treatment program
- Not require 24-hour skilled nursing care, although they may need rest, supervision, and/or assistance by nursing staff, as well as some skilled nursing care
- Have adequate help and support for care at home
- Have prior approval from payer source for the program or have met the criteria and been approved for free care through Sister Kenny Institute's free-care fund

The core services provided through the day hospital include physician supervision and referral to specialists as required, case management and coordination, rehabilitation nursing, social services, nutritional assessment and education, escort service, physical therapy, occupational therapy, neuropsychology, psychological counseling, speech and language therapy, vocational service, and therapeutic recreation. Other services, such as diagnostic testing in the radiology department, laboratory service, and ambulatory surgery, are available as required. Transportation to and from home is provided for all patients.

Prior to admission to the day hospital, the Sister Kenny Institute admissions coordinator determines, in consultation with the medical director of the day hospital, whether the patient meets the admission criteria. The admissions coordinator also obtains preauthorization for payment in the program; initiates prescheduling of the services the patient requires; works closely with the social services department, which arranges transportation to and from the program; assigns a Sister Kenny Institute physician, who evaluates the patient either prior to or on the day of admission; requests written referral information; and coordinates the admission of the patient with the nursing staff.

A patient admitted to the program from the community, rather than from the hospital or institute, must provide a physician's order before or on the day of admission. Each day hospital patient is required to have a supervising physician who is on the Abbott Northwestern/Sister Kenny Institute medical staff. If the patient does not have one, a Sister Kenny Institute physiatrist is assigned after consultation with the patient and his or her referring physician.

Patients admitted to the day hospital have a patient conference, which includes the patient and his or her care givers, if possible, prior to or shortly after admission to develop the goals and establish a schedule for the patient's day at Sister Kenny Institute.

A day hospital chart is established that includes the physician's orders, transfer form, history, physical, evaluation conference report, social services evaluation, acute care discharge summary, if appropriate, and any X-ray or special diagnostic reports that are needed to provide follow-up care.

At the start of each day, the patient is given a copy of his or her daily schedule. Each patient's daily schedule varies depending on individual needs. A typical day includes the following:

- The patient is picked up at his or her home between 7:30 a.m. and 8:30 a.m.
- The patient arrives at Sister Kenny Institute between 8:30 a.m. and 9:30 a.m.
- The patient is greeted at the Sister Kenny Institute entrance and escorted to the day hospital area unless a family member assists the patient or the patient has reached a sufficient level of independence to require no escort.

  Some patients will begin with breakfast and activities of daily living (ADL) supervision by the occupational therapy staff. (Activities of daily living include such everyday tasks as bathing, dressing, and feeding oneself.) Others will begin their daily therapy schedules. Still others will remain in the day hospital space and receive their nursing care and supervision. The therapy schedule includes:

–One to two hours of physical therapy
–One to two hours of occupational therapy
–One hour of speech and language therapy
–One hour of neuropsychological testing and evaluation followed by psychological counseling
–One to two hours of rehabilitation nursing
–One hour of vocational counseling
–One hour or less of therapeutic recreation
–Appropriate time with the social worker

- The patient returns to the day hospital area for lunch. More independent patients have lunch in the cafeteria, accompanied by staff. Lunch is followed by a rest period, nursing treatments, patient education, and more therapy as appropriate.
- The patient returns home between 3:00 p.m. and 5:30 p.m.

Because this program provides a bridge between acute care and independence, discharge planning for the patient begins at admission, when the social worker determines specific plans for each patient. The patient, family, and care givers are involved in this planning. Social services staff members maintain weekly contact with the family and the patient to provide support and assist with any difficulties in the home setting and to ensure that the discharge plans continue to be appropriate. The patient, the family, and the care givers are encouraged to attend progress rounds. The referring physician, if he or she has not been involved in the treatment plan, is also notified of anticipated discharge date and plans.

The discharge criteria were established early in the development of the program and have continued relatively unchanged. The criteria for discharge are:

1. The goals of the treatment plan as established by the patient and treatment team are met.
2. The patient chooses to end participation in the program.
3. The patient's medical condition prohibits further participation.
4. The patient's condition no longer requires the integrated, comprehensive services of the day hospital program.
5. Reimbursement and/or free-care funds for the services are no longer available.

The day hospital program was originally funded by a three-year federal grant. The program operates under the supervision of Sister Kenny Institute's director of social services.

The program was designed to share space and staff with the adult day-care program for persons with multiple disabilities. Patients in the adult day-care program required some nursing care, but primarily required diversionary activities rather than rehabilitation therapies, counseling, and medical care.

Combining the two programs provided initial gains in staffing and space efficiency, but it created confusion among referral sources. Many did not understand the difference between day care and day hospital care. The two programs were separated in 1986.

The program was designed to accommodate a small patient group that could be treated efficiently, would require no physical plant changes, and could easily be integrated into other Sister Kenny Institute outpatient programs. Currently, only five or six patients are in the facility at a given time. The number reflects our break-even point. Because we try to keep the number of patients low, we do not market the program to patients outside Abbott Northwestern/Sister Kenny Institute.

In 1986, the program was located in one of the hospital nursing stations, and nurses were assigned to each patient based on levels of acuity and independence. Each patient was assigned a room for rest periods. The common space was used for group activities and meals.

The program is now housed at Sister Kenny Institute in a large, open, multipurpose room that includes some specialized equipment, chairs that recline into beds (for patients who need to nap during the day), and examination and treatment areas. Medical treatments and examinations are performed in the appropriate hospital area on an outpatient basis.

Staffing

The program was staffed originally by a full-time licensed practical nurse and a full-time social worker. Recreational, physical, and occupational therapists, a psychologist, and a speech–language pathologist were used. All were full-time Sister Kenny Institute employees.

As the program has evolved, we have depended more on hospital staff, rather than maintaining a dedicated staff. The program is now coordinated by a social worker, and the nursing and therapy staff are assigned based on the patient's inpatient treatment examination. We try to maintain continuity of the staff for treating patients.

Many volunteers also participate in the program and have kept our staffing requirements low. Some of the volunteers are graduates of the program; others come to us through the Sister Kenny Institute volunteer program.

Financial Issues

All payments for treatment are preauthorized. Most of our patients are covered by HMOs and private insurance. Those who are on Medicare must pay for their own transportation to and from the program, because Medicare does not pay these fees. In other instances, Sister Kenny Institute funds the patient because care can be provided more efficiently in the day hospital.

We weigh enrollment in the day hospital against the costs of continued hospitalization.

Evaluation and Future Directions

Over time, our focus has changed somewhat in that we have all but eliminated the day-care aspects of the program in favor of a day hospital approach. This shift has occurred partly in response to competition. When we began the program, it was the only such program available in the Twin Cities. By 1987, 21 geriatric day-care centers had opened.

In the meantime, however, patients who were not part of the geriatric population but who clearly could have benefited from our services were being referred to us. Multiple sclerosis, brain injury, and arthritis patients in their forties, who would otherwise have had to remain in acute care, were obvious candidates for the program, as were children undergoing selective rhizotomy.

The day hospital patients generally have more flexibility in their home settings than do geriatric patients and can thus receive great benefit from our counseling programs. The fact that nursing homes, which constitute the only other alternative besides continuing hospital care, are not appropriate solutions for these patients increased the attractiveness of this program to them.

We continue to focus on patients referred from Abbott Northwestern/ Sister Kenny Institute and, because of transportation logistics, only patients in the Twin Cities area. However, what began as a geriatric day-care program is now moving toward a day hospital program for specific patient groups, regardless of age.

References

1. U.S. Bureau of the Census, Decennial Censuses of Population, 1900–1980 and Projections of the Population of the United States: 1982–2050 (Advance Report) Current Population Reports, Series P-25, No. 922, Oct. 1982. Projections are middle series.
2. Institute of Medicine. *Toward a National Strategy for Long Term Care of the Elderly.* Washington, DC: Institute of Medicine, National Academy of Sciences, Apr. 1986.

Chapter 15

Pediatric Rehabilitation at the Rehabilitation Institute of Pittsburgh

Judith H. Nagy

Introduction

The Rehabilitation Institute of Pittsburgh, a private, not-for-profit, 128-bed facility, has been providing specialized care to persons with disabilities for almost 90 years. The Rehabilitation Institute of Pittsburgh encompasses an accredited specialty hospital, a regional comprehensive rehabilitation facility, and a private day school. It is located in a primarily residential section of central Pittsburgh, Pennsylvania; is convenient to several university-affiliated hospitals; and is easily reached by car or public transportation. Its patients are drawn primarily from the surrounding and outlying areas and nearby metropolitan areas.

The Rehabilitation Institute of Pittsburgh was founded in 1902 by a group of philanthropic women as the Industrial Home for Crippled Children. It offered long-term domiciliary care with the goal of educating children with disabilities and providing whatever vocational training was possible to not only strengthen their bodies, but also to maximize their potential to become self-supporting.

During the 1940s, selected staff members and patients at the Industrial Home for Crippled Children participated in Dr. Jonas Salk's development of the polio vaccine, and during the 1940s and 1950s, the Home was one of the nation's major postpolio convalescent centers.

In the 1950s, the center moved into comprehensive rehabilitation. In 1957, it changed its name to the Home for Crippled Children. In 1966, it was designated a regional comprehensive rehabilitation center for children (and young adults) who had been disabled by any cause (for example, cerebral palsy, spina bifida, arthritis, traumatic head injury, and high-risk infancy).

In 1972, the Home for Crippled Children was accredited by the Joint Commission on Accreditation of Hospitals as a specialty hospital. In that same year, the school program was formalized into a private day school and was recognized by the state department of education. It currently serves about 200 day students, who spend time in both the classroom and therapy.

In 1981, in recognition of its move toward provision of more outpatient services and more services to adults, the name of the facility was changed from the Home for Crippled Children to the Rehabilitation Institute of Pittsburgh (TRI). In 1983, TRI formally established an outpatient services department, which serves children and an increasing number of adults, as a separate administrative unit. Today, TRI provides rehabilitation services to children in three capacities:

1. As inpatients
2. As students at its day school, where they receive special education and specialized therapy services
3. As outpatients

This case study focuses on the third group, the pediatric outpatients.

Program Development

The Rehabilitation Institute of Pittsburgh has long offered pediatric outpatient services as part of its continuum of care. Often after discharge, inpatients would need continuing rehabilitation services, which TRI had always provided to continue its support of its patients. Also, as the day school program expanded, TRI found that it was delivering what were in effect outpatient services to the students, who received occupational therapy, speech and language therapy, physical therapy, vocational counseling, and psychological counseling in addition to their regular academic or school program. Outpatient care, however, was not acknowledged as a separate division, and outpatients were not differentiated from inpatients. For example, a cerebral palsy outpatient was "lumped in" with other cerebral palsy patients, regardless of whether he or she was an inpatient, a day school patient, or an outpatient. In addition, outpatients shared billing, scheduling and appointment services, and medical recordkeeping services with inpatients.

In the early 1980s, a number of factors had coalesced to persuade TRI's administration to increase its efforts to provide outpatient care and formalize its delivery of outpatient services into a separate department:

- The emphasis in health care delivery was shifting from inpatient services to outpatient services, with a resulting decrease in both the inpatient census and revenues generated by inpatient services.

- At the same time, the demand for outpatient services was rising, providing new patient opportunities. However, TRI was finding that its existing organizational structure was not enabling it to encourage and increase direct referrals for outpatient care.
- Because pediatric outpatient care is one-on-one intensive and requires extensive case management and because outpatients as a group have different needs from inpatients (for example, in terms of scheduling, an outpatient will need back-to-back therapy appointments, whereas an inpatient can have intermittently scheduled appointments), it was difficult to provide proper case management without differentiating outpatients from inpatients administratively.
- Increasing numbers of adults began seeking outpatient services from TRI, and it was difficult to serve this new and growing patient population under the existing structure, which was oriented toward pediatric inpatient services.

As an institution, TRI was committed to providing outpatient services. In 1983, the administration approved the formalization of outpatient care by officially designating a department of outpatient services. The new department would be decentralized in terms of billing and accounting, scheduling and appointments, medical records, and case management, but would utilize the same clinical staff that served the rest of TRI's patient population. Outpatient services was not a new venture for TRI, and the move to decentralize in 1983 was not a diversification strategy. Rather, establishment of the new department was a formalization of services that already were being provided, an affirmation of the institution's commitment to serve outpatients, and the recognition that, in the face of rising demand for outpatient services, decentralization would best serve the needs of both TRI and the patients.

Program Implementation

Because this was not a new venture for TRI, no market needs, financial, or internal capabilities analyses were done. The organization's administration knew that there was a need for outpatient services and that the organization could provide them, because it was already doing so. Thus, once the decision was made to decentralize, implementation was fairly straightforward. Recruitment of the director did not prove to be a problem. An MPH candidate (and registered nurse) who was doing her administrative residency at TRI and who had already made well-received contributions to TRI's delivery of outpatient care agreed to head the new department. A speech-language pathologist who was already on staff became the program coordinator (there will be more on this role later). As already stated, the outpatient department would utilize TRI's clinical staff. A support staff was hired that included two billers, a receptionist/appointment scheduler, and a medical records manager.

The new department did not need a new location; the staff simply set up their administrative shop near the pediatric treatment areas, carving out a registration area from what had been a dental clinic. The Rehabilitation Institute of Pittsburgh's 145,000-square-foot facility stretches across a city block and is an amalgamation of three different building programs. The pediatric outpatient program is based in the main building. There are two pediatric treatment areas, one on the second floor and one on the third. The reception area is on the second floor, around the corner from the treatment area. The entire facility is accessible to persons with disabilities. There are two parking areas, although, as is to be expected in a primarily residential area, parking is limited.

Program Elements

In the 1950s, when TRI was still the Home for Crippled Children and an inpatient facility, its administrators created the program coordinator model for case management and delivery of care. In this model, a program coordinator serves as a team leader, pulling together and monitoring all aspects of a patient's treatment program, coordinating the activities of the various professionals (physicians, physical therapists, occupational therapists, speech pathologists, social workers, and so forth), helping with financial arrangements, and serving as the patient's advocate. The Institute originated the model because, previously, there had been no one on staff or outside to "pull it all together" for children with disabilities and their families. It was clear that this kind of coordination of services reached far beyond the medical aspects of a patient's case. Thus, the concept was born of a program coordinator who was a generalist rather than a physician. The program coordinator remains the key element of TRI's delivery of care to all patients, whether they are inpatients or outpatients, children or adults.

The institutional hierarchy has four senior program coordinators who are equivalent in rank to vice-presidents: two serve the inpatient program, one serves the day school program, and one serves outpatients. Reporting to them are the assistant coordinators. There are four assistant coordinators in the outpatient services department who oversee services for patients who have had head injuries or who need vocational rehabilitation, orthopedic, poststroke, or pediatric services.

The assistant program coordinator may come from any of the relevant professional disciplines. For example, one program coordinator has a master's degree in social work, another is a registered nurse with a master's degree in rehabilitation counseling, and another has a master's degree in vocational training. The pediatric coordinator has a master's degree in speech–language pathology.

In the pediatric outpatient program (and throughout TRI), the program coordinator serves four major functions:

1. As *internal advocate* for the child, the program coordinator manages the team of clinicians to ensure that the care that has been ordered is delivered.
2. As *financial advocate* for the child, the program coordinator makes financial arrangements and works out the best compromises with family resources. For example, it is possible to arrange a sliding scale for fees based on family income.
3. As *information manager,* the program coordinator gathers previous medical, educational, and treatment records and information. This is extremely important, because most pediatric rehabilitation is now done on an outpatient basis and most patients have been treated elsewhere at an acute care facility or rehabilitation hospital. The Institute's clinicians will need to see a child's previous medical records before they make their evaluations.
4. As *service marketing coordinator,* the program coordinator keeps parents and referral sources well informed of a patient's treatment progress.

The program coordinator assembles a treatment team for each patient on a case-by-case basis. The Rehabilitation Institute of Pittsburgh does not use designated teams, which means that it can tailor a program to a child's individual needs, rather than admit the child to a preordained program. For example, some patients may not need speech therapy, and others may need unusually extensive physical therapy.

The physician is a coequal member of the treatment team, not the team leader or "tiebreaker." This is not to say that the medical aspects of patient care are downplayed; the medical expertise of TRI's physicians is second to none, and every child in the program is under prescriptive treatment. However, the children need more therapeutic management than medical management. They have chronic conditions, and their medical profiles may not change, except developmentally. The Rehabilitation Institute of Pittsburgh's treatment program maximizes the residuals of the underlying medical conditions. The mission of the pediatric outpatient program is to muster its resources in the child's best interests in order to maximize his or her functions and return the child with the best gains possible to the least restrictive environment.

Once the program coordinator has assembled a team of therapists for a child, those therapists stay with the child throughout treatment. This allows a continuity of care for the child. However, as already stated, it is not a permanently designated team in the sense that the next time a child with similar functional compromises is admitted, he or she will be treated by those same team members.

As mentioned earlier, the outpatient services department does not have its own clinical providers. Instead, it utilizes TRI's 107-person staff of physical therapists, occupational therapists, speech pathologists, physicians (primarily physiatrists), social workers, dietitians, orthotists, and psychologists. Each of these professional disciplines has its own department head, who recruits and supervises the clinicians. Hours of operation for the outpatient program are from 7:00 a.m. to 8:00 p.m., Monday through Friday.

The pediatric outpatient case mix, which TRI analyzes in terms of acuity, has remained fairly consistent over the years. Patients are grouped into one of three categories:

- Type I, which involves substantial handicapping conditions and requires multiple services on a daily basis (usually five or more services provided five times a week) over a long term
- Type II, which involves less complex conditions that require fewer services delivered fewer times a week (usually three services delivered three times per week) over a shorter term
- Type III, which involves one or two services delivered one to three times per week for a relatively short term

Table 15-1 shows the patient mix for the years 1985 through 1990. The smallest percentage of patients (less than 5 percent) over the years fall into Type I; Type II accounts for 20 to 50 percent of the patients; and the largest percentage of patients (49 to 75 percent) fall into Type III.

The number of direct outpatient referrals has grown along with overall outpatient volume. When the outpatient services department was formally designated in 1983, the majority of pediatric outpatients were internal referrals. In 1989, the majority were referred by outside sources. The pediatric inpatient census in 1989 averaged only about 35 patients, so direct outpatient referrals should continue to be the major source of patients.

Table 15-1. Patient Mix by Acuity, Pediatric Outpatient Services, The Rehabilitation Institute of Pittsburgh

Disability/Services	1985	1986	1987	1988	1989	1990
Type I Substantial disability/multiple services daily	5%	5%	5%	4%	3%	1%
Type II Less serious conditions/fewer services, fewer times	20%	30%	30%	40%	40%	50%
Type III Short term/1 to 2 services, 1 to 3 times per week	75%	65%	65%	56%	57%	49%

Marketing and Promotion

Marketing and promotion of the pediatric outpatient program focuses on the outcome of the services provided and the effectiveness of the coordination of care. The program produces excellent functional and developmental results. The child's progress is communicated by the program coordinator to patients' families, third-party payers, and sources of referral. These outcomes and cost savings through early intervention and prevention are the program's most effective marketing tools. The program's sources of referral include:

- School districts
- Physicians
- Social workers
- Therapists
- Psychologists
- Families

As already described, the program coordinator is the key element in marketing the program as well as in the patient care program.

In addition to service-marketing to sources of referral, which is centered on individual patients, more general promotional efforts for the pediatric outpatient program include:

- Brochures
- A billboard campaign
- Advertisements in local periodicals
- Public relations campaigns
- Participation in the Children's Miracle Telethon Network

Pricing and Other Financial Issues

The Rehabilitation Institute of Pittsburgh's administration and chief financial officer are sensitive and responsive to input from the director of outpatient services and the outpatient staff with regard to the setting of fees for the program's services. A number of years ago, the director of outpatient services requested a reduction in fees because she found that the existing fee structure was noncompetitive. After surveying fees charged by other facilities, the chief financial officer agreed to the reduction. In 1989, the chief financial officer sought to raise fees, but before doing so he presented his research to and sought the advice of the outpatient services director and her staff. The sensitivity and responsiveness of TRI's administration in this area applies to its patients as well as its staff: TRI provides a great deal of unreimbursed care. As much as $2.5 million of its $19 million budget provides unreimbursed services. Although the cost of all services continues to increase, the application of a sliding scale and free services reach many in need.

The majority of pediatric outpatients are covered by private insurance, and payers are divided equally among Blue Cross/Blue Shield, major medical, and commercial carriers.

Despite the rapid growth and continued success of the pediatric outpatient program in terms of increase in patient volume, development of outside referrals, and good patient outcomes, pediatric rehabilitation is not a profit-making undertaking, nor should it be expected to be. Pediatric rehabilitation is very one-on-one intensive, and the individualized care and attention provided by TRI's program coordinator model for delivery of care makes the process even more costly and labor intensive.

The Rehabilitation Institute of Pittsburgh's pediatric outpatient program is heavily subsidized by the institution. However, TRI remains committed to the provision of pediatric outpatient rehabilitative services, which it feels are an essential part of the continuum of care it offers, and provides important and irreplaceable services to patients, their families, and the community. The Institute stays current in its knowledge of federal and state funding for services and community programs.

Problems Encountered

The rapid growth of the pediatric outpatient department has dramatically increased the caseload of its program coordinator, who is responsible at any one time for as many as 200 children. Financial constraints make it unlikely that another patient coordinator will be hired any time soon. Fortunately, the program coordinator is extremely skilled and dedicated and has strong institutional support, so she has managed to maintain high standards of patient care despite a burdensome work load. However, her case management duties leave her with no time for program development, which will be essential to the future growth of the program.

Another problem, which is relatively minor by comparison, is one faced by any facility located in a residential area—parking. Fortunately, TRI's administration has been responsive to the problem and has arranged for two designated parking areas, which has greatly improved matters.

A third problem is that of space for the rapidly growing outpatient services department. The institute's building program calls for a new structure to be completed in 1992. Adult services will move into the new building, leaving more space for pediatric services.

Evaluation

The pediatric outpatient program has experienced rapid growth since its decentralization in 1983, confirming TRI's belief that there is an ever-increasing market for pediatric outpatient rehabilitation services. In 1983, the program treated an average of 60 to 75 patients; in 1989, there were 200 active cases.

Despite the rapid increase in patient volume with no accompanying increase in the number of pediatric outpatient program coordinators (a single program coordinator serves all 200 patients), the department has been able to maintain its high standard of patient care and its excellent outcomes. This is because of an unusually talented and dedicated staff and a high degree of cooperation from the various professional departments who provide clinical services.

It is likely that patient demand and volume for pediatric outpatient rehabilitative care will continue to increase. Nationwide, the demand for outpatient services, from patients and payers alike, shows no signs of abating. In the area of pediatric rehabilitation, demand will be especially strong because as medical advances increase the rate of survival from accidents, birth trauma, and premature birth, the number of children with some function compromised will increase. The number and frequency of services will extend over a longer time because of earlier identification. In addition, success in this area increases demand: the greater the number of good outcomes produced by facilities such as TRI, the greater the number of parents of children with compromised function who will seek rehabilitative treatment.

Future Directions

As mentioned earlier, any future growth for pediatric outpatient services will require program development. Until the program coordinator can turn some of her attention away from her heavy caseload, specific planning for the future will have to remain on the back burner. Current "back-burner" items include expanding services to burn patients and a day-care center that would mix employees' children with children with disabilities.

The expected growth in demand for existing services will provide a continuing challenge, and the expected physical expansion of pediatric services in 1992, when the new building opens, will offer opportunities for enhanced services as well as increased space.

The Rehabilitation Institute of Pittsburgh is extremely proud of the superb care that its pediatric outpatient program provides and the excellent outcomes it has achieved. It continues to be committed to the provision of pediatric outpatient rehabilitation services, and expects that patient volume will continue to increase and provide ongoing challenges and rewards to the staff.

Chapter 16

BackBuilders, Operated by St. Lawrence Rehabilitation Center

Sister Janet Henry and Janice G. Cunningham

Introduction

St. Lawrence Rehabilitation Center is a 116-bed, not-for-profit hospital located on a 35-acre campus in Lawrenceville, New Jersey. It is owned and operated by the Catholic Diocese of Trenton and serves Mercer County and, to a lesser extent, six other counties in the central New Jersey area.

St. Lawrence is the only inpatient facility in the area. In 1971, it was licensed as a skilled nursing facility and emphasized rehabilitation. In 1976, it was licensed as a general rehabilitation center, treating orthopedic patients, stroke patients, amputees, brain-injured patients, and the like.

In 1986, when the emphasis in health care delivery was shifting from inpatient services to outpatient services, Dr. Robert Carabelli, a staff physiatrist at St. Lawrence, approached the hospital with an idea for a fully comprehensive outpatient treatment and rehabilitation program for people with back and neck pain, whether chronic or the result of accident or injury. Dr. Carabelli was convinced that such a program, whose ultimate goal would be to treat patients before they get to the stage of chronic pain, provided the best results to back pain sufferers.

The Board of Trustees of St. Lawrence, which makes policy decisions for the hospital, was receptive to the concept, and after three years of planning, development, and implementation, the program, called BackBuilders, opened in August 1989.

Program Development

The hospital board's first step was to hire a consultant to do market research and explore the program's potential in two target counties of the hospital's service area. However, a feasibility study of potential users proved to be problematic. It was difficult to gather good data for several reasons:

- The perception of back pain is subjective and thus difficult to quantify.
- Relatively few centers do back rehabilitation.
- Patients generally do not seek treatment for back pain unless it is severe.

However, the consultant was able to extrapolate from national statistics to determine that 80 percent of the population would suffer some degree of back pain at some time in life.

Dr. Carabelli; Sister Janet Henry, the chief executive officer of St. Lawrence; and St. Lawrence's planning and development committee assessed the feasibility of undertaking the new program. They determined that the program was a good risk because of the following considerations:

- Back pain sufferers made up a substantial population that St. Lawrence was not tapping fully.
- No significant competitors in the area offered comparable services, nor were there plans for any.
- This was the type of pioneering effort that St. Lawrence was interested in pursuing.

They were also aware that there probably would be some shifting of outpatients from St. Lawrence to the new program, but they thought that the influx of new patients the innovative program would attract and St. Lawrence's financial interest in the new program would offset any negative impact.

Once the decision was made to go ahead with the new program, the next step was to determine how the new venture would be structured. Dr. Carabelli had provided the concept and could provide the medical expertise and some financial resources. St. Lawrence could provide additional financial resources as well as administrative functions.

The two parties decided that the best way to minimize potential competition between St. Lawrence and the new program, maximize benefits to each party, and facilitate future expansion was to enter into a joint venture agreement. To obtain additional financial resources, they decided to include a third party, St. Francis Medical Center, in the joint venture. St. Francis, which is part of the Franciscan Health Systems, is a 350-bed acute care center located in Trenton, New Jersey. The administrators of the two hospitals knew one another and felt that they could work well together, and the involvement of a third party diluted the financial burden.

Hammering out a contract that proved satisfactory to all parties and would allow for future expansion (a kind of "franchising" of the BackBuilders program) was quite time-consuming; all in all, it took about 18 months. One factor in this process was the difficulty of assigning a reasonable market value to the trademark and modus operandi brought to the venture by Dr. Carabelli; this value, of course, would determine the additional financial commitment he would have to make to the venture. Another factor was the rapid rise in costs and salaries during this period, with the resultant difficulty in determining how much start-up capital would be needed.

Ultimately, the contract terms were agreed on and the three partners—Dr. Carabelli, St. Lawrence, and St. Francis—formed a corporation, Lawrence Medical Associates, which owns the BackBuilders concept. In addition to being an equal partner, St. Lawrence is also the provider; it leases back from the corporation the right to run BackBuilders at its satellite location 5 miles from the hospital. If and when the corporation expands, the St. Lawrence–operated program will serve as the model; future programs can be run by other providers.

The new director's first assignment was to find a delivery site. The planning and development committees had in fact entered final-lease negotiations for a rental property while the director was being recruited, but those negotiations fell through before she was hired.

Finding an affordable and appropriate site was no easy task. Mercer County is a very expensive area, and the site selected had to be fairly close to St. Lawrence and easily accessible by car and public transportation.

The site finally chosen is in a small strip "mall" in Ewing Township, New Jersey, near three major roadways. It is about a 10-minute drive from St. Lawrence and is near heavy industrial areas (industrial injuries were projected to be a major source of patients). Although most patients arrive by car (the mall location offers ample free parking), the site is easily accessible by public transportation. There are about 10 other tenants in the mall, which is a "business services" center (that is, the tenants are service-oriented businesses such as corporate car-leasing agencies and furniture rental stores, rather than convenience and clothing stores).

The space occupied by BackBuilders is 4,290 square feet. When Lawrence Medical Associates signed the lease in February 1989, the space was little more than a shell, and the landlord was amenable to remodeling as necessary.

An architect who had done work for other tenants in the mall was hired, plans were drawn, and bids were solicited from contractors. The contractor selected was familiar with the building, which was an asset, but had not done work on health care facilities, which was a potential liability because he was not familiar with codes and regulations for such facilities. However, the director's knowledge and experience and the contractor's willingness to research the codes and regulations ensured that the work proceeded smoothly, and the renovation was completed in about 100 days.

About half the space of the completed facility is devoted to an open exercise area. There is a desk in the exercise area from which staff members can observe patients using the equipment. The rest of the space consists of a reception area, private treatment cubicles, the physician's office, the director's office, two examining rooms, a conference room, two locker rooms with showers (one for each sex), and storage space. The facility was designed to be very comfortable and pleasant for patients and has the ambience of a health club, albeit one with highly sophisticated equipment.

Staffing

The staff for the new center was projected to consist of:

- 1 physician (Dr. Carabelli)
- 1 director (who would be involved mostly in operations to start with, but who as time went on would devote about 50 percent of his or her time to marketing)
- 1 licensed physical therapist with special training in back rehabilitation (with plans to hire a second physical therapist as patient volume increased)
- 1 exercise physiologist
- 1 registered nurse (who, in addition to playing a clinical role, would assist the director with administrative work)
- 1 receptionist/secretary

Only the director would be hired during the implementation stages, so that he or she could:

- Identify suitable delivery sites
- Supervise the renovation
- Negotiate contracts
- Recruit staff
- Prepare marketing materials

The search for a qualified director took six months. The candidate chosen, Janice Cunningham, is an occupational therapist with experience running outpatient rehabilitation programs and expertise in marketing. She was hired in June 1988.

As the renovation neared completion, the director and the physician began recruiting additional staff members. Although many staff members at St. Lawrence had the requisite experience with back patients, they wanted to remain in the more generalized physical therapy clinic. However, after running advertisements, Ms. Cunningham had little difficulty recruiting qualified staff members. Salaries and benefits are comparable to those for similar positions at St. Lawrence, and BackBuilders staffers were helping to create a new program, both of which were strong drawing cards.

Program Elements

BackBuilders offers two levels of programming:

- Program A, an intensive program for treating patients who are in good overall health but who have serious back pain as a result of industrial injuries or automobile accidents
- Program B, a less intensive program for people who have developed chronic back pain over the years through chronic misuse of their bodies

Program A, for which treatment is usually covered by workers' compensation or personal injury insurance, is priced at a package rate, whereas the less intensive Program B is fee-for-service. For both programs, the fee structure was determined by costing out staff time and equipment time used and by assessing what other physical therapy and rehabilitation programs across the country charge for similar services. The fees for physical therapy are in line with the fees charged by St. Lawrence.

Programs A and B may differ in intensity, but they share the same goals:

- Getting patients off medication, which only masks pain but does not eliminate it
- Treating the physiological cause of pain
- Helping patients to again become fully functioning family members and employees
- Giving patients the knowledge to maintain their state of well-being and avoid further back pain and injury

For patients in both programs, the procedures followed are more or less the same, although the length and intensity of the treatment will be different. The stages are as follows:

1. The medical director does a complete physical examination (including a medical history), orders any necessary tests (MRI, CAT scan, X-rays, electromylogram, nerve conduction, and so forth), and prescribes a

treatment program. The physician notes any special treatments (for example, hot packs) or any special precautions (for example, cardiac problems) that a particular patient requires.

2. Prior to the first meeting with the physical therapist, the patient's insurance is verified via telephone and a follow-up letter, which the insurance company must sign. Patients whose insurance will cover part of the costs of treatment (usually 80 percent) are billed for the balance. Patients without coverage are referred to St. Lawrence on a case-by-case basis to work out a payment plan.
3. At the first appointment with the physical therapist, there is a thorough evaluation that may take anywhere from one hour to several hours, depending on the patient's needs.
4. The patient meets with the registered nurse and completes a survey to determine whether there are psychological or other causes of the back pain, such as job-related stress, poor nutrition, poor sleeping habits, poor overall fitness, or smoking.
5. The patient proceeds with treatment. Treatment for patients in Program B consists almost entirely of physical therapy. In the more intensive Program A, however, patients meet weekly with the registered nurse, who provides psychological support and makes appropriate referrals if there are underlying psychological problems that are interfering with treatment. Patients in Program A are much more likely than their Program B counterparts to have experienced interference in their ability to function as family members and employees as a result of their back pain, and the nurse's support is helpful in returning these patients to their normal work and home functions as quickly as possible.
6. The patient has a follow-up visit with the medical director, the timing of which varies from patient to patient and condition to condition. In addition, patient progress is reviewed at regular staff conferences, and insurance companies and employers are kept informed of patient progress.
7. After treatment has been completed, the patient is offered a five-part back education program consisting of:
   - A general overview of common conditions and misconceptions, given by the medical director
   - An overview of anatomy and functional body mechanics (explaining, for example, the proper way to sit in a chair or lift a box), given by the physical therapist
   - A discussion of how to make your environment work for the patient, given by a consultant who specializes in ergonomics
   - A session tailored to the needs of a particular group, such as discussions of relaxation techniques, smoking, or obesity, given by the registered nurse
   - A "relay race" during which patients, in addition to having fun, demonstrate their knowledge of proper techniques for stretching, lifting, and the like

The back education program is included in the package for Program A and is available to Program B patients for a fee.

8. A follow-up program is available for an annual fee that entitles patients to continue to use the exercise equipment under staff supervision.

The hours of operation were from 8:00 a.m. to 4:30 p.m. on Monday, Wednesday, and Friday, and 11:00 a.m. to 7:00 p.m. on Tuesday and Thursday, to provide a balance of early and late hours. However, after a couple of months of operation it was clear that it would be necessary to add a half-day on Saturday because:

- Many patients need to come three times a week; consequently, Mondays, Wednesdays, and Fridays tended to be extremely busy, whereas Tuesdays and Thursdays tended to be slow.
- Many patients are employed and need expanded hours to accommodate their work schedules.

Financial Issues

As the partnership agreement was being worked out, the planning and development committees from St. Lawrence and St. Francis did the pro forma, using data from the consultant's feasibility study and their own knowledge and research.

Because the St. Lawrence campus was being used to capacity, it was clear that the new program would have to be located off-site. It was decided to rent an existing structure rather than build a new facility because renting would:

- Minimize capital outlay up front
- Involve only a three-to-five-year commitment
- Allow the corporation to get a clear idea of the potential for success without making a large investment

Because the BackBuilders program offers total body conditioning, it was projected that the cost of the necessary equipment would be the largest expense, even larger than the cost of any renovation of the rental space that might be needed. This projection proved to be accurate.

The planning committees projected that start-up costs for BackBuilders would be $208,445, broken down as follows:

- $100,000 for equipment and furniture
- $60,000 for rental and renovation costs
- $15,000 for promotion and marketing (brochures and so forth)
- $33,445 for preoperational salaries, legal fees, consulting fees, and insurance

These projected costs proved to be fairly accurate, the major variation being that renovation costs were about $8,000 more than projected.

As predicted, equipment costs were the biggest outlay for BackBuilders. BackBuilders provides total body conditioning, and the 17 pieces of Cybex/Eagle equipment in the exercise area are designed to work every muscle of the body. Other equipment includes:

- Free weights
- Cuff weights
- NordicTrack
- Upper-body ergometers
- Schwinn Aerodyne
- DMG 2000
- Exercise bicycles
- Ultrasound
- Hot and cold packs
- Mats
- Treatment tables

In addition, there is a crash cart on the premises, and all staff members are trained in cardiopulmonary resuscitation.

Marketing and Promotion

BackBuilders' goal is to be the first-choice treatment for people with back pain—to get to people before they have gone through the medical mill. To accomplish this, the staff has worked hard to establish and maintain an excellent reputation in the medical community, with the general public, and with payers.

The overall marketing plan has a strong educational component, in addition to its public relations aspect. BackBuilders wants to educate the general public, employers, and the medical community about the efficacy of its comprehensive outpatient rehabilitation program.

Even before BackBuilders opened, brochures were mailed to likely sources of referral: physicians, hospitals, insurance companies, and local businesses and industries. In the early months of operation, there were numerous referrals because of Dr. Carabelli's excellent reputation.

As the director is able to turn more of her attention away from operations and toward marketing, she will attend orthopedic staff meetings at area facilities and make cold calls on likely sources of referral. She also plans to develop an advertising campaign, attend local health fairs, and contact the health and science editors of local print and broadcast media. For the immediate future, the director has a target goal of 13 to 14 new patients per month.

BackBuilders is keeping accurate statistics on patient progress so that case studies and articles can be produced. The statistics will also aid future expansion by demonstrating the need for and efficacy of the BackBuilders program.

Evaluation

Since its opening in August 1989, BackBuilders has exceeded projections of patient volume and gross revenues. In its first quarter, the program treated about 80 patients and was handling between 12 and 16 patients per day, about twice the number that had been projected. About one-third of the patients were Program A (package rate), and two-thirds were Program B (fee-for-service). By the end of the first quarter, gross revenues were already covering basic operating needs. Original projections anticipated that the facility would be self-supporting by its third year of operation.

Relatively few problems have been encountered. A potential staffing problem, the need for Saturday hours, was resolved by using contract staff for the new hours until patient volume justifies the hiring of another permanent staff member. Storage needs have been greater than anticipated, but the problem is not pressing enough to require immediate resolution.

Future Directions

A long-term future goal of BackBuilders and the parent corporation, Lawrence Medical Associates, is to "franchise" the BackBuilders program to other providers. The original BackBuilders team will assist with program design and implementation, set standards and criteria, and offer ongoing support and monitoring.

Shorter-term goals include carrying out the marketing plan discussed earlier, starting a patient support group, and, as patient volume increases, adding another full-time licensed physical therapist.

St. Lawrence Rehabilitation Center, the partners of Lawrence Medical Associates, and the staff of BackBuilders are pleased with the patient volume, gross revenues, and smoothness of operation of BackBuilders' first months of operation. Clearly, there is a demand for this kind of comprehensive outpatient back rehabilitation program, and patients, sources of referral, and payers have been pleased with the high quality of the treatment offered. The future looks bright for the program's ongoing success and future expansion.

Chapter 17

Outpatient Rehabilitation at the Mayo Clinic

Gudni Thorsteinsson, M.D.

Introduction

Several years ago, the officers of the Mayo Clinic in Rochester, Minnesota, concluded that, despite its continued sound operation and medical practice, the Mayo Clinic would have to adjust to a number of changes in the health care industry at large, including changing competition, such as health maintenance organizations (HMOs); changing regulations, such as diagnostic-related groups (DRGs); changing technology, such as magnetic resonance imaging (MRI); and changing patient needs.

In preparing to respond to these changes, Mayo went through an analysis of its strengths and weaknesses. The strengths of the institution were seen as the following:

- People
- Reputation
- Coordinated practice
- Role in medical education
- Tradition of research
- Tradition of sound financial planning
- Political knowledge of its governing board and administration

The following weaknesses were identified:

- Location
- Small population base
- Complacency
- Overconcentration of service in one location

From this analysis, a new strategy was devised at Mayo—*diversification.* For the Mayo Clinic, diversification was not a series of strategies, such as plans to alter the facility's mission or satellite programs, nor was it related directly to short-term seasonal fluctuation in capacity/demand ratios. Instead, diversification was and is (1) a series of plans to ensure the long-term future of Mayo Medical Center within a health care environment that is dynamic, rapidly changing, and uncertain; (2) a multifaceted broad-based effort; and (3) a recognition that concepts are evolving and some may take years to develop. The strengths and weaknesses revealed by this analysis have been the basis for some of the recent changes:

- Opening of group practices in Jacksonville, Florida, in 1986 and Scottsdale, Arizona, in 1987
- Development of the Mayo HMO (local)
- Consolidation of the Mayo Clinic, St. Marys Hospital, and Rochester Methodist Hospital into the Mayo Medical Center in 1986
- Creation of a reference laboratory service, Mayo Medical Laboratories, in 1971, in Rochester, that receives specimens from all over the world
- Publication of *Mayo Clinic Health Letter* for the general public, with a national and international circulation in 1990 of 300,000
- Distribution of *Mayo Clinical Update* (to the medical profession in the contiguous states), with a circulation in 1990 of 100,000
- Provision of helicopter transportation for emergency cases
- Certification for the rehabilitation unit at St. Marys Hospital by the Commission on Accreditation of Rehabilitation Facilities (CARF)

The approximately 16,500 people who make up the staff of the Mayo Medical Center include about 950 physicians and medical scientists; 867 physician residents; 7,842 administrative and paramedical personnel; 59 clinical and research associates; 377 students (medical students and health-related science trainees); and more than 6,200 other persons affiliated with the hospitals, including nursing and paramedical personnel.

The programs available at the Mayo Medical Center span the entire spectrum of services needed for comprehensive health care delivery. The Mayo Medical Center market region is somewhat restricted: 80 percent of the patients are from within a 500-mile radius, and of these, half are from Minnesota. Only 2 percent come from outside the United States. Since the current registration system began in 1907, more than 4 million patients have registered at the Mayo Clinic. In 1989, the clinic had 289,561 patient registrations. About 7 percent of the patients came without advance appointment. Of the total annual outpatient visits, 20 percent required subsequent hospitalization.

This chapter focuses on the department of physical medicine and rehabilitation (PM&R), development and implementation of outpatient programs and services, marketing of new programs, and evaluation of the results and possibilities for the future.

Department of Physical Medicine and Rehabilitation

Figure 17-1 shows the organizational structure of the Department of Physical Medicine and Rehabilitation (PM&R). The department is under the Board of Governors and the Clinical Practice Committee of the Mayo Clinic, and it works in close contact with the two hospitals, Rochester

Figure 17-1. Organization of the Department of Physical Medicine and Rehabilitation

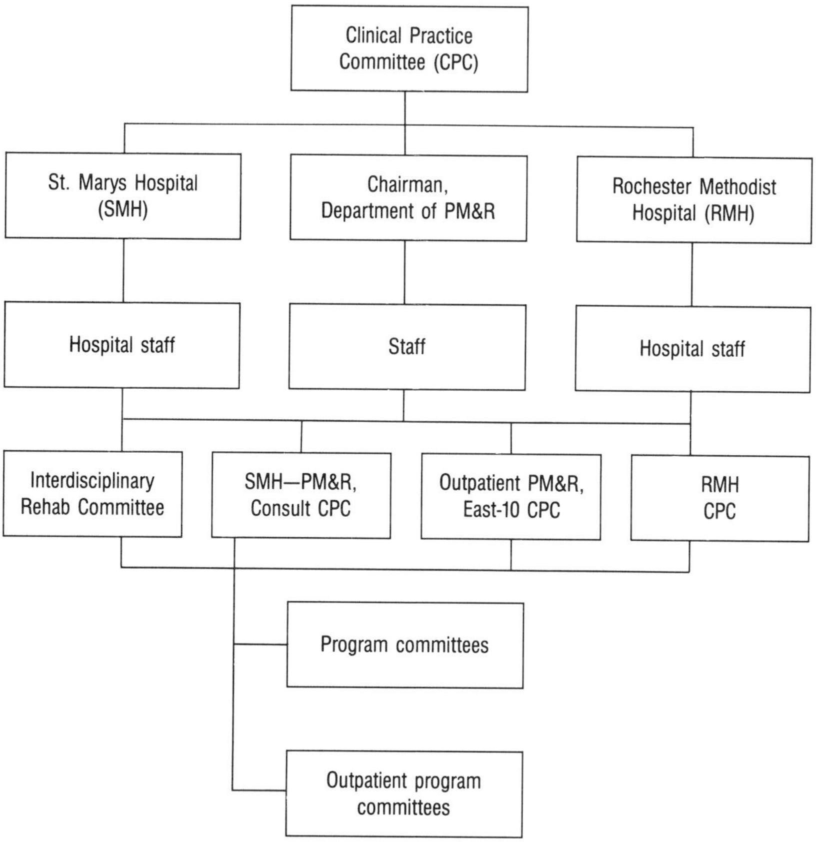

Methodist Hospital and St. Marys Hospital. All programs, services, and administration come under the chairman of the department, and the practice is provided or supervised by medical staff. The operation is divided into several sections by location and, to some degree, function. Each of these sections has a medical director who is directly responsible to the chairman of the department. The responsibilities of the director include coordination of practice, facilitation of development of new programs, and cooperation with the administrative assistant regarding financial, personnel, and administrative matters. The department head has the final say with regard to finances, personnel, and space.

Figure 17-2 shows the organization of programs within the PM&R department. Each program has a committee that is responsible for the program's development, coordination, and maintenance at all locations. This structure avoids duplication and maximizes utilization of services, space, and expertise. These program committees are responsible to the chairman of the department, and their function is closely coordinated with the same programs in the Mayo Medical Center through Mayo Medical Center committees, for example, patient education, quality control, and spinal cord injury program.

The major programs within the department are concerned with spinal cord injury, brain injury, stroke, pediatrics, amputation, hand, cardiac, acute care (community medicine and musculoskeletal problems), sports fitness, back, rheumatology, cancer, functional work evaluation, work hardening, and general physical medicine and rehabilitation programs. Other programs that are a part of the comprehensive activity of the PM&R department include bladder training, spasticity control, and bowel training.

The department functions mainly in three roles: inpatient rehabilitation service, hospital consultation service, and outpatient physical medicine and rehabilitation.

The medical director at each location is responsible for integrating the two organizational concepts—inpatient care and outpatient care—into a coordinated flow of practice. Flexibility and availability are basic goals in coordinating programs and services. As a result, personnel, space, and activities are not fixed in one program but, rather, are shared and varied depending on variations in demand. This, of course, means that the specialist also has to manage "general conditions." This concept is applied across the board in the department (and in the Mayo Clinic as a whole), not only to physicians but also to therapists and other personnel. Although we maintain a requirement for this practice, we also encourage specialty training and support this through program committees. However, there is a constant tendency to want to steer into the comfort of subspecialization, and this tendency has to be controlled by the medical director.

Figure 17-2. Programs within the Department of Physical Medicine and Rehabilitation

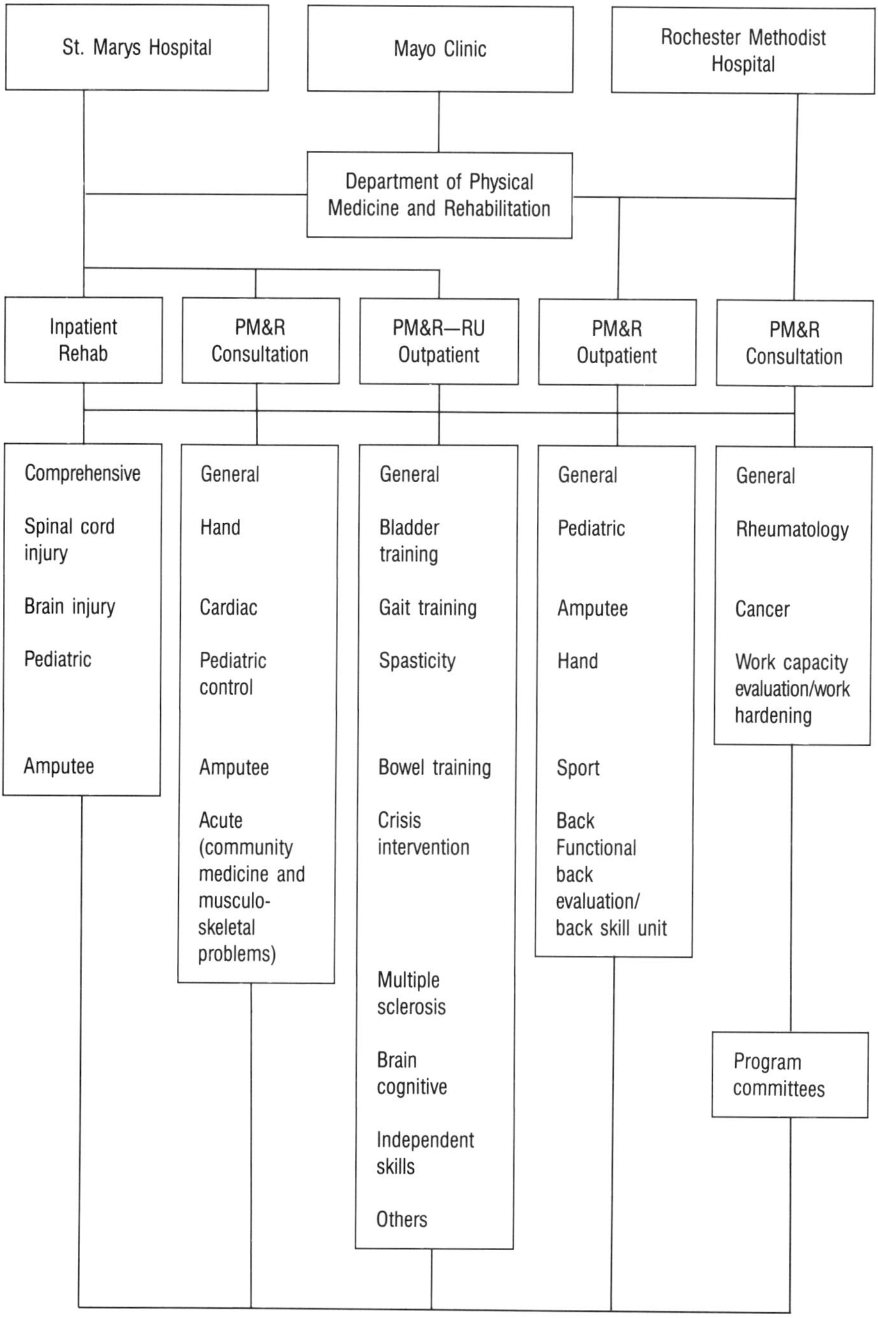

Coordination is essential. In our complex operation, with multiple sections and programs, the direction and integrity of the organization must be maintained. The chairman of the department directs the overall programs and sees to the maintenance of missions, goals, and objectives. Finances, personnel, disciplinary action, and space all come under the chairman, so that loopholes and conflicts of interest can be avoided. The medical director coordinates the clinical practice in an individual area. For some programs, program coordinators are needed to oversee daily operations that involve interdisciplinary teams so that protocols and procedures are maintained and patients entering the program obtain services effectively and efficiently.

The space that the PM&R department has is far too small. Major building projects are under way. The ultimate goal is to have most of the operation of the inpatient and outpatient programs in one place. Some of the consultation services will still have to be at the hospitals. The outpatient clinic, usually referred to as East-10 PM&R, consists of 11,350 square feet: 2,800 square feet for physiatric consultation, 6,000 for general physical medicine, 1,700 for the sports fitness center, 350 for the back skills unit, and 500 for hand therapy. The space occupied by each program fluctuates with program requirements. Occupational therapy (1,200 square feet) is provided mainly at the Rochester Methodist Hospital. Splinting in relation to hand surgery is performed at the main outpatient clinic, on East-14 (400 square feet), but some modification of splints is also done in the hand therapy clinic at East-10 PM&R.

The distribution of personnel within the PM&R department is summarized in table 17-1. Because the distribution of personnel depends on the type of practice in each section, it is quite variable and depends on a number of factors. One factor is therapist involvement in patient evaluation. In the outpatient area, the therapists do the patient evaluation 25 percent of the time. Other factors are severity of illness, whether the physiatrist is the primary physician, whether group therapy is used, and the source of patient referral (for example, orthopedics or neurology). Many of the available services are provided by other departments. For example, speech pathology, nutrition, and vocational rehabilitation are provided on referral.

Development of Outpatient Services

One factor in development has been whether to develop satellite clinics with a basic general program, services, and personnel to which specific programs or services can be attached or to have specific clinics away from the general program with fixed programs, services, and personnel. Because Mayo's experience with fixed clinics has not been good, new programs are built from the general program. This concept has proved

Table 17-1. Personnel in the Department of Physical Medicine and Rehabilitation, Excluding Hospital Staff

Category	Mayo Clinic E-10	Rochester Methodist CS	St. Marys Hospital 1-D	St. Marys Hospital RU
Medical director	1	1	1	1
Physiatrist[a]	10.7	2	2	6
Residents[b]	(varies)	2	2	6
PT supervisor	4	4	3	3
Physical therapist	32.5	7	13.5	13
PT assistant	4	3	2	0
PT student	6	5	6	5
OT supervisor	0	1	0	1
Occupational therapist	1	4.5	4	11
OT assistant	2	1	1	1
RT supervisor				1
Recreational therapist		3		
RT assistant			1	
Patient and family education coordinator				1
Psychologist				2
Social worker[c]				4
Secretaries	6	1	1	4
Aides and desk attendants	16	4	4	6

Abbreviations: E-10=outpatient Physical Medicine and Rehabilitation (East-10 PM&R); CS=Physical Medicine and Rehabilitation Consulting Service at Rochester Methodist Hospital; 1-D=Physical Medicine and Rehabilitation Consulting Service on 1-D; RU=Physical Medicine and Rehabilitation inpatient rehabilitation unit; PT=physical therapy; OT=occupational therapy; RT=recreational therapy.

[a] Including chairman and medical directors.

[b] Distribution varies according to off-service rotations (total of 8).

[c] Consultations available by referral.

much more beneficial in financial terms and the utilization of personnel, space, and services.

There are various reasons for developing new rehabilitation programs. The first is needs assessment. The process of needs assessment can be facilitated significantly by ongoing documentation of practice. For each patient, we document the referral source, who evaluates the patient, in which section the patient is seen, the physical medicine and rehabilitation diagnoses, the regional diagnoses, and so forth. This information is entered on a computer card for each patient after each evaluation.

Documentation of referral sources (see table 17-2) may indicate variations or stability in sources. Documentation of clinical conditions, as shown in tables 17-3 and 17-4, may indicate variations or the need for more efficient and effective concentrated effort to handle certain conditions, for example, development of specific programs and special expertise (such as back, shoulder, and multiple sclerosis programs). Table 17-3 shows the need for a concentrated arthritis team, which was recently established, and the need for a coordinated follow-up program was also

Table 17-2. Referral Sources for Outpatient Clinic, East-10 PM&R, 1985

Referral Source	1st Quarter	Rank	2nd Quarter	Rank	3rd Quarter	Rank	4th Quarter	Rank	Total
Surgery	1,020		821		834		1,176		3,851
Orthopedic	941	2	733	2	745	3	780	2	3,199
Neurologic	28	5	24		18		23		93
Other	30		54	5	26		24		134
Hand clinic	21		10		45	5	349	4	425
Medicine	3,424		3,479		3,400		3,400		13,817
Rheumatology	538	4	494	4	517	4	426	5	1,975
Neurology	695	3	775	3	747	2	673	3	2,890
Other	2,191	1	2,210	1	2,250	1	2,301	1	8,952
Primary PM&R	431		528		526		484		1,969
	4,875		4,828		4,874		5,060		19,637

Table 17-3. Summary of Clinical Conditions Seen at East-10 PM&R in 1985: Arthritic

Condition	1st Quarter	Rank	2nd Quarter	Rank	3rd Quarter	Rank	4th Quarter	Rank	Total	Rank
Periarthritis	59		48		78		61		246	19
Rheumatoid	123		138		144		68		473	13
Ankylosing spondylitis	23		18		28		17		86	
Juvenile rheumatoid	6		11		10		6		33	
Miscellaneous	35		22		36		32		125	
Psoriatic	5		7		6		4		22	
Systemic sclerosis	12		17		22		6		57	
Polyarthritis (other)	2		8		4		6		20	
Degenerative	1,845	1	1,780	1	1,759	1	1,885	1	7,269	1
Total									8,331	

evident. The high frequency of tendinitis shown in table 17-4, mainly reflecting shoulder problems, has been the reason for ongoing development of a specific shoulder program. The frequent referrals with the diagnosis of tension myalgia indicate the need to update equipment (biofeedback) and develop expertise (therapist certification) in this field. The total number of conditions, about 29,000 per year, is seen equally from quarter to quarter, approximately 7,000 per quarter.

The age distribution of the patients in the outpatient program, especially the 700 under 17 years old who are seen per year, indicates a need to shift some of the residency training to the outpatient department instead of concentrating all of it in the inpatient program. The paucity of referrals from the emergency department indicates a need for internal marketing to this potential referral source.

A demand for a new program is not always evident from data collection within an established program. Sometimes demand comes from outside, as a result of new programs in other departments or new regulations or trends (for example, arthroplasties and fitness centers). New procedures and techniques may create demands for new programs, such as prosthesis management, spasticity control, strengthening techniques, and shoe fitting (runner's shoe clinic). The need for programs can also become evident from recognition of social trends, for example, early intervention for multiple sclerosis patients and their families to prevent psychosocial breakdown or shoulder programs for the increasing number of women in the labor market.

When developing new programs, the organization has to consider the benefits for both patients and the organization. The problem is to

Table 17-4. Summary of Clinical Conditions Seen at East-10 PM&R in 1985: Miscellaneous

Condition	1st Quarter	Rank	2nd Quarter	Rank	3rd Quarter	Rank	4th Quarter	Rank	Total	Rank
General			821		834		176		3,851	
disability	29		30		32		37		128	
Infection	5		2		3		10		20	
Burns	1		2		1		2		6	
Cardiac rehabilitation	1		0		0		6		7	
Nonpsoriatic dermatitis	2		2		5		5		14	
Acute disc disease	21		18		10		20		69	
Genitourinary	23		18		28		34		103	
Muscular dystrophy or atrophy	11		14		24		17		66	
Other muscle problem	185	9	208	7	265	6	496	5	1,154	6
Myopathy	6		6		6		23		41	
Psychiatric	51		39		45		63		198	22
Respiratory	2		3		0		4		9	
Tendinitis, bursitis[a]	496	4	396	4	435	4	518	4	1,845	4
Tension myalgia	1,057	3	808	3	883	3	892	3	3,640	3
Ulcer	6		7		2		7		22	
Total									7,322	

[a] Reflects mainly shoulder problems.

find the proper balance. Patients benefit from expertise, efficiency, and effective programs. The organization benefits from higher patient satisfaction, marketing by word of mouth (and thus bringing in more patients), higher revenue, and better use of personnel by streamlining the delivery of services. Also, better use of space is achieved by concentrating the functions used in programs and services in one area.

The drawbacks of a new program would be evident from underutilization of personnel and space. This situation can happen to programs and services that are too specialized and therefore sensitive to fluctuations in patient flow. This emphasizes the importance of flexibility and backup by the general program. If not backed up by a general program, the special program may not be able to meet temporary increases in demand, leading to dissatisfied patients. If a clinic is too remote from the referring sources, it is not as visual and, therefore, constant marketing is necessary until referral becomes routine.

There has been a definite trend toward specialty programs within the PM&R department in recent years. Following is a list of recently developed programs and the basic reasons for their development:

- *Hand therapy clinic:* This was first developed as a satellite on the orthopedics floor in response to a recognized need combined with a lack of referrals from the orthopedic surgeons. It later was moved to East-10 PM&R because of the therapists' dissatisfaction, especially with fluctuations in load, overtime, and lack of actual supervision by a physiatrist.
- *Sports medicine clinic:* This developed from needs created by the fitness craze that has spread throughout the country. It has been extremely successful.
- *Amputee clinic:* This developed from the provision of better services and follow-up for amputees, and the provision of better training for the PM&R residents. This program has been successful in meeting those needs.
- *Functional work evaluation:* This developed in response to changes in workers' compensation rules that created a need for reliable documentation.
- *Arthritis clinic:* This developed to improve communication to the referral source, to stabilize follow-up, and in response to the lack of space at the outpatient department and a decline in patient load in the PM&R consulting services at the hospitals. This program was set up in the Rochester Methodist Hospital consulting service.
- *Referral:* Referral of community patients with acute musculoskeletal problems to St. Marys Hospital consulting service was instituted to relieve the outpatient department at East-10 PM&R and also to replace declining patient load.

- *Functional back evaluation and back skill unit:* This was needed to meet the heavy referral load of patients with back pain and at the same time render more effective and efficient service and evaluation.
- *Miscellaneous programs:* These include biofeedback, temporomandibular joint, and osteoporosis programs. They developed from the need for more efficient and effective programs.

The following is a summary of the methods used in the department of physical medicine and rehabilitation at the Mayo Medical Center for development of all new programs:

1. For needs assessment, collect fundamental data on referral sources, clinical conditions, and so forth.
2. Expand the new program from existing programs.
3. Emphasize personnel flexibility—specialist versus generalist.
4. Emphasize space flexibility.
5. Maximize availability.
6. Comply with the rule of relationship between the specific programs and the general program. This means those working in a specific program will first take care of referrals to the specific program and then pick up referrals to the general program.

Each rehabilitation program, whether outpatient or inpatient, has to fit into and follow the basic standards of the patient care processes in the Mayo Medical Center and the PM&R department, including the following:

- All new protocols, procedures, and forms have to fit into the parent system.
- Each patient has a single medical record, which is delivered from one area to another within the Mayo Medical Center as the patient moves from service to service.
- Each patient has a primary physician who coordinates all the care for that patient.
- One central appointment desk coordinates all appointments within the Mayo Medical Center.
- The scheduling desk for the PM&R department schedules appointments within each section (program, services, modalities).
- A service record by the provider is completed after each patient contact. The patient does not move within the system until the service record is completed.
- The dismissal procedure for patients (forms used, communication channels, and so forth) is standard.
- Follow-up procedures are standardized.

Some differences in procedure exist between the rehabilitation unit and the outpatient program. For example, the inpatient rehabilitation unit has more Medicare and medical assistance patients than does the outpatient department. However, this situation would probably not be the case for an inner-city medical center.

The outpatient rehabilitation program in the rehabilitation unit has been developing recently in response to changes required by DRG rules. It represents a step between the inpatient program in which multiple services are needed and the outpatient clinic at East-10 PM&R. The patients served in this rehabilitation program do not need all the inpatient services, but do need more intensive rehabilitation than is provided in the outpatient programs. They especially need more intensive rehabilitation nursing and patient and family education.

Marketing

The PM&R department at the Mayo Medical Center is in a unique position because 90 percent of its referrals are from within the medical center. So the department does most of its marketing internally. One exception to this is the increasing number of direct referrals to the sports medicine clinic, which come mainly from the local area.

External marketing has also been necessary. Accreditation by CARF of the rehabilitation unit at St. Marys Hospital was a part of external marketing.

The development of the sports medicine program showed the PM&R department the importance of needs assessment analysis and marketing. Needs assessment indicated that the potential patient population was different from that of other programs in terms of age, geographic area, and general health status. The patient origin for the program would be predominantly local, 85 percent from Minnesota compared to 50 percent for the general program, and the patients would be younger. The needs assessment also indicated a need for different devices (due to the higher incidence of knee injuries), special services such as the runner's shoe clinic, and extended hours because of the patients' school and work requirements. The medical center also identified a need to survey the competitors in the area to be certain that the center matched what they had to offer.

Evaluation and Future Directions

Changes in rehabilitation medicine are bound to occur. The best way to cope with them is to document the past and try to make predictions according to observed trends. In 1981, documented growth and past trends were used to make predictions regarding personnel, programs, space, education, and research. The actual experience has been close to those predictions.

Over the years, Mayo Medical Center has been evaluating the growth of the department of physical medicine and rehabilitation. Compared with that of the Mayo Medical Center as a whole, the department has shown a larger increase in registration of patients, number of new consultants, number of new residents, and assigned floor space (table 17-5). This trend indicates higher demand and better recognition. Rehabilitation medicine at Mayo Medical Center will continue to grow.

Table 17-5. Growth in Mayo Medical Center and the Department of Physical Medicine and Rehabilitation

		% Increase	
Factor	Years	Mayo Medical Center	Department of PM&R
Patient registrations	1960–1970	3.91	4.3
	1970–1980	1.95	4.7
	1980–1985	2.07	5.8
Consultant staff	1960–1970	4.45	5.38
	1970–1980	3.94	7.23
	1980–1985	2.30	3.25
Assigned space	1960–1970	1.48	0
	1970–1980	4.00	3.24
	1980–1985	0.21	5.20
Residents in training	1960–1970	1.87	9.87
	1970–1980	0	7.12
	1980–1985	4.30	12.7

Chapter 18

Behavioral Health and Rehabilitation at Advanced Rehabilitation Management

Jerry Strum

Introduction

In 1985, Advanced Rehabilitation Management, Inc. (ARM) entered into a partnership agreement with a group of physicians to develop and operate an outpatient comprehensive pain service in Orlando, Florida. This service was based on a highly successful program that has been in operation in California for the past 14 years.

Advanced Rehabilitation Management is a wholly owned, not-for-profit subsidiary of Casa Colina, Inc. (CCI), based in Pomona, California. It provides outreach services to hospitals and physicians interested in implementing rehabilitation programs, and consulting services for business plan development, program development and management, and unique joint ventures. The corporation also operates a case management program that serves persons suffering from catastrophic injury or illness and their families, physicians, and insurers. These services include recommendations, cost analyses, long-term or life planning, and cost projections. The chronic pain program described here was joint-ventured under ARM. Advanced Rehabilitation Management operates with a relatively small governing board, which permits rapid decision making without a lengthy bureaucratic process.

The physician joint venture was the first of its kind for ARM. The thrust of the program is to provide rehabilitation services to industry. The patient caseload in the programs in both California and Florida comprises a high percentage of workers' compensation patients. The physician partnership was developed for the program in Florida.

Prior to 1981, the organization consisted of Casa Colina Hospital for Rehabilitative Medicine, which is the flagship component of the business. It is a 66-bed freestanding acute rehabilitation facility located in

Pomona, California. In 1986, the hospital celebrated 50 years of service to rehabilitation patients. The present facility evolved from a 10-bed convalescent home for polio-stricken children. It has no medical-surgical component; rather, its emphasis is on treatment and rehabilitation of patients with severe disabilities such as stroke, brain injury, spinal cord injury, and neuromuscular conditions. The delivery system is organized clinically under a programmatic design. The hospital also operates outpatient services, including a children's services center that focuses on assessment, treatment, and individualized programs for children with physical, neurological, or related problems in development.

Casa Colina is the parent holding company that oversees the development and operations of its eight subsidiary corporations. Its primary mission is to advance the development of high-quality, cost-effective rehabilitation services. The Casa Colina Foundation provides fund-raising and charitable support to the organization.

A physically separate outpatient service at CCI is devoted to the comprehensive back services program. The program, begun in 1973, is one of the first such endeavors in the nation. It has been shared with many hospitals and is one of the leading models for back programs in the United States.

The hospital also owns and operates a motel for outpatients and residential transitional living centers for brain-injured and spinal cord–injured adults. This program offers cost-effective alternatives to long-term institutional placement. Residents work toward individual rehabilitation goals in a supervised home setting. The center maintains four residences and has plans for expansion.

Casa Colina Skilled Rehabilitation, Inc. (CCSRI) operates skilled nursing rehabilitation services. A pilot business, Peninsula Rehabilitation Center, was acquired in 1982. The 48-bed facility offers inpatient and outpatient services for persons disabled by stroke, orthopedic problems, and brain injury, as well as a technologically sophisticated ventilator-dependency rehabilitation and coma-stimulation program. The center's stroke program is recognized as a high-quality, cost-effective alternative to rehabilitation in an acute care hospital.

Casa Colina Career Development Center, Inc. (CCCDC) provides vocational rehabilitation to disabled and disadvantaged adults. It provides vocational counseling, work evaluation, work adjustment, work hardening, skills training, on-the-job training, transitional employment, job-seeking skills development, and placement services in competitive industry. Within the center are two subdivisions—Casa Colina Industries and Casa Colina Clerical Training Center.

Padua Village, Inc. (PVI) was organized to provide supervised residential living for developmentally disabled and brain-injured individuals. This business is designed to develop an alternative to long-term institutional placement. Currently, PVI owns and operates two homes, one in Claremont and one in Lucerne Valley, California.

Casa Colina Comprehensive Outpatient Rehabilitation Services, Inc. (CORS) was formed to develop and operate satellite outpatient services for rehabilitation patients. The corporation focuses on restorative day hospital services, day health care, Alzheimer's disease services, and respite and day-care programs. These services permit earlier discharge from acute inpatient rehabilitation and enable patients to continue living in their home communities.

Program Development

One of the reasons CCI began considering joint venturing was in response to the changes that were and still are occurring in the health care industry. Prior to 1980, many hospitals were not interested in outpatient rehabilitation. However, Medicare prospective pricing and rehabilitation's exemption stimulated development of outpatient rehabilitation services. Similarly, there has been a movement in the health care industry toward vertically integrated systems of patient care and diversification of service delivery to ensure good patient outcomes.

Significant changes occurring among physicians also stimulated interest in joint venturing with hospital providers. Hospitals are competing with physicians and physician groups for everything from outpatient services to diagnostic services. Private physicians are competing with multispecialty groups. Well-capitalized, freestanding outpatient centers are also competing with individual physicians. Physicians are experiencing price competition and increasing consumer choice about where to receive medical treatment. Finally, the freedom of physicians to move about in the health care market has been restrained by federal and state health planning laws. All these factors have created an environment that makes joint ventures between hospitals attractive because such arrangements are mutually beneficial. These changes, in part, stimulated CCI to consider physicians as limited partners in the venture.

The popularity of joint ventures was also increasing and continues to increase. Many hospitals and physician groups have entered into joint ventures as vehicles to increase utilization of health care services and solidify referral systems. This type of arrangement can be mutually beneficial to both types of health care providers.

In 1985, Ernst & Whinney conducted a national survey to evaluate trends in joint ventures by health care providers.[1] More than 700 hospital executives volunteered to participate in the study. The types of ventures that were most prevalent were in ambulatory care. Many hospitals also expressed interest in developing joint ventures in alternative delivery systems. About 24 percent were considering joint ventures in medical office buildings, laboratories, laundry facilities, and alcoholic rehabilitation centers. The partners of choice by hospitals were physician group practices (about 48 percent). Multihospital systems were most likely to already be involved in a joint venture.

The legal mechanism for the joint venture that the provider chooses deserves special attention and expert advice. The choices are the partnership model (limited and general), the corporate model, and the contractual model. The type of legal vehicle will in part be dictated by tax implications and management and liability issues. Not-for-profit organizations should be particularly sensitive to implications that may arise from joint ventures. The Internal Revenue Service (IRS) has ruled that a tax-exempt organization can jeopardize its exempt status if it becomes the general partner in a limited partnership. Although the IRS has reversed this position and now permits tax-exempt organizations to participate with taxable entities or private investors, individual providers are encouraged to seek outside counsel for each venture. The IRS will also closely scrutinize tax-exempt organizations with respect to unrelated business income.

In addition, if the joint venture includes physicians, the arrangement should be carefully evaluated under Medicare fraud and abuse provisions. The fundamental provisions prohibit payment for any kind for patient referrals.

In early 1985, CCI was contacted by a group of physicians interested in developing an outpatient comprehensive pain service. They had become familiar with CCI's program through the scientific literature published by the organization. The group consisted primarily of orthopedists who were interested in developing the program for the benefit of their patients and practice.

When the contact was first made, CCI decided to undertake the consideration of a joint venture under Advanced Rehabilitation Management. This subsidiary was historically organized to permit this type of arrangement, and ARM had already entered into joint venture arrangements with hospitals. The governing board of ARM approves these arrangements only if they are financially viable. A classical business plan was expected, which the management of ARM developed. The following sections review the components of the business plan and the actions taken to implement it. These components included the business description, the market analysis, the definition of rehabilitation product lines and requirements, regulatory requirements, marketing and promotion strategies, management and organization, financial implications, and an implementation schedule.

Business Description

The business description section of the business plan described the purpose of the joint venture from a business perspective. The objective of the new business was to develop a comprehensive pain service that was patterned on the program successfully operated by Casa Colina Hospital for Rehabilitative Medicine. The narrative focused on the clinical aspects of the program (medical versus psychosocial), the types of patients expected to benefit from the program, and the implications of focusing on a strictly outpatient model in contrast to a blend of inpatient and outpatient services.

Market Analysis

The purpose of the market analysis section was to carefully evaluate the market to determine the potential need for chronic pain services. This information was needed to prepare the operating budget and determine the project's feasibility. The analysis contained several key elements.

The investing physicians were surveyed to determine their historical caseloads according to the types of patients who would be appropriate for the program. Under normal circumstances, ARM would have surveyed the physician community at large. However, there was sufficient representation and caseload potential irrespective of the general community. The potential caseload survey to physicians revealed a heavy reliance on workers' compensation as a payment source. This was not a surprise, because many pain patients have experienced vocational injuries.

Generally, the health care industry has three distinct consumers: patients, physicians, and third-party payers.

To fully evaluate if third-party payers would use the program, a survey was conducted of insurance carriers who operated in the state. It was constructed to evaluate the volume of patients currently being handled by the claims reviewer. Of equal importance was a compilation of the insurance carriers' views about the quality of programs that currently existed. They were asked to identify the programs and to quantify how satisfied they were with their accessibility, cost, continuity of care, and the patient outcomes. This process served a dual role: first, it helped identify potential competition within the market; second, it served to quantify the strengths and weaknesses of existing programs.

The market survey would normally also include surveys of hospitals in the market area and, in particular, their discharge coordinators, social services staff, and therapy staff. However, most chronic pain patients experienced their acute episode some time ago in the past; therefore, this component was eliminated. However, a local hospital in the immediate service area was contacted to determine if it perceived the development of the program as a threat to any of its services. This hospital did not see the program as a threat.

The physicians and insurance carriers had identified competition. The potential competitors were further researched and plotted on a service area map. Researchers at ARM also collected information about the scope of the services provided by the competitors as well as a profile of charges for their services. Additionally, profiles of other providers outside the service area were developed. The primary objective of this research was to assist in the development of revenues in the financial feasibility section of the study.

Finally, this section of the study clearly defined the service proposed by ARM in the context of services already furnished to the community. A description of the target consumers was provided, and the competitive edge that ARM's services might have was presented. At the conclusion of this section of the business plan, the corporation's management had a clear understanding of the program's market potential, potential caseload, competitive position, and the extent to which the program would need to be marketed to third-party payers once it became operational.

Definition of Rehabilitation Product Lines and Requirements

This section of the business plan focused on how the services were to be delivered: who, what, when, and where. The objectives of the program from a clinical perspective were provided in detail, including what the patient census objectives would be and why they were established (what). Similarly, based on the census objectives, a profile of the staff needed was developed (who). For this profile, the staff objectives were determined to include a medical director, a clinical psychologist (Ph.D.), a program coordinator, and clerical staff. This section also included productivity objectives of therapeutic staff, targeted when a liaison nurse would be added, and described how physical therapy and biofeedback therapy would be added.

Fortunately, the physicians already owned a building that could be leased to the partnership to provide space for the program. The particulars of the lease arrangement were negotiated, and a functional space program was developed. A specialist from corporate headquarters visited the property and developed a schedule and budget for leasehold improvements, which were then incorporated into the lease documents. This transaction required that the lease arrangement be negotiated at fair market value. Market research was completed for similar space and compared with the lease terms to ensure that this test had been met.

At this point in the development of the business plan, ARM's management was able to compile an equipment list based on the potential patient volume and the functional space program. Because the therapeutic program was based on an existing clinical design, this effort was not difficult. A budget was developed for equipment in excess of $500 (to be depreciated) and equipment less than $500 (to be expensed during the first month of operation).

Because space availability was a determining factor in when the program would start, at the conclusion of this section of the plan, ARM's management could develop a target date for the project to become operational.

Regulatory Requirements

Because the health care industry operates in a highly regulated environment, this section of the business plan focused on the regulatory requirements that had to be met in order to implement the project. These were generally centered on licensure, certificate of need (CON), and Medicaid and Medicare reimbursement.

The Florida State Department of Health was contacted to determine if the outpatient service needed to be licensed as a business. Although the program itself was not required to be licensed, the treatment staff was. The requirements for licensed personnel were requested and incorporated into this section of the plan, along with objectives for licensure compliance.

In many states, this new type of operation would require CON review. Initial discussions with the state planning agency revealed that a CON was not required. (Had a CON been required, this section of the business plan would have incorporated the CON law, capital expenditure thresholds, the sections of the state plan that provided needs assessment for the service, the CON criteria that would need to be met for compliance, and the procedural implications [time line] that might influence the targeted start-up date.) Because a certificate of need was not required, a program description was sent to the state agency, along with a request that the agency respond in writing that a CON was not required. This document was incorporated into the business plan.

The program, as planned, showed little or no reliance on Medicaid or Medicare funding. Consequently, regulatory requirements for Medicaid or Medicare funding were not incorporated. Had the program needed certification from these agencies, the certification requirements would have been reproduced in this section of the plan along with objectives, how certification would be met, specifications regarding who would be assigned accountability for compliance, and a budget of the expenses related to certification.

Marketing and Promotion Strategies

Generally speaking, the health care industry has only recently come to value the benefits of a marketing strategy for health care product lines. Health care providers have learned that marketing health care can be as effective as marketing any other business.

The development of a marketing strategy for the business proposed was of particular importance to ARM—and a particular challenge. The business was proposed for Florida, yet ARM's management was located in California. In its California operation, ARM relies heavily on services provided by the marketing division of Casa Colina, its parent company. Marketing staff were asked to develop a marketing strategy, with measurable objectives and accountability.

Preparation of a classical business plan permits easy implementation of a marketing program. The market research section of the plan had already revealed physicians and insurance carriers who showed an interest in the program's development. Therefore, a list of potential consumers of the program was already in place.

The specific marketing strategy was to invite these persons to an open house, and the expenses for such an open house were budgeted. Other marketing costs for brochures, direct-mail expenses, and advertising (yellow pages, Chamber of Commerce, newspapers) were developed, and accountability was assigned. The marketing strategy, costs, and accountability were incorporated into this section of the business plan and segregated by pre–start-up activity and costs and post–start-up activity and costs.

Management and Organization

Decisions related to management and organization were incorporated into this section of the business plan. This included the organization of the new Florida operation as well as how the organization related to its parent companies, ARM and CCI.

This section of the business plan presented a unique challenge to the management of ARM. First, the organizers were certain that they did not want to enter into a project as passive investors. Because the program was patterned after one in which ARM could demonstrate management skills, a decision was reached to enter into a joint venture in which ARM was general partner with the physicians as limited partners. Further, ARM was designated in the partnership agreement as the managing general partner. Second, a decision was needed as to the governance of the operation. A partnership does not normally have a governing body, yet ARM's other business operations were subject to governance. To overcome this problem, ARM's governing body was named in the partnership papers as responsible for governance and approval of capital expenditures and operating budget approvals. Thus, proposals are presented to ARM's board, and minutes of these meetings are given to the limited partners.

There was also a need to articulate reporting relationships within the new satellite and define how its manager would report to ARM. Initially, the program's psychologist was designated program manager. Subsequently, another individual was named manager.

The distance between the parent company and the satellite created some unique organizational problems. To overcome the distance, a report was designed to help ARM management track the most important variable of the program—patient census. This report is now sent to ARM on a weekly basis and reports on referrals, evaluations, admissions, discharges, and the budgeted census. The actual census is compared to budgeted census and the program manager explains the differences, if any. The report also includes the number of hours spent on marketing against marketing objectives and reports on income. The report also requires comments on the quality of accounts receivable and the changes in accounts receivable. Variances from budgeted expenditures require explanation. This report serves as an early warning system for the overall performance of the business and permits the tracking of key variables that may require intervention by ARM management.

The partnership documents require that ARM management designate the responsibility for keeping the financial records and books, and CCI was given that responsibility. Revenues and expenses are collected in Florida and sent to California. The corporate accounting staff presents monthly financial statements to the management of ARM, along with the operating budget and variances.

The partnership document contained an extensive section that addressed allocations of profits and losses. This section was written by an attorney to comply with Medicare fraud and abuse laws and regulations. Other provisions, such as transfer of partnership units or interest and dissolution, were clearly described to protect both the general and the limited partners.

Job descriptions for the staff of the Florida project were also prepared and incorporated into this section of the plan along with reporting relationships. This section also included the results of a Florida salary survey and the salaries targeted for the positions for which job descriptions were written. The basis for compensating ARM for management expenses was outlined and presented in this section and incorporated into the legal documents.

Financial Implications

At this point, sufficient information had been collected to do an operating budget. The known variables were the potential patient census, program prices, salary profiles of staff, addition of staff as a function of census, a marketing budget, equipment to be bought, management expenses, the depreciation schedule, and lease expenses. Using zero-based budgeting, the remaining operational expenses were estimated and a monthly operating budget was prepared.

A start-up expense budget was also developed. The plan was to recruit staff locally (in Florida) and to put this staff through a training program in Pomona, California. The expenses related to this training (airfare, ground transportation, and per diem) were budgeted along with a charge from the corporation conducting the training. Security deposits and prepaid rent were also included in the start-up plan. Legal expenses were estimated in consultation with outside counsel.

In the original research with insurance carriers, the claims managers were asked to estimate the length of time needed to process a claim and pay the bill. This information was used to determine the cash flow position of the new business. All these elements were included in the start-up budget. The combination of the operating statement, which showed net cash flow, aging of the accounts receivable, the equipment budgets, and the start-up budget, provided an estimate of the money needed to capitalize the business. These documents were incorporated into the partnership papers as an exhibit.

A return-on-investment (ROI) was calculated based on the forecasted operating budget. Because a usable building already existed, this particular project did not require heavy funding for property, construction, building, and improvements. The ROI before consideration of reserves was estimated to be in excess of 35 percent.

Implementation Schedule

An implementation schedule was also prepared and incorporated into the business plan. This schedule listed key dates for implementation procedures and designated accountability for space planning, equipment acquisition, personnel recruitment and training, capital formation, and implementation (quality assurance, performance audit, business licensure, acquisition of tax identification numbers, filing partnership documents, insurance purchasing, policy and procedure manuals, and so forth). The marketing time schedule, prepared earlier, was also incorporated into this section.

Once the business plan was finished, the program was implemented. The program elements are described in the next section.

Program Elements of Chronic Pain Service

The treatment of chronic pain can be one of the physician's most unrewarding tasks. The inability to effect a cure for the chronic pain patient denies many physicians the professional rewards they can get in other areas of their practices.

The national costs of chronic pain are staggering. Frequently, chronic pain patients are subjected to years of misdiagnosis and unsuccessful treatment. The patient becomes pain-centered and suffers losses in quality of life, job opportunity, personal relationships, and self-esteem. For example, in August 1986, the U.S. Department of Health and Human Services published a monograph from *Vital and Health Statistics* of the

National Center for Health Statistics. It uses findings of the National Ambulatory Medical Survey. These data are based on visits made to nonfederal, office-based physicians practicing in the United States over a two-year period, from January 1980 through December 1981. During this period, there were 73 million chronic pain visits. These data include patients with a pain problem with a duration of three months or longer. The highest frequency in any category was back pain patients. They represented 17 percent of all visits in the chronic pain sample universe.[2]

In a study by Clark and others, low back pain alone has disabled an estimated 7 million Americans and accounts for more than 8 million physician office visits yearly in the United States.[3] A report by Chapman noted that patients seen at the University of Washington pain clinic have experienced as many as between 20 and 25 surgical operations to help alleviate pain.[4] A communication from the American Pain Society indicated that about 800 pain clinics nationwide are coping with chronic pain syndrome.[5] That number has no doubt climbed in recent years.

Casa Colina has operated a comprehensive pain program for nearly two decades. The program serves both inpatients and outpatients. A motel adjacent to the hospital is frequently used as an alternative to patient placement in the inpatient services of the hospital. This approach provides a noninstitutional setting for patients and saves money for insurance carriers in that the more costly inpatient rooms are not used.

When the program began, the corporation decided to capitalize a research component. This element performs longitudinal studies on the patients who undergo treatment. The research is made up of more than 600 data elements that are collected annually and analyzed. From this, scientific papers that, among other things, demonstrate the efficacy of the service are published every five years. The result has been that the organization has assembled a body of evidence demonstrating that the program works. These papers have proved to be one of the program's more effective marketing tools. Anyone planning a comprehensive pain program is encouraged to develop a research component.

Pain programs in the United States can generally be grouped into two categories: the *medical* model and the *psychosocial* model. The medical model includes implementation of traditional medical techniques in response to demonstrable tissue damage. The psychosocial model involves a multidisciplinary team of behavioral specialists. This program is designed to alter behavioral consequences and thus reduce tissue damage and pain. Under the psychosocial model, the physician maintains medical management of the patient, and a team of behavioral specialists manages the therapeutic program. In the medical model, medical intervention assumes that the pain is a symptom of physical injury. Treatment is directed at the injury with the expectation that the pain will go away. However, the medical model may fail to recognize that the brain is involved in the perception of pain. Also, a number of factors *other than* the injury may reinforce the behaviors associated with the pain. Casa Colina uses the psychosocial model in its chronic pain service.

In recent years, pain has been seen as a complete psychological phenomenon that involves cognitive and emotional components. The psychosocial design provides a comprehensive program of treatment designed to modify a variety of factors contributing to back pain disability that function as deterrents to vocational rehabilitation. This program includes several types of intervention, including biofeedback training and assertiveness training as well as cognitive and behavioral techniques for pain management.

The essential emphasis of the psychosocial program is on the patient's roles in his or her own recovery. Patients are encouraged to view themselves as primary agents in their recovery process, rather than as passive respondents to cures that only the therapist or physician can effect. All patients are expected to give up the invalid role, reduce dependence on medicine, and learn to manage their bodies and their pain.

The types of patients in the chronic pain program include those with recent injuries (such as strains and sprains), prechronic patients, support and maintenance patients, and chronic patients. Prechronic patients are those who are not benefiting from physician intervention and are developing psychological systems that may lead to a chronic pain syndrome. The chronic patient is one who has had repeated surgeries and medical intervention and has been disabled for a period in excess of six months. Chronic patients are no longer candidates for surgical intervention.

Evaluation and Problems Encountered

The program was implemented in 1986. It did have a bit of a rough start and has since undergone some major restructuring.

One problem was the staffing structure. Initially, a clinical director was in charge of the administrative duties. This was not working well, so the clinical director was replaced by an office manager who has proved more effective in this role.

Another problem was stiffer-than-expected competition from another, similar program. That program was subsequently acquired by CCI and consolidated into its program.

New federal regulations that went into effect shortly after the program started limited many relationships between physicians and nonphysician groups. As a result, in 1987, CCI bought out the physicians' shares. The program now operates under the name Behavorial Health and Rehabilitation.

The Orlando program has also been gradually modified to respond to patient concerns and the desire of insurance carriers for a less expensive program with suitable patient outcomes. That process is continuing today.

References

1. Ernst & Whinney (now Ernst & Young). *Health Care Joint Ventures, Survey Results* (No. J58589). Cleveland: Ernst & Whinney, E&W , 1985.
2. Koch, H. *The Management of Chronic Pain in Office Based Ambulatory Care: National Ambulatory Medical Survey* (NCHS Advance Data, no. 123). Washington, DC: U.S. Department of Health and Human Services, 1986.
3. Clark, M., Bosnell, M., and Shapiro, D. The new war on pain. *Newsweek,* Apr. 25, 1977, pp. 48–58, 89.
4. Chapman, C. R. A behavioral perspective on chronic pain. Paper presented at the annual convention of the American Psychological Association, Montreal, Canada, Aug. 1973.
5. Turk, D., Meichenbaum, D., and Genest, M. *Pain and Behavioral Medicine.* New York City and London: The Guilford Press, 1983, p. 73.

Chapter 19

The Diversification Strategy of Casa Colina: A Chronology of Change

Dale E. Eazell

Introduction

Casa Colina Rehabilitation Center was established in 1936 to serve children stricken with polio. With the development of the Salk polio vaccine in 1953, the original purpose for which Casa Colina was founded was less viable, and the board of directors began to look at other rehabilitation options.

Rehabilitation services had proved successful in facilitating the return of injured persons to productive involvement in the community, as was particularly evidenced by injured veterans returning from service in World War II. Recognizing the growing need for and value of rehabilitation services, in 1960 Casa Colina's board of directors broadened the services of this 66-bed acute care licensed hospital to include rehabilitation for persons with stroke, spinal cord injury, traumatic brain injury, and general traumatic injury and illness. This case study details the chronology of the diversification strategy developed at Casa Colina.

Organizational Structure and Change (1960–1973)

From the beginning, the organizational structure of the new operation posed some problems. From 1960 through 1973, the board of directors retained a dual reporting relationship to itself, represented by an administrator and a medical director. Every two to three years during this period, administrative leadership often alternated between the medical director and the administrator. Because of this, the focus of Casa Colina's programs periodically vacillated between quality-of-care issues and fiscal restraint issues. This "Ping-Pong process" had several effects: (1) no growth and/or sustained rehabilitation service innovation; (2) fiscal disaster with operating losses of 5 to 10 percent on a gross of $1 million annually, including donations; and (3) demoralization of staff, which resulted in high turnover and an unfocused mission.

With the encouragement of the medical director, the board of directors concluded that the organization could not be managed by a dual reporting relationship. This conclusion was overwhelmingly supported by organizational research in management literature. As a result, a chief executive officer (CEO) was sought through a national search. Board and staff members contacted rehabilitation health care facilities and executives throughout the United States. Interviews with candidates were conducted by key staff and board members after reaching a consensus on the skills required and the demonstrated performance characteristics of the executive sought. Those characteristics included demonstrated history and experience with medical and vocational rehabilitation, innovation in program development, the capacity to work with employees in achieving a balance between patient and referring agent goals, and financial solvency. The educational background required included graduate work in business or rehabilitation, with a preference for the latter, backed by a strong business performance history in rehabilitation facility leadership.

The executive chosen to lead Casa Colina demonstrated a national performance record in turning around rehabilitation corporations, both medical and vocational. Further, the executive was connected with both state and national rehabilitation trade associations in leadership roles. The CEO was retained in 1973 and continues to serve the organization today in that same capacity.

Since 1973, Casa Colina, now located in Pomona, California, has grown into a corporation providing $50 million in rehabilitation services annually. It has grown from 60 employees to nearly 1,000; from 1 location to nearly 20, with 2 to 4 new services introduced annually; from losses to gains that nearly approximate all of the 1973 gross revenues on a quarterly basis and to a balance sheet that can support a credit line equal to its gross revenues. It has developed from the services of a general acute care hospital specializing in rehabilitation to a continuum of services, including acute and subacute (skilled nursing) rehabilitation services, day hospitals, transitional living centers for persons with head injury, adult day health programs, home rehab, long-term residential, and vocational rehabilitation services.

Issue Discovery (1973–1975)

Two main processes were implemented by the CEO upon arrival at Casa Colina: interviewing staff to determine issues requiring change or further study, and developing plans to implement changes to spur growth.

The first process was to interview *all staff* (approximately 60 medical, paraprofessional, and support staff members) to determine the issues that prevented successful achievement of the organization's mission and to assess staff interest in helping implement necessary changes. During the interview process, certain issues emerged more frequently than others; those issues with the highest incidence required more immediate plans for action.

The principal issue that emerged from the interview process was a lack of consensus regarding the corporation's mission, strategies, and goals. And related to this was each individual's vague understanding of his or her role in the organization's plan, as well as a dissatisfaction with his or her ability to achieve a performance result. Another, related major issue was the sense that there was a lack of leadership. Staff indicated that whether or not they agreed with a leader's direction, consistency of leadership was a critical element in satisfying their needs. They characterized this leader as someone who would listen, evaluate, decide, mobilize, and lead the resources of the business (space, equipment, dollars, and human energy) in a set direction.

Interviewees were also evaluated as to their readiness for accountable participation in issue resolution. To do this, the CEO conducting the interview used various strategies to determine each interviewee's attitudes toward being accountable for and effecting change. The characteristics of *accountable* behavior versus *victimhood* behavior are generally easily observable in an interview. Persons who illustrate victimhood behavior generally look outside themselves—to others, to circumstances beyond their control—for the cause of an issue's lack of resolution. These people usually have great difficulty in accepting responsibility for problems or explaining how they could help in problem or issue resolution. This type of individual seeks the comfort and support offered by social situations in which he or she can complain to colleagues about difficult relationships or issues and provide several reasons why these difficulties cannot be resolved. Called coffee klatching, this technique enables the individual to reduce his or her stress by "bending the ears" of sympathetic colleagues. It is relatively easy to identify those people who are on either end of the "accountability curve"; however, the vast majority of people fall within the curve's normal limits. On occasion, all of us fall into victimhood behavior. The question is, Are we playing the role of victim so intensely that we cannot effectively work with an accountable team of people, to begin to adopt a "let's-fix-it" attitude. This is what the interviews were used to determine.

Of the 60 staff members interviewed, only 4 perceived themselves as helpless when it came to accountability. The balance of staff were committed to being personally successful and part of an organization that was providing high-quality services and achieving good financial performance. Of course, the degree of commitment for accountability varied from person to person, but generally a positive search for issue resolution, goal development, and performance result was evident. Of the four unable or unwilling to view their and Casa Colina's condition as workable, none was terminated by management. Within six months, all resigned for different reasons. Two of these four employees submitted letters of resignation with the expectation that their influential positions would cause management to negotiate their decision to resign. However, management's philosophy was to respect and accept all resignations submitted, recognizing that the time to discuss the pros and cons of organizational participation and value is before a resignation is submitted, rather than after. The other two employees left for other employment.

The second process—developing action plans—was implemented within the first six months. The major issues raised by the interviews were converted into action plans. The following plan was implemented with regard to the lack of planning and consensus: Staff at senior- and middle-management levels were invited to a retreat to brainstorm and develop goals and plans for setting new directions. With goals developed, assignments made, and progress in assignment checked on at periodic intervals, a new focus and level of consciousness-raising emerged. The critical issue was that leaders and managers had to understand and be personally responsible for the plan and its rationale. From this effort, time-quantified, measurable objectives led to resolution of the issues raised. The net result was that financial break-even was achieved within 12 months. This was the result of increased productivity yielding increased revenue through more focused attention on improved patient care.

One example of this outcome was that the physical, occupational, speech, and psychological therapists increased patient hours billed by 15 percent through improved productivity and without additional staff, which resulted in increased revenues amounting to several hundred thousand dollars. The same decision today would not improve the bottom line due to Medicare and contractual HMO and PPO reimbursement methodology. However, the involvement of individuals (in this case, the therapists) in resolving issues that affect them and their clients continues to yield effective performance for the corporation, even in today's cost-restrained environment.

Another problem that was resolved concerned trust relationships between policymakers and senior staff. Several staff and board members had social relationships wherein corporate performance might be discussed outside the boardroom. Frequently, the CEO would be confronted at board meetings with corporate performance concerns for which management response was ill prepared. Agreement was reached that no further communication regarding the organization would occur between staff and board members at informal sessions. Line authority would be respected, subject to disciplinary action by management and the board. Improved communication, well-prepared proposals regarding performance issues, and trust between parties were the results.

During this same period, the interview process was broadened beyond staff to include consumers and referring physicians. The discovery was that neither consumers nor physicians understood which disabling conditions were best served by rehabilitation. Accordingly, rehabilitation services were redefined by the disability group served, including programs for stroke, spinal cord injury, traumatic brain injury, and back pain. The rationale for this was that persons disabled by stroke would better understand their referral to a stroke rehabilitation program than to a rehabilitation hospital. Further specialization in that "service line" by staff would yield more effective patient outcomes. The redefining of rehabilitation was not an event, but a process. The inquiry process of patients was conducted by research staff. Staff members would contact former patients to follow up on postdischarge needs and advise the program managers of program elements that required improvement. Rehabilitation nurses (liaison nurses) would contact acute care hospital discharge coordinators and physicians, both referring and nonreferring. The approach was not to tell and sell, but to inquire how services could be improved, find out what was wrong with programs, and discover what the unmet needs were. These persons not only valued being asked, but appreciated Casa Colina's response even more when a service was improved or a new one was introduced as a result of the inquiry.

Finally, third-party payer advisory committees were established for the sole purpose of determining what Casa Colina was missing and how it could improve.

With the power of opinion from creditable outside agents, the need to change behavior was not directed from "the boss," but from the market. It was clear to most staff that if referring agents were not happy, there would be no more referrals, and if there were no more referrals, there would be no more Casa Colina. This process invited the community to become a significant part of the corporation's program development and change. Every opportunity was taken to show appreciation for the ideas shared for Casa Colina's improvement.

The result of this effort in program redesign and inquiry was an increase in patient referral of between 20 and 30 percent, depending on the program.

New Program Diversification (1976–1984)

Between 1976 and 1984, ongoing interviewing of physicians, internal staff, third-party payers, patients, and families showed that the hospital had several unmet needs. These included the need of the target market for vocational rehabilitation and the opportunity to offer choices for earlier discharge from a costly inpatient setting to a less sheltered, less costly, and more clinically appropriate outpatient setting. A strategic planning group was developed to respond to the need for change and to develop diversification strategies.

The composition of Casa Colina's strategic planning group varied over the years with representation from line-, middle-, and senior-management positions; the CEO was always represented. Several small work groups representing different rehabilitation specialties and interests met over two-day periods to focus their thinking on three different future scenarios. From the beginning, the organizational positions represented in the strategic planning group were less important than the fund of knowledge about rehabilitation and the variance in how each group member viewed the world. Three categories were selected as bases for discussing future strategies: possible futures, probable futures, and preferred futures.

- *Possible futures:* The first scenario was to present and discuss ideas as though resources were unlimited. Because the resources required to implement these ideas were not considered relevant, the group had complete freedom to dream.
- *Probable futures:* This type of discussion contemplated the dollar implications of the ideas; trends and competitive forces; human resources availability; and space, equipment, and their management. Verification of marketplace responsiveness to the ideas was also discussed and later reality-checked.
- *Preferred futures:* From the previous discussions, a chosen or preferred future was developed. This future was one that each group member could personally buy in to. From that personal ownership, time-quantified and measurable objectives were developed that identified *what, who, how, where,* and *when* objectives would be achieved leading to the preferred future.

The different work groups forwarded their preferred futures to be considered by senior management, and ultimately the board of directors, for inclusion in the corporation's strategic and annual business plans.

During this planning period, the CEO was invited to attend a training session by a group of staff who especially valued a leadership training program and thought the CEO would find it useful. The three-day training pointed up four different personality styles or views of the world, all of which must be reasonably represented in a planning effort if the strategic plan is to be completely successful. If a corporation is dominated by only one style, that corporation and its effort risks not having balanced services, effective public relations, and/or long-term viability. The general population is reported to be evenly distributed among the four views, which are as follows:

1. *Promoter style:* Characteristically, the people who represent this type of management style collect information intuitively. Their ideas are generally more expansive and less encumbered with the details necessary for implementation strategies. Typically, they are idea people, characterized by others as eternal optimists. They focus their efforts on working with people and relationships, enjoy brainstorming, and have little patience with working out the nitty-gritty.
2. *Controller style:* This style of leadership is task focused. People in this group perceive employees as instruments needed to carry out a plan. Empirically validated data, substantiated conclusions, and a focus on how objectives are arrived at are important to this group. Brainstorming, without supportive data, is commonly perceived as a waste of time by the people in this group. Controllers would perceive promoters as people who seldom get the job done, who have bright ideas but no follow-through, or who are flakes. On the other hand, promoters would view controllers as emotionless machines who are steeped in detail, have the only truth, and are unreceptive to the important and subtle needs of the marketplace.
3. *Analytical style:* The individuals who represent this leadership style characteristically observe, collect, and analyze data about the world with great neutrality. They are not swayed by emotionally laden presentations commonly made by promoters. This group gathers enormous amounts of data but seldom is comfortable using the data to make decisions for fear that the data may be insufficient.
4. *Supporter style:* The people who fall into this leadership style are commonly the workhorses of any organization, as long as there is clear direction. Without such direction, supporters tend to be dissatisfied with the job. Confrontation with differing views (conflict) is not comfortable for these people. Loyalty and commitment to the assigned task is exceptional among supporters, and feedback regarding performance is more critical to this group than to any other.

It is interesting to note that each style is inclined to *judge* the others as having less value. Management encouraged staff members with different views of the world not to stand in judgment of each other, but rather to acknowledge the strengths that different views can bring to issue review, evaluation, or resolution.

A dominant leadership style can bring disaster to a business purpose. Our intention was to keep some balance over time in our planning and implementation efforts. We selected our management staff based on performance results and related experience, with the secondary intention of having a mix of the four views of the world as much as possible. The task was to capitalize on each style's view of the world in order to achieve a balanced strategy and a focused planning effort.

The result of having divergence in view and consensus for plans yielded more effective implementation efforts. From such views and planning efforts, a case-managed continuum of care evolved.

Alternatives were designed to meet the needs for less sheltered and less costly (than inpatient) outpatient settings, including comprehensive outpatient rehabilitation facilities (CORFs) with a day hospital component (same staff as a rehabilitation hospital but without beds) and an adult day program (designed to provide an alternative to a skilled nursing facility). A vocational rehabilitation division was developed to facilitate patient transition from activity in the medical rehabilitation setting to activity that focused on return to work. Using subcontracted work from industry and payment for work according to productivity, the consequence was the facilitation of persons back to work. Another program included the provision of subacute rehabilitation care within a skilled nursing facility, providing outcome results at half the cost of traditional acute inpatient care for a majority of persons with stroke or orthopedic problems and for ventilator-dependent patients.

With the clinical and pricing point choices in rehabilitation services (from $25 per day for service in adult day health care to $250 per day in the outpatient day hospital, to $450 per day in subacute rehabilitation care, to between $700 and $1,000 a day for acute services), patients, referring agents, and buyers/payers had a number of options.

The array of services grew from one rehabilitation hospital to over 50 programs in many locations, at a rate of approximately 20 percent per year over a 17-year period. Gross revenues increased from $1 million to over $50 million annually, and the number of employees from 60 to over 1,000. The balance sheet on 30 different measures are in the top quartile for 28 out of 30 measures when compared to comparable facilities. The two lower ratings have to do with the average age of the building and how foundation income is reported.

In part, this growth occurred at Casa Colina because management encouraged representation of diverse views in planning, listened to those views nonjudgmentally, was willing to take risks, and planned for the future.

In 1978, a national trend emerged to create health care delivery systems under more than one corporate vehicle. At the time, this trend was supported in part by the opportunities available to maximize reimbursement under several corporate structures.

During this period, Casa Colina developed a parent holding company that held the only corporate vote for the subsidiary corporations it created. Three powers were held by the parent corporation over the subsidiaries: (1) election of board members; (2) approval of capital, operating, and pro forma cash flow annual budgets with business plans; and (3) final authority in liquidation of assets. Corporate organization was developed along product lines. The advantage to this was that it focused on each respective business by retaining both competent senior management experienced in the product line and policymakers with interest in and commitment to that product line. The organizational structure that evolved included a parent corporation and a foundation:

- *A parent corporation* with accountability for strategic planning, financial resource allocation, and operational audit of subsidiary business plans that are written and quantified annually.
- *A foundation* with accountability to raise funds for program development, free care, and cutting-edge rehabilitation research. This foundation not only had a board of directors committed to this singular purpose, but also a subsidiary group of geographically dispersed trustees, volunteers, and auxiliaries who would represent fund-raising programs in the different geographic regions in which Casa Colina programs were represented.

A hospital corporation, a skilled nursing corporation, a comprehensive outpatient rehabilitation services corporation, a vocational rehabilitation corporation, and a long-term residential corporation all emerged from the reorganization. These subsidiaries assumed their own tactical planning, quality assurance, and operational accountability. Finally, a corporation that was developed to assume accountability for growth and diversification strategies was later converted to a for-profit corporation, the only one among all the Casa Colina corporations.

Although growth, development, and performance were enhanced by the reorganization, the efforts of both management and the board to serve all the varying needs of each corporation proved time-consuming. The CEO of the parent corporation maintained line authority by sitting on each subsidiary corporation board and retaining authority to hire and fire over each subsidiary's chief operating officer. This line authority ensured that everyone knew who was boss and enhanced communication, planning, and execution among the senior management of all the subsidiaries. The parent corporation also provided management information systems; financial, environmental, and facility planning; and marketing, research, and human resources support systems to the subsidiary groups.

After approximately 10 years of separate corporate operation under this scenario, the service operation corporations were consolidated into a single corporation called Casa Colina Centers for Rehabilitation. This corporation was represented by one board of directors having accountability for the hospital, skilled nursing, vocational rehabilitation, comprehensive outpatient rehabilitation services, and residential services corporations. The rationale for the consolidation included saving both management and policymakers time, establishing more mature corporate support systems, and enforcing greater communication between senior-service line management and policymakers in order to provide more effective continuity of patient care.

By broadening the conceptual base of rehabilitation through the introduction of new programs to meet consumer needs, several factors emerged that enhanced Casa Colina's market share and capacity to compete:

- *Profitability improved:* Broadening the service base with additional services improved the gross contribution margin by spreading general and administrative expenses over a broader base, and provided the opportunity to keep profit, accelerate growth, or maintain a pricing competitiveness in the marketplace.
- *Market share increased:* By providing new services that met the needs of existing patients, Casa Colina attracted other patients not usually served by its programs.
- *Pricing points were established:* The new services established pricing choices for third-party payers by having alternatives for inpatient rehabilitation programs that were one-third to one-half the cost of traditional inpatient services. Further, this factor enhanced Casa Colina's reputation among third-party payers as an organization implementing cost-effective behaviors in a cost-conscious environment.

However, support for diversification was not universal. For example, medical staff were interested in enhancing inpatient services in which their time and earned income would be most enhanced. Management and policymakers from the community were more interested in and supportive of developing rehabilitation alternatives. The end result of the diversification was to satisfy all parties concerned by providing a broader base of financial support and a more clinically relevant continuum of care for patients served. This enabled the organization to grow and attract more sophisticated and qualified staff to compete in the marketplace. Even in today's environment, Casa Colina is experiencing less of a shortage in professionals or management candidates than seems apparent in other programs.

Accelerated Growth Period (1984–present)

Prior to the most recent period, Casa Colina studied the nature of patient outcomes via their functional status at admission, discharge, and 90-day follow-up. Comparisons were made between stroke patients served in acute and subacute settings. The populations showed reasonable measures of comparability and functional status outcomes. Accordingly, we believed that this subacute treatment strategy could have a very positive impact on the costs involved in treating stroke patients in our community and the nation. Further, over a three- to four-year period, the ambulatory and subacute centers were making more money than they spent, although initially persuading third-party payers of their value was an uphill battle. However, the more the nation pressed for cost containment, the more attention focused on the subacute model.

Having shown the ability of the ambulatory and subacute programs to produce clinically relevant patient outcomes, and having gained market acceptance by showing financially sound returns on investment, it was now time to invest resources to accelerate program growth. Accordingly, the board of directors approved and encouraged accelerated investment.

The *financial capacity* to fund accelerated growth was developed through two primary methods. The first was to hold management accountable for producing more revenue than expense so that the financial data worksheets showed the capacity to pay debts. This expectation was introduced early in the 1970 development period. The result was a fund balance that enabled investment in new services.

The second method was to research nationally proven fund-raising techniques and implement a successful program at Casa Colina. Identifying the proven methods of fund-raising was rather simple; finding skilled fund-raisers proved more difficult. Turnover was extraordinary in that leadership role and the length of employment was approximately two years. In frustration, Casa Colina's CEO, using a delphi-type strategy, interviewed those fund-raisers rated by their peers as practitioners to emulate.

A search began. The CEO knew he had the right person when, in the interview, the candidate asked the CEO how much he gave to Casa Colina's purpose. Proudly, the CEO revealed the dollar amount. The candidate replied that the CEO was *not* modeling appropriate giving behavior and specified an amount that would meet that definition. Within a year, the CEO increased his contribution to set the standard for appropriate giving behavior. The candidate had demonstrated principle number one of fund-raising: Give personally an amount that purges the soul before you ask anyone else to give. The candidate was hired and remains with the corporation, having now generated millions of dollars over seven years and outperforming health care giving nationwide by over 800 percent compounded growth.

A delphi-type interview process might be productive for other chief executive officers to learn the five or six principles of fund-raising; however, be aware that it will personally cost you. Between 1981 and 1988, this fund-raising program generated financial support from the community that enabled research and free care for some patients, and provided program development funds comparable to venture capital sought from Wall Street investment firms.

The problem of finding the *human resources* needed to implement the accelerated growth was resolved by bringing in talented managers with specialties in acute inpatient rehabilitation, subacute rehabilitation in skilled nursing facilities, comprehensive outpatient rehabilitation services, transitional and long-term residential programs, and comprehensive back injury rehabilitation services. In addition, training programs were developed internally to promote existing talent to management levels. Four-week to three-month orientation and management internship programs were developed to broaden the choices for future management talent.

A *marketing strategy* evolved that was based on the premise that sole ownership of a program by Casa Colina in a new community was not as attractive as a joint-ventured relationship with an established health care institution or a physician group. Accordingly, sales, research, and public relations activity focused on identifying community physician groups and health care institutions that had sufficient patient activity, as well as a positive and established image to ensure program success.

The *method to establish new programs* followed the usual steps of any market research and implementation plan. Upon contact and interest expressed by a party in rehabilitation services, the joint venture group would screen for patient volume, joint venture interest, positive image, and financial capacity criteria. This screening was followed by jointly funded market research of the community to be served. Research areas included the incidence in the community of the disability for which the program was intended; physician interest and referral patterns; competitor analysis; and licensure, regulation, and accreditation requirements. From that research, market share goals and strategies were developed, an organizational structure was considered, and risks were analyzed. The final process was development of pro forma capital, operating, and cash flow scenarios from which a go/no-go decision would be reached between parties.

Future Directions

Future opportunities in our accelerated growth mode will likely yield a rehabilitation corporation in the year 2000 that has more affiliations and locations throughout our targeted geographic markets. However, with the managed care environment so prominent in the southern California area, growth will require enormous strategic and tactical changes.

The specifics to achieve the aforementioned growth in today's competitive environment are not yet clear. Suffice it to say, we are listening carefully to those who pay the bills. We are encouraging increased outreach by senior and middle management and interested staff to ask the questions, "How can we improve?" and "Will you help us meet your needs?" Casa Colina has found that being a distance apart from those who pay the bills will lead to loss of program relevance/utilization. Its management believes that real value or behavior change occurs out of economic necessity. There is a powerful economic message being sent by those who pay the bills, and it is: "Do it better for less." Health care executives and staff, along with the consumer and buyer, have the ability to change the future and render continued relevance and leadership for this country's health, illness, recovery, and rehabilitation care systems. However, it will likely be provided at less cost and with the consumer and buyer involved in the service delivery design.

Annotated Bibliography

Ambulatory Care and Rehabilitation

General Overview

American Hospital Association, Section for Rehabilitation Hospitals and Programs, Department of Special Surveys, and Hospital Data Center. *Survey of Medical Rehabilitation Hospitals and Units in 1988.* Chicago: AHA, 1990.

Prepared by the Hospital Data Center, Department of Special Surveys, in conjunction with the Section for Rehabilitation Hospitals and Programs.

Barone, W., Costante, P. A., and Ennis, R. S. The challenge to adapt. A specialty care facility refocuses its services to promote continuity of care. *Health Progress* 70(5):50–56, June 1989.

Because clients now spend less time than before in acute care hospitals, specialty care institutions have had to modify and expand their services to meet new needs. They must not only provide new kinds of care, but they must also assist clients and their families in making the often confusing transition from acute care to rehabilitation and, finally, to the community. In the past few years, the St. Lawrence Rehabilitation Center, Lawrenceville, New Jersey, has been making just such changes. In response to a systematic review of its services, the center established its social work services department in 1987. Seven program managers are the core of the department. They encourage patient and family participation in St. Lawrence services, advocate for them in a variety of contexts, help define treatment goals, and ensure that clients, families, and treatment teams keep these goals in mind. St. Lawrence has also updated its admissions process, creating an admissions team whose role is to locate appropriate referrals and expedite patient admission to the center. Whereas the earlier process typically took several weeks to complete, St. Lawrence now has an intake system capable of a 24-hour turnaround. The center has also expanded its outpatient services and established an orientation program that keeps outpatients abreast of the services available to them at St. Lawrence.

Davis, D., and Hobbs, G. Measuring outpatient satisfaction with rehabilitation services. *Quality Review Bulletin* 16(6):192–97, June 1989.

Rehabilitation services department staff at University Hospital-UBC site (Vancouver, British Columbia) conducted a patient satisfaction survey in 1987 to measure outpatient satisfaction with the care received. Fifty completed surveys, which represented approximately 10 percent of the outpatient population discharged during the study period, indicated that outpatients were primarily satisfied with the actual care and services provided and least satisfied with environmental factors, such as parking, waiting area conditions, and directions to treatment facility.

Fazio, S. M., and Fralish, K. B. A survey of leisure and recreation programs offered by agencies serving traumatic head-injured adults. *Therapeutic Recreation Journal* 22(1):46–54, 1st Quarter 1988.

This article describes a study conducted to determine the status of leisure and recreation programs currently being offered to head-injured individuals participating in postacute rehabilitation programs. Lack of funding and staff shortages were the most common reasons cited for nonexistent recreation and leisure programs. The recreation and leisure education goals that were viewed as most important included social skills development and reduction of inappropriate behaviors in order to promote successful community reintegration. Assessment tools and a list of leisure skills/activities for the head-injured population were the types of assistance recommended by respondents. This study is the first national survey that has examined existing recreation programs in head injury rehabilitation settings.

Market scan: ten leading trends for rehabilitation in the 1990s. *Hospital Strategy Report* 2(10):1, 4–7, Aug. 1990.

This article lists the top 10 trends that will affect rehabilitation in the 1990s. These trends include projected growth rates of ambulatory rehabilitation, based on the aging population and rising demand for services. Other trends include the increase in specialty niches such as brain injury and amputee programs; the increased focus on service line management; and the need to gain an edge over competitors through service excellence. The article briefly discusses the implications of each trend.

Wallace, C. Rehabilitative care moving to lower-cost treatment centers. *Modern Healthcare* 18(3):32–33, Jan. 15, 1988.

Specialists in the rehabilitation field point out that rehabilitative care is moving from acute, inpatient treatment settings into such growth areas as transitional living centers and lower-cost treatment centers. Several experts from investor-owned chains counter these arguments by saying the demand for inpatient rehabilitation will continue for several years. However, the field of rehabilitative care is entering a new phase of development. The article discusses the route hospitals, nursing homes, and entrepreneurs are using to access the rehabilitation market. In particular, through interviewing specialists in the field, the article provides an "up-close" perspective on the organizational and financial nuances in the rehabilitation market.

Zafiratos, C. A continuum of rehabilitative care. A day hospital extends patients' lifeline to the medical center. *Health Progress* 71(9):55–57, Nov. 1990.

Alexian Brothers Medical Center in Elk Grove Village, Illinois, carries out its commitment to a continuum of care through the Alexian Brothers Rehabilitation Center and its Physical Rehabilitation Day Hospital. The day hospital treats patients who need rehabilitation but do not need around-the-clock hospitalization. The day hospital individualizes its intensive comprehensive, pulmonary, and arthritis programs. An important component of these outpatient programs is education and preventive techniques to reduce the need for repeat treatment. Only medically stable patients are transferred to the rehabilitation center, where an interdisciplinary team helps them achieve the maximum function possible within the limits imposed by their disabilities. The rehabilitation center sponsors a community support group for young adults who have sustained head injuries and a group for alumni of the center. Through its home health care program and its adult day-care program, the medical center offers a variety of treatment delivery methods that enhance the center's continuum of care.

Cardiac Rehabilitation

Gutin, B., Prince, L., and Stein, R. Survey of cardiac rehabilitation centers in New York City. *Journal of Community Health* 15(4):227–38, Aug. 1990.

Outpatient cardiac rehabilitation centers in New York City were surveyed in order to determine current practices. All 24 centers operating as of May 1987 were sent questionnaires; 16 responded, for a return rate of 67 percent. In general, practices of the centers were in accordance with guidelines of the American Heart Association (AHA) and the American College of Sports Medicine. The incidence of medical complications in the centers was quite rare, perhaps accounting for the failure of centers to follow all of the American Hospital Association's emergency guidelines, such as daily testing of the defibrillator. The major aim of the centers was to enhance physiological status, rather narrowly defined as aerobic fitness and cardiovascular function. Little attention was paid to nutrition, body composition, and strength, even though the value of broadening the concept of fitness to include these parameters is becoming evident. Lifestyle counseling to help in long-term rehabilitation was also rare. Third-party payers should be encouraged to support such components of a rehabilitation program so that centers will more likely incorporate them.

Comprehensive Outpatient Rehabilitation Facilities

England, B. A winning combination in rehabilitation. *Business and Health* 5(5):26–31, May 1988.

This article discusses a return-to-work strategy implemented on an outpatient basis that not only prepares the client to get back to work earlier, but also helps him or her maintain and possibly increase functional ability after resuming work. The article provides useful information on program development specifically examining provider selection, program evaluation, and client orientation. The article emphasizes that successful outpatient rehabilitation coordinates the needs of employer, provider, and employee.

Grass, R., and Weinstein, E. CORFs (comprehensive outpatient rehabilitation facilities): an emerging health care system for brain-injured patients. *Journal of Ambulatory Care Marketing* 2(2):67–78, 1988.

This article follows the development of comprehensive outpatient rehabilitation facilities (CORFs) as they emerged from the day hospital concept into a new health care delivery system. The structure, requirements for stature, reimbursement considerations, and potential problems associated with CORFs are discussed. Issues relating to the care of patients with brain injuries are presented, and an innovative model of an institute that individualizes a program of techniques to arouse comatose patients and trains and supports families during the process of arousal from coma is described. The article goes on to explore the problems and potentials of a CORF serving as a cost-effective, efficient health service delivery system for brain-injured patients with long-term rehabilitative needs.

Geriatric Rehabilitation

Applegate, W. B., Miller, S. T., Graney, M. J., Elam, J. T., Burns, R., and Akins, D. E. A randomized, controlled trial of a geriatric assessment unit in a community rehabilitation hospital. *New England Journal of Medicine* 322(22):1572-78, May 31, 1990.

This article describes a randomized trial in a community rehabilitation hospital to determine the effect of treatment in a geriatric assessment unit on the physical function, institutionalization rate, and mortality of elderly patients. Functionally impaired elderly patients (mean age, 78.8 years) who were recovering from acute medical or surgical illnesses and were considered at risk for nursing home placement were randomly assigned to either the geriatric assessment unit (n = 78) or a control group that received usual care (n = 77). The two groups were similar at entry and stratified according to the perceived risk of an immediate nursing home placement.

Ardron, M. E., and Finneston, A. Use of rehabilitation apartments for elderly patients. *Age and Ageing* 19(3):195–98, May 1990.

Sixty-three admissions to rehabilitation apartments were studied. In almost half of the patients, the actual outcome on discharge disagreed with the occupational therapy assessment after they used the apartment. Patients who were placed in the apartment to help them gain insight into their disabilities remained unconvinced, the majority returning home despite advice. Although rehabilitation apartments may improve patient morale, they should not be used to predict ability to survive at home or to dissuade patients who seem likely to fail from returning there.

Cassak, D. Medical rehabilitation: tapping into a growing alternate site market. *Health Industry Today* 51(3):52–60, Mar. 1988.

This article is based on an interview with James Hoover, a leading expert in the rehabilitation field and an analyst for the San Francisco–based investment firm of Robertson, Colman, and Stephens.

In the article, Hoover discusses growth trends in the rehabilitation marketplace, the provider's role in developing rehabilitation facilities, the different types of rehabilitation facilities, and the role of physicians in this geriatric rehabilitation market. Additionally, the article provides numerous perspectives regarding financing CORFs and skilled nursing facilities, reimbursement policies, corporate involvement in the field, and the relationship between medical technology and advances in rehabilitation therapy. As Hoover states, medical rehabilitation can play an important role in cost-effective treatment and reduction of productivity losses and disability costs due to injury and illness, as well as address the whole area of workers' compensation claims.

Dacher, J. E. Rehabilitation and the geriatric patient. *Nursing Clinics of North America* 24(1):225–37, Mar. 1989.

The true challenge in the care of the elderly is to keep people at home, in the community, with a high degree of functional ability. This is beneficial to the individual and, from a financial point of view, to the community and the public. Maintenance and restoration of function are best accomplished within a framework that considers the psychosocial and developmental needs of the geriatric patient and in a setting specifically intended for the geriatric rehabilitation patient.

Kondis, C. L. Healing and hope. A multiservice health care provider gives elderly patients a chance to return to the mainstream. *Health Progress* 71(9):42–45, 59, Nov. 1990.

Responding to a mission commitment to serve the elderly, Mercy Medical, Daphne, Alabama, has developed a multiservice rehabilitation program that includes inpatient and outpatient care, as well as residential and home health services. The Mercy Medical staff assumes that even elderly patients who have suffered catastrophic injury or illness can return to mainstream life, if they can participate in an effective medical treatment program. The Mercy Medical philosophy is to encourage patients to take an active role in their treatment programs and to stress from the beginning that patients are expected to recover. The staff also encourages patients to take risks that might speed their recovery, and the staff itself is willing to experiment with more effective ways of increasing patients' functional ability. Like most rehabilitation programs, Mercy Medical uses an interdisciplinary approach, with a physician heading a staff team that includes nurses; social workers; pharmacists; and physical, occupational, and respiratory therapists.

Smith, M. E. The organization, delivery, utilization and financing of rehabilitation care for the elderly. *DRG Monitor* 7(6–7):1–12, Feb.–Mar. 1990.

In order to meet the needs of a large, elderly disabled population in the 1990s, the inevitable close linkage between the hospital and postacute care providers will place increased demands and responsibilities on the hospital management team and its hospital practicing physicians for patient care decisions along the continuum of care for the elderly.

Legal Issues

Johnson, C. P. Relationships between CORFs and long-term care facilities. In: T. C. Fox, editor. *Long-Term Care and the Law.* Owings Mills, MD: National Health Publishing, 1986.

This article represents an address delivered at the National Health Lawyers Association's Tenth Annual Symposium. It discusses the legal issues behind the management of CORFs, specifically examining Medicare regulations, accounting practices, leasing arrangements, staffing, and corporate structuring.

Watson, P. G. Rehabilitation legislation of the 1980s: implications for nurses as healthcare providers. *Rehabilitation Nursing* 13(3):136–41, May–June 1988.

Laws enacted for the benefit of persons with disabilities establish the parameters around which various health care services can be provided. This article discusses the federal rehabilitation legislation of the 1980s. The significance of this legislation is put in perspective by comparing it with the legislative accomplishments of the 1970s. Attention is directed to the current status of rehabilitation in the United States as governed by statute. In addition, the article provides a glance into the future of rehabilitation legislation and its impact on both providers and users of rehabilitative care. The article also provides a framework through which nurses can work to advocate for the health care needs of persons with disabilities.

Marketing

Martin, J. Problem analysis: application in the development of market strategies for health care organizations. *Journal of Health Care Marketing* 8(1):5–16, Mar. 1988.

The problem analysis technique is an approach to understanding salient customer needs that is especially appropriate under complex market conditions. The problem approach provides information to health care providers that is directly applicable to strategic decisions such as gaining and retaining patronage, increasing usage and diversification, and supporting rapid competitive reactions. After an overview of the rationale and nature of problem analysis, the methodology of an empirical study is explained. The author demonstrates the use of the approach in segmenting markets and conducting competitive analysis for positioning strategy decisions in health care.

Pediatric Rehabilitation

Burkett, K. W. Trends in pediatric rehabilitation. *Nursing Clinics of North America* 24(1):239–55, Mar. 1989.

The definition of pediatric rehabilitation has expanded to include the care and treatment of children with congenital and acquired disabilities. The pediatric rehabilitation nurse is challenged to keep abreast of new developments in the field while seeking and implementing innovative ways to assist the child and the family in their adjustment to the child's disability. A knowledge base of normal growth and development is essential when assessing abnormal patterns in the child with a disability. Complete assessment of the child with a disability includes a parent–child interview and physical assessment, with particular focus on the child's developmental age, movement patterns, and functional activities of daily living.

Ireys, H. T., and Eichler, R. J. Program priorities of crippled children's agencies: a survey. *Public Health Reports* 103(1):77–83, Jan.–Feb. 1988.

This article represents the findings of a survey undertaken to determine the programmatic priorities of crippled children's agencies. The authors surveyed all state crippled children program directors, obtaining a response rate of 92 percent. The questionnaire included a list of 27 specific activities whose importance directors were to evaluate in terms of achieving their agencies' goals. The key findings indicated that coordinating patient care services, team conferencing on individual cases, developing and disseminating standards of care, reviewing or reworking eligibility criteria (or both), and collecting payments were the activities most frequently judged very important. In addition, the findings suggested that not enough time is being allocated to such things as staff continuing education, developing alliances with private-sector providers, and developing new ways of financing care, although these three activities were among the top in importance. Overall, the article puts into perspective the need to garner both organizational and financial support to fulfill and broaden the missions of crippled children's agencies.

Page, C. M., Bornhoeft, D. M., and Barcome, D. F. Providing outreach services in a rural setting utilizing a multidisciplinary team: the CARES Project. *Rehabilitation Literature* 46(9–10):264–67, Sept.–Oct. 1985.

The CARES (Coordinated Rehabilitation Evaluation Services) Project presents a model that appears workable to provide multidisciplinary services for children in rural settings who have multiple disabilities. The project is a three-stage process leading to the eventual establishment of an ongoing, locally based program of coordinated rehabilitation services. This article provides background information on the components of the model as well as data to illustrate both the evolution and present performance of the program. Nearly 400 children with multiple disabilities have received services through the CARES Project.

Productivity

Blodgett, C., and Pekarik, G. Program evaluation in cardiac rehabilitation IV: efficiency evaluation. *Journal of Cardiopulmonary Rehabilitation* 7(10):466–74, Oct. 20, 1987.

In this article, the authors discuss the role of efficiency measurement in program evaluation. Addressing the efficiency of rehabilitation services requires knowledge of the number of service units provided and the total cost of delivering these services. In addition, for cost-benefit or cost-outcome analysis, knowledge regarding the outcome of the service is required. The article provides detailed information on how efficiency evaluation can be operationalized in a rehabilitation setting, specifically focusing on a discussion of the data elements needed, a definition of psychosocial interventions, and the steps taken in designing a workable evaluation scheme. Evaluation of a hypothetical rehabilitation program is provided to illustrate how efficiency evaluation can be effectively designed and implemented.

Boyd, S. D., Coven, B., and Kurth, E. Productivity considerations in the development of a new program and the ongoing management of an outpatient rehabilitation center. *Journal of Ambulatory Care Management* 11(1):34–40, Feb. 1988.

St. Joseph Hospital and Health Care Center in Chicago established and transferred outpatient rehabilitation referrals to the Rehabilitation and Fitness Center, a freestanding facility affiliated with the hospital. The facility provides physical therapy, occupational therapy, and cognitive rehabilitation. In order to meet the goal of attaining maximum productivity at the hospital and the center, a monthly productivity system was integrated via the hospital patient charging system. This article describes the productivity system developed and implemented by the facility. It discusses the impetus behind the creation of the freestanding facility, the monitoring and control of staffing as they relate to the productivity system, how the productivity system was developed and implemented, evaluation and refinement of the system, and how the facility determines future staffing, facility, and equipment needs.

Ventrone, J. M., Zanotti, M., and Heidtman, M. M. Dressing for success: measuring productivity can ensure continuing success. *Healthcare Financial Management* 42(8):30–32, 34–38, 40, Aug. 1988.

Both managerial and financial benefits can be gained by implementing and monitoring productivity standards in the health care organization. However, to be effective these standards must be reasonable and acceptable to both management and staff. By implementing a logging system to determine actual daily activity, Elizabethtown Hospital was able to develop reasonable productivity standards that allowed department managers to manage their operations more efficiently.

Quality Assurance

Carey, R. Integrating case management, program evaluation, and marketing for inpatient and outpatient rehabilitation programs. *Advances in Clinical Rehabilitation* 3:219–49, 1990.

This article discusses the integration of case management, program evaluation, and marketing for inpatient and outpatient rehabilitation programs.

Schurman, B. A. Durable data. A rehabilitation center collects and distributes information for functional assessment and program evaluation. *Health Progress* 71(9):52–54, Nov. 1990.

As physical rehabilitation services have expanded nationwide, both payers and providers have increasingly felt the need for adequate outcome data. In 1988, organizers at Marianjoy Rehabilitation Center, Wheaton, Illinois, launched the Center for Rehabilitation Outcome Analysis, a service for rehabilitation facilities that want to develop in-house functional assessment and program evaluation systems. The center has focused on meeting three major needs of rehabilitation providers: outcome data analysis and reporting, education, and research. It uses the Patient Evaluation and Conference System for a variety of needs from planning programs to establishing functional outcome expectations. The center also educates participants on the use and meaning of outcome data. In addition, it has enlisted the help of the profession's behavioral scientists, evaluators, and statisticians to scrutinize and enhance program evaluation and measurement models.

Verhey, S., and Upton, B. Evaluation system assesses rehabilitation. *Health Progress* 69(9):48–50, 53, Nov. 1988.

The program evaluation system has evolved into a valuable tool for improved management of patient programming and accountability, providing objective assessment of patient functions. Each program states primary objectives, measurements, and expectancies to determine how well it has met the objectives. The objectives deal with areas that reflect the patient's overall function, which ultimately determines what level of care the patient will need after discharge. The functional assessment scale (FAS), an ordinal rating scale of values ranging from total dependence to total independence, is used to measure the objectives within the parameters and to assess the severity of the disability, progress, and outcome. Concurrent evaluations enable physicians, therapists, and administrators to identify where problems occur in the individual's program and to change treatment accordingly. The FAS generates quarterly management reports that demonstrate achievement of the objectives using the measurements and goal expectancy and that facilitate pattern analysis. The system easily integrates with the facility's current operations, including quality assurance.

Reimbursement

Batavia, A. I. *The Payment of Medical Rehabilitation Services: Current Mechanisms and Potential Models.* Chicago: American Hospital Association, Section for Rehabilitation Hospitals and Programs, 1988.

This book evaluates the major alternative approaches to payment for rehabilitation services against a specific set of criteria. It clarifies the nature of the choices and probable consequences. It offers an agenda for research and evaluation of payment systems specific to medical rehabilitation services.

England, B., compiler. *Medical Rehabilitation Services in Health Care Institutions.* Chicago: American Hospital Publishing, 1986.

Reimbursement for rehabilitation therapy is lacking in consistency and universality among public and private insurers. Lack of acceptance among medical and allied health professionals and third-party purchasers is due primarily to the lack of understanding of what is possible in this field. Chapter 8, "Insurance and the Rehabilitation Program," puts into perspective the various dilemmas facing rehabilitation providers in securing reimbursement for their services. In addition, it discusses what insurers expect from rehabilitation, the effect on cost of claims when rehabilitation is included as a benefit, what insurers look for in a rehabilitation facility, and what rehabilitation programs can do to attract insurers and persuade them of the benefit of rehabilitation programs.

Jacobs, P. Financial management in ambulatory care: which problems? which tools? *Journal of Ambulatory Care Management* 11(2):81–89, May 1988.

As the ambulatory care sector continues to expand, managers will be required to handle an increasingly greater share of financial and budgetary concerns. Tasks such as controlling costs, setting budgets, managing assets, and capital financing will occupy more and more of the administrator's time. Consequently, a more in-depth understanding of financial management theories and applications will be a requisite for profitability and success. This article provides an overview of three disciplines related to financial management: managerial finance, managerial economics, and managerial accounting. For each of the areas addressed, the author discusses the orientation and tools used in each discipline and how the literature supports the utilization of such tools.

Sports Medicine/Fitness

Marsey, A. Strategy at work—from rehab to fitness centers. *Texas Hospitals* 43(5):26–27, Oct. 1987.

This article traces the development of the decision of All Saints Health Care, Inc., to expand a freestanding center for outpatient cardiac and pulmonary rehabilitation into a full-fledged fitness center. In order to attract potential users to the facility, public relations/advertising/marketing was charged with developing and executing a plan to achieve the desired level of utilization. The article specifically addresses the decisions made to change the name of the facility, analyze the competition, develop scheduling and staffing patterns, develop new products, and create an advertising plan.

Sports medicine: where do we go from here? *The Physician and Sports Medicine* 16(6):170–77, June 1988.

This article presents a spectrum of views from sports medicine practitioners about where sports medicine has been and where it is headed. It discusses the role various aspects of the medical profession will take in advancing the theories and practice of sports medicine. At the same time, it illustrates the obstacles facing medical care practitioners in advancing sports medicine and integrating it into the health care delivery system. It specifically analyzes the role that preventive medicine, pediatrics, women's health practitioners, and orthopedics will play in the future sports medicine market. Safety in sports, the drug problem in sports, innovations in research, and exercise potential for the aging problem are also presented as critical components in the evolving field of sports medicine.

Tonti, D., Trudeau, T., and Daniel, M. Linking fitness activities to rehabilitation. *Business and Health* 4(9):23–27, Sept. 1987.

Reducing the number of employee injuries and the time it takes to recover from them can have a significant financial impact on a company. This article provides a description of one corporation's decision to implement an in-house health maintenance and injury prevention program. The objectives of the program were to establish a cost-effective, in-house rehabilitation/fitness program for all employees, promote a rapid rate of recovery for disabilities, reduce the associated financial impact on both the employee and the corporation, and continue to enhance employee relations and strengthen the company's image as a socially responsible employer. The article discusses the specifics of the training program, including staffing, equipping, and designing the program to meet the fitness and rehabilitation needs of its employees.

Weisman, E. Sports medicine attracts a young, healthy market. *Hospitals* 64(22):49, Nov. 20, 1990.

This article focuses on the opportunities for hospitals to attract young and healthy patients via a sports medicine program. The program should establish a presence in the community, especially with schools. The article also advises planners to target the right markets and provide a facility that is upbeat and seems more like a gym than a hospital.

Strategic Planning and New Business Development

Beltramini, R., Fullam, C., and others. Utilizing the strategic planning process in the development of innovative hospital-based programs. *Journal of Professional Services Marketing.* 1(1/2):135–47, Fall 1985, Winter 1985–1986.

The changing business environment in the health care field has made the role of strategic planning and marketing in the development of new product or service lines increasingly important. This article follows one hospital's utilization of the strategic planning process in the development of a new program. It specifically addresses such issues as environmental analysis, the definition of the hospital's mission, marketing opportunity analysis, and the objectives of the market study.

In addition, it illustrates how this process was implemented in the hospital's attempt to survey the community to determine the viability of a proposed new service. The final step of the marketing plan employed by the hospital was to prepare operating policies and develop evaluation procedures.

Ziegeler, D. Product-line management outside the hospital. *Health Care Strategic Management* 6(2):12–13, Feb. 1988.

This article illustrates how one health care corporation maintained a continuum of care for its patients by applying product-line management to services provided on an outpatient basis. CliniShare provides prehospitalization and posthospitalization technologies for all payers and is a for-profit subsidiary of Health West Foundation. Historically, CliniShare consisted of nine operating units grouped under three major divisions, with each unit functioning independently. Seizing on the opportunity to bundle programs and treat specific ailments comprehensively, the corporation set out to replicate hospital product-line management on an outpatient basis. The author describes the approach taken to solve the problem of fragmented posthospital care for diabetes, which led it to acquire Sugar Fill Centers, a supplier of diabetes products, health food, and education and training programs.

Vocational Rehabilitation

England, B., compiler. *Medical Rehabilitation Services in Health Care Institutions.* Chicago: American Hospital Publishing, 1986.

Chapter 7, "Legal Concerns of the Rehabilitation Program," contains information concerning the legal environment in which a rehabilitation facility operates. It specifically evaluates the legal issues that must be considered in the patient care process, documentation, allocation of financial resources, and payment for services. In addition, it provides an in-depth discussion of the facilities' legal obligations to facilitate a patient's transition from the facility to home, as well as its liability regarding patient suicide – a concern of all rehabilitation facilities. The special nature of rehabilitation creates concerns that must be considered in addition to the usual legal concerns of a general hospital service. As the chapter emphasizes, a rehabilitation program should strive to maximize patient functioning and reimbursement payments while simultaneously minimizing potential liability associated with patient care.

England, B., Glass, R. M., and Patterson, C. H., coauthors and editors. *Quality Rehabilitation: Results-Oriented Patient Care.* Chicago: American Hospital Publishing, 1989.

Working from the principle that health care providers must develop the capability to prove that they achieve good outcomes to anyone who wants to know—including patients, families, third-party intermediaries, risk managers, and professionals providing care—the book's 26 contributors describe what the rehabilitation community has done and is doing to monitor and measure the quality of care patients receive.

Hamilton, S. Implementing a successful quality assurance program in the rehabilitation setting. *Journal of Nursing Quality Assurance* 2(1):49–57, Nov. 1987.

Accrediting agencies such as the Joint Commission on Accreditation of Healthcare Organizations have specific quality assurance (QA) standards. Joint Commission standards state that as part of the hospital's QA program, the quality and appropriateness of the patient care provided by the nursing department/service should be monitored and evaluated, and identified problems should be resolved. To accommodate the unique QA needs in a rehabilitation setting, the author discusses development and implementation of an effective QA program for rehabilitation nursing. The article discusses the role of the QA committee and its position in the nursing department's organizational chart; its interface with other departments involved in rehabilitation; and unit, divisional, and departmental QA responsibilities. In addition, the author points out the need to have definitive and accurate documentation and how a facility can use this information to evaluate the quality of patient care in a rehabilitation setting.

Koch, C. A task of orientation. *Business and Health* 5(5):23–25, May 1988.

A total disability management system includes both functional and systems management. Functional management refers to any independent policy, procedure, or action taken to reduce costs or improve the quality of service on an individual claim or cause of an injury or illness. Systems management takes a coordinated approach to managing disability claims by focusing on reducing the cause, frequency, or severity of aggregate groups of illness or injury, thereby improving the quality of service and reducing costs. This article discusses the differences between functional and systems management, specifically focusing on the reasoning behind the use of each, organizational structuring of the disability program, management commitment, and the use of performance measures in evaluating the program.

Newkirk, W. L., and Jones, L. D., editors. *Occupational Health Services: A Guide to Program Planning and Management*. Chicago: American Hospital Publishing, 1989.

The 11 chapters in the first half of the book provide an in-depth examination of the components that can be included in the occupational health services product line. The next 10 chapters focus on operational issues, progressing from developing a marketing plan through nuts-and-bolts issues. Concluding chapters present a case study and a discussion of trends for the future.

Olsheski, J., and Growick, B. Industrial rehabilitation in the public sector: the Ohio experience. *Journal of Rehabilitation* 54(2):46–48, Apr.–May–June 1988.

The state of Ohio maintains a rehabilitation division within its Industrial Commission that is charged with responsibility for helping individuals with work-related injuries to access their rehabilitation centers. These centers, which were created by the Industrial Commission, offer comprehensive services of a multidisciplinary nature for injured workers who need specialized treatment in order to return to work. The state of Ohio is unique in that it provides industrial rehabilitation services entirely through the public sector. This article describes the industrial rehabilitation philosophy of the state of Ohio and how its policies and practices differ from those of most other states.

Watson, S. Independent living options: helping disabled workers. *Business and Health* 5(2):23–25, Feb. 1988.

Independent living programs (ILPs) are not-for-profit organizations providing a variety of services to help persons with disabilities live as independently as possible. Taking advantage of the various programs afforded by ILPs can help employers avoid costly duplication of counseling, workplace accommodation, and other services already available in their community. This article traces the development of ILPs, the philosophy underpinning their creation, and the types of services typically provided. It provides illustrations of operational ILPs and how they are being accessed by employers to help their workers with disabilities to maintain their independence in the community and eventually return to work.